Mother and Child Health

DELIVERING THE SERVICES

Third Edition

Cicely D. Williams, M.D., D.C.H.
was Adviser in Maternal and Child Health
World Health Organization

Naomi Baumslag, M.D., M.P.H.
Clinical Professor, Department of Pediatrics
Georgetown University Medical School
and President, Women's International Public Health Network

Derrick B. Jelliffe, M.D., D.C.H..
was Professor Emeritus of Public Health and Pediatrics
Schools of Public Health and Medicine
University of California, Los Angeles

New York   Oxford
OXFORD UNIVERSITY PRESS
1994

Oxford University Press

Oxford   New York   Toronto
Delhi   Bombay   Calcutta   Madras   Karachi
Kuala Lumpur   Singapore   Hong Kong   Tokyo
Nairobi   Dar es Salaam   Cape Town
Melbourne   Auckland   Madrid

and associated companies in
Berlin   Ibadan

Published by Oxford University Press, Inc.,
200 Madison Avenue, New York, New York 10016

Oxford is a registered trademark of Oxford University Press

Library of Congress Cataloging-in-Publication Data
Williams, Cicely D.
Mother and child health : delivering the services /
Cicely D. Williams, Naomi Baumslag, Derrick B. Jelliffe. — 3rd ed.
/ edited by Ruth Tamara Yodaiken.
p. cm.   Includes bibliographical references and index.
ISBN 0-19-508148-X (cloth :).
ISBN 0-19-508149-8 (paper)
1. Child health services.   2. Maternal health services.
3. Community health services.
4. Child health services—Developing countries.
5. Maternal health services—Developing countries.
6. Community health services—Developing countries.
I. Baumslag, Naomi.   II. Jelliffe, Derrick Brian.
III. Yodaiken, Ruth Tamara.   IV. Title.
RJ101.W54   1993
362.1′9892—dc20   93-16378

1 3 5 7 9 8 6 4 2

Printed in the United States of America
on acid-free paper

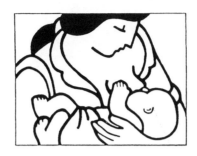

To my dear friends and colleagues Cicely Williams and Dick Jelliffe, who did not live to see the third edition of this book published but who throughout their lives worked for the betterment of the world's mothers and children. May the spirit of their work live on.

And to health workers who, despite almost insuperable obstacles under trying conditions, strive unselfishly to lessen suffering and prevent death and through improvisation, innovation, and a spirit of inquiry bring hope and new solutions.

CONTENTS

PREFACE TO THE THIRD EDITION

The changing global scene of recent years has had both beneficial and harmful effects on the health of women and children, and necessitated a third, revised, edition of this book. Ecological, biological, and social situations have been drastically altered in many parts of the world. These situations are characterized by increasing poverty, urbanization (with overcrowded cities), disrupted families, altered dietary patterns, and war and refugees, as well as by changes in climate and environment. There has been an increased potential for food scarcity and famine, malnutrition, stress, drugs and altered behavior, and the recognition that gender violence is a serious health problem. In addition, there has been a resurgence of some old infections, such as malaria and tuberculosis, and the emergence of new diseases, most notably AIDS. The management of some infections has become more difficult and uncertain with the development of drug-resistant bacterial strains, as in tuberculosis, leprosy, and malaria. Furthermore, the social and emotional support of the family has often been ignored. All of these circumstances affect health either directly or indirectly.

On the positive side, increased worldwide use of national programs employing effective and appropriate technology have often produced spectacular results. These include the use of oral rehydration in diarrheal disease, multiple immunizations against childhood communicable diseases (notably measles, whooping cough, diphtheria, and neonatal tetanus), an understanding of the true significance and prevention of fetal iodine deficiency, and a simplified practical approach to the diagnosis and treatment of different forms of acute respiratory infections.

The last decade has seen declarations, summits, and world congresses called by a consortium of international organizations requesting political commitment and resources, and directing the global effort to abolish world hunger, make motherhood safer, promote breastfeeding as a birthright and a positive resource, and prevent micronutrient deficiency.

Global programs and policies to improve the health of women and children have been altered in recent years as a result of the experience, international guidance, and leadership from WHO and UNICEF. Modern ideas concerning health surveillance and health education have improved as a result of newer insights into motivation (including the need for cultural involvement), communication skills, and social marketing.

Examples of specific changes abound.

These include an appreciation of the role of vitamin A as an anti-infective nutrient, as well as its long-recognized role in eye pathology; the ever-clearer significance of the health of women throughout their life cycle on the well-being and nutrition of both women and infants; adaptive methods for newborn care when resources are limited; and the worldwide effort to promote breastfeeding.

Successful vertical programs, however, pose questions about affordability, long-term effects, and sustainability. Until these interventions are combined with horizontal programs that improve the quality of life of the population, such as child spacing and provision of basic services, they will have only a temporary impact. Given the shortage of available resources, the need to prioritize and evaluate the effectiveness of programs has become more essential, as has the need to develop human resources and involve the community at all levels.

Many new terms, such as "structural adjustment" and "development with a human face," have been bandied about, but the poorest of the poor—women and children—are still unserved, and the gap is widening as privatization of medical care increases. Drug companies and food companies continue to exploit the fears of the people and to promise more than their products can deliver. Preventive measures are undermined for profit, for example, with the promotion of cigarette smoking and drinking alcohol. Environmental exposures of women and their infants to toxic chemicals remains uncontrolled in many parts of the world and may increase with the expansion of worldwide "free" trade. Health care workers will have to organize on issues, not just provide health education.

Probably the most significant change in this book is an emphasis on women rather than on mothers. This emphasis reflects the fact that females bear tremendous and often underappreciated burdens from birth through childhood and adolescence, both during and between pregnancies, with added problems stemming from childbearing.

In maternal and child health services, the women who have given birth are often viewed as appendages or simply child-care providers. However, the woman is the key to any successful change, and unless her health and status throughout her life cycle are given major resources, the beneficial effect of services on family health will be negligible in the long run. The health sector must consider how best to extend services to women instead of making impractical demands on them as mothers.

It should be noted that many of the studies and examples cited in this book are classic pioneering efforts, which are only now being recognized and replicated in many countries with local adaptation.

Likewise, the work of Cicely D. Williams and Derrick B. Jelliffe is as relevant today as it was fifty years ago. Training local women as community health workers was started by Williams in 1929. Community health workers called *promotoras* were trained in Mexico twenty years ago. Only recently has this been done in the United States to reach the rural poor and urban needy. In January 1992 a promotora program was started for poor rural women in New Mexico to assist them with a wide variety of services including transport to clinics, antenatal care, health education, immunization, referral, and information on sources for financial assistance and other resources. Health authorities in the region have proclaimed the initial pilot program cost-effective. Preventive health measures used in developing countries are beginning to be introduced in the United States and other industrialized countries so that basic health services can also reach the poor and needy and hold down escalating health care costs.

Throughout this book we have been able to record the experience and wisdom of health workers in many different settings. Some of the main themes in the book underscore the importance of breastfeeding and nutrition (e.g., cuddles are as important as calories; food shortage is often not the root cause or only cause of malnutrition). The book also stresses the importance of preventive care; that birth control begins with death control; services must be community based and extensive, not just intensive; the importance of training community health workers; health education begins with listening; that services must be woman-centered; that parents matter; and that the increasing number of aged must not be left out. The World Development Report 1993 recommends much of what is in this book for improving health care globally. The approach recommended includes fostering an environment that enables households to improve their own health, promoting the rights and status of women through legal empowerment and legal protection against abuse; reducing inequitable health services; improving access to quality health care to the poor and unserved; making more money available for common debilitating diseases and prevention; increasing use of funds for the most cost-effective interventions best delivered at low level facilities; reducing inefficiency and waste and making the most use of national natural resources. These and other suggestions have been advocated in the book and they are most timely. Although Williams and Jelliffe both died before the printing of this edition they have left us with a legacy of wisdom and common sense, spirit, and dedication to build on.

1994   N. Baumslag

PREFACE TO THE FIRST EDITION

The vulnerability of mothers and children, although traditionally well appreciated in all cultures, received little emphasis in health planning in less developed areas of the world until very recently, and even then attempts to deal with the often huge and complex problems raised were too frequently made by means of imposed or imported, and often inappropriate, services and ill-adjusted methods.

All aspects of a society, whether it is relatively static or in a stage of dramatic upheaval, affect the health of every member of the family and of the community, and especially of its most physiologically and culturally vulnerable groups—mothers and young children. Thus, alterations in the level of maternal and child health (MCH) will result from changes in environmental situation, from cultural attitudes, from multifarious methods and standards of education, from changes in mores and values, from fluctuations in national and individual economics, from the effects of world trade or agricultural production, and from innumerable other aspects of life, including wars and civil disturbance, which profoundly affect the health and nutrition of mothers and their children.

This is not intended to be an inclusive textbook, nor to give details of programs or clinical management. It does not attempt to cover the complete literature in its field nor to analyze the details of all the techniques, systems, and procedures that have so far been tried in the development of MCH services in different regions. It sets out rather to present a point of view, some examples of diversity, and a practical philosophy. Little is presented in the way of clinical details, except insofar as these help to illustrate certain situations. For, basically, MCH services have to be tailored to local circumstances. Universal solutions are an illusion, and the "blueprint" export of services from one part of the world to another is rarely valid; in the past, it has too often led to levels of confusion suggestive of Lewis Carroll.

The traditional tendency of classical "tropical medicine" to concentrate on major communicable disease control programs has increased human survival and longevity. But such programs do not automatically provide for a higher standard of health or education. Moreover, many regions are in urgent need of a more understanding and responsible attitude toward fertility. These aims may be sought through improved MCH services.

The main concerns of such improvements would be to establish priorities, to adapt scientific principles of varying ecologies, and above all to devise and construct an interlocking network of MCH services, and to establish truly appropriate training—both "classical" and experimental—in the economic, educational, cultural, and geographical realities of the particular region, for the personnel urgently needed to man the maternal and child (or family or community) health services in both rural and urban areas.

Furthermore, recent developments in North America and Europe have already highlighted the facts that there are significant areas of economic, educational, and technical underdevelopment in these apparently affluent, largely industrialized continents and that there are more parallels to be found between the problems of administering MCH services in Bombay, Birmingham, and Baltimore than was previously appreciated.

There is a close similarity between these problems and the strategy needed for their solution, whatever the latitude. Thus, in a recent study of newborn babies visited at home in Leeds, England,* it was found that for one-tenth the help of the health visitor, the children's officer, the National Society for the Prevention of Cruelty of Children, or the police had to be sought, even in 1966; in the assessment of overcrowding according to the 1957 Housing Acts, no account is taken of children under 1 year; 15 percent of children are admitted to hospital for "social" rather than somatic reasons; and the total number of children admitted to hospitals has still to be ascertained. How can planners and administrators, humanists and doctors afford to remain aloof or to engage in demarcation disputes? It is surely time for doctors to comprehend their responsibilities from a humane viewpoint.

The need for family care, community health measures, and the practice of so-

cial medicine is now universally recognized. Whatever name is given to it, care of mothers and children (MCH) will engage the most time and attention. The more sophisticated countries developed their curative services (doctors and hospitals) years ago. But it was only at the beginning of the twentieth century that the personal preventive services were developed, and then under the title "public health," and separate from the hospitals and other curative services. For traditional European and North American training in MCH ignores the curative services, or else regards them as separate bodies, an attitude which is reflected in both national and international organizations.

Although the need for integration of the curative and preventive services is now admitted, there is little guidance as to how this should be carried out. The distribution of "simple medicines and food supplements" is not enough by itself. Neither prevention nor cure is worthwhile unless there are also good diagnosis, effective treatment, and follow-up. Simplification—yes, but palliatives—no. Sulfur ointment, for example, is cheaper and often more useful than benzyl benzoate, but it is first necessary to diagnose the scabies for which this should be used. It is only after the effective integration of hospitals, health centers, and home care that patients may be observed, investigated, treated, and educated. Hospitals often fall under the aegis of the government health services, and MCH centers under that of the local authorities. Thus, those who concentrate on "public" health may find it difficult to appreciate the needs of a service that is essentially for individuals. Whether or not this administrative separation persists, it is the function of the MCH personnel to ensure collaboration, for it is only at an individual level that services can identify cases of high risk, and the multifarious natures of those risks.

Health depends, first, on a person's

---

* Quoted from a book review of the article "A New Look at Child Health" (1966) by M. Joseph and R. C. McKeith in the *Lancet*.

ability to regulate his or her own habits and environment and, second, on the availability of good medical care. MCH services should help to ensure both. They can provide help to individuals and contribute to the educational and economic progress of the community, at minimum cost.

Avant-garde economists in the United Nations Second Development Decade, as well as youthful hippies, are realizing increasingly that people cannot live by GNP alone, and that the quality of life is as important as economic advancement, and, indeed, is an integral part of it.

"The survival of the fittest" is now an outworn cliché. Conditions that kill off the weaklings will also damage those who would otherwise be strong, and the ultimate objective of the MCH services is therefore not only to reduce mortality and morbidity but also to reduce the incidence of violence, crime, drug taking, alcoholism, inadequacy, and neglected and unwanted children. The principles discussed in this book may therefore merit as much consideration in the slums of Glasgow, Harlem, or Lisbon, and in the Appalachians, or rural Montenegro, as in the *favellas* of Rio or the *manyatta* of the Masai.

1972

C. D.W.
D. B. J.

ACKNOWLEDGMENTS

The authors had the privilege of living and working in more than a hundred countries, not only as visiting specialists or consultants but also at the grass-roots level, and met large numbers of babies, children, and their parents. We worked with many doctors, nurses, and other health-related workers and have been able to discuss problems with experienced and dedicated people in the field who have been most generous with their time, suggestions, and comments and revision of this book. They are too numerous to be thanked individually by name, but many are quoted in the text. In particular we thank Myrna Zelaya; Claire Senseman, Esther Kazilimani, and Jean Larsen (Georgetown University Medical School) for research; Fred Zerfas, Douglas Mackintosh, and Ben Ocheng for technical expertise; and Blanca Keogan and Gloria Haws for clerical assistance. UNICEF, PAHO, the World Bank, and Gayle Gibbons and Virginia Yee, APHA Clearinghouse on Mothers and Children, were most helpful in providing information and publications. And special thanks to Ruth Tamara Yodaiken for her editing and to Edith Barry and Jeffrey House at Oxford University Press for their assistance and recognition of the importance of this book.

Mother and Child Health

1

General Introduction

*If in this world of misery we must exist, so be it; but let some
little loophole, some glimpse of possibility at least, be left, which
may serve the noble portion of humanity to hope and struggle
unceasingly for its alleviation. . . . Fate has allowed humanity
such a pitifully meagre coverlet, that in pulling it over one part
of the world, another has to be left bare.*
RABINDRANATH TAGORE, 1983

Throughout the world, poor women and children are the most vulnerable and least serviced. In the last decade, despite the increasing recognition of the needs of the poorest of the poor and despite massive vertical programs targeted at them, the effect globally has been less than satisfactory. While the concept of Health for All was revolutionary, its implementation has been limited by the complex interrelationship of health with economics and the environment. This limitation has led to the development of the more attainable goal of death control through programs aimed at child survival. Simplistic solutions in catchy packages sold by international agencies have come and gone. However, the problems of the poor, especially poor women, have not only remained, but the gap between the "haves" and "have-nots" has widened in spite of good intentions (Babbs et al. 1993; Sanders 1985).

The problems are massive. Refugees, displaced persons, and street children make up large segments of the populations of developing countries. Famine affects millions every year. New diseases, such as AIDs, and the recurrence of resistant old ones, such as tuberculosis and malaria, are unsolved problems. The reappearance of cholera has challenged some long-held concepts about disease transmission and the effectiveness of vaccination and the cordon sanitaire. Environmental conditions—a deficient water supply and poor sanitation, poor hygiene, contamination of food, and lack of planning—lead to rapid spread of disease, densely populated human settlements, and poor health infrastructure (Pub. Hlth. News 1991). Children may be saved in infancy from death and their mothers from death in childbirth, only to struggle for survival (King 1990).

Largely as a result of poverty, one out of five persons in the developing world are malnourished; 192 million children under 5 suffer from protein energy malnutrition, and more than 2,000 million have micronutrient deficiencies. Globally more than 1,000 million are at risk for iodine deficiency. Iodine deficiency is particularly prevalent in mountainous and flood-prone areas, where over 200 million people have goiters, 26 million have mental defects, and 6 million are cretins. All of these conditions are preventable. It has been estimated that worldwide, 40 million people lack sufficient vitamin A. In addition, diet diseases, such as obesity, cardiovascular disease, diabetes, and some forms of cancer, are emerging as public health problems in many countries (ICN 1992).

The magnitude of environmental problems and their impact on health is only now being realized. Lead is one of them. This major environmental contaminant causes mental retardation and neurological damage in children, and its effects on the developing central nervous system are devastating. Although it affects children in industrialized societies as well as developing countries—in the United States 3 million to 4 million schoolchildren have abnormal blood lead levels—the condition is more prevalent in very poor areas. The prevention of lead poisoning depends on the will of the community to affect regulation of the major sources of contamination: lead pipes, lead paint, and lead in the soil (Katz March of Dimes 1992, personal communication).

Workers in undeveloped areas are being exposed to toxic levels of chemicals not acceptable in Western countries, and the number of birth defects reported in some areas is cause for concern. Mercury, for example, a toxic chemical used in certain industries, has been found to double the risk of spontaneous abortion if the father's urine mercury is more than 50 micrograms per liter (Cordier et al. 1991). Furthermore, these chemicals for production and profit are being dumped with no regard to people or vegetation and are contaminating the air, crops, and the water supply.

THE VULNERABLE

In the less technically developed areas of the world, disease and death take their highest toll among mothers and children, who make up over two-thirds of the population. Perinatal mortality may be as much as ten times higher than that of infants born in technically developed countries; the infant mortality rate may be six to twenty times greater than in the industrialized regions of Europe and North America; the death rate among preschool children is up to ten times as high (Table 1.1). In technically underdeveloped countries, half of the total mortality may occur in children below 5 years of age, compared with only 5 percent in countries such as the United Kingdom and Sweden (McDermott 1966; UNICEF 1992).

This pattern of death and ill health extends to women not only in the form of maternal mortality, but also in the form of morbidity. Mortality reaches as high as 1,000 per 100,000 live births in developing countries compared with 5 to 30 per 100,000 in industrialized countries. Women who do not die in childbirth suffer from a number of debilitating conditions including maternal depletion. This is the result of a number of causally related factors such as pregnancy at an early age, cultural subservience, continuous cycles of pregnancy, inadequate diet leading to anemia or malnutrition, and an onerous workload resulting in premature aging, disease, and early death. Apart from the effects of depletion on the mother, the fetus, and her dependent children, the economic consequences may also be considerable. When women are too compromised in their health to perform important tasks within the village, including the production of food and the collection of fuel and water, the entire community suffers. Attention to optimal growth and development in childhood, by means of good nutrition and health protection, represents an investment in future health and national productivity.

Table 1.1. Comparisons of Extreme Levels of National Maternal and Child Mortality Rates

	Least developed countries	Developed countries
Perinatal mortality[a]	91	5–9
Infant mortality[a]	119	14
Under-5 mortality[a]	198	18
Maternal mortality[b]	737	34

Sources: WHO (1987, 1992).

[a]Per 1,000 live births.

[b]Per 100,000 live births.

Overall Pattern of Disease

There are marked differences between developed and developing countries (Fig. 1.1). Although there are local variations throughout the world, the overall pattern of ill health seen in children and mothers in developing countries who are living in poverty bears a remarkable similarity.

More than half the deaths of children under age 5 in these countries are the result of a combination of acute respiratory infections (ARI) (33 percent) and diarrheal disease (24 percent), largely preventable.

Among the newborn, grave problems are caused by infections, particularly neo-

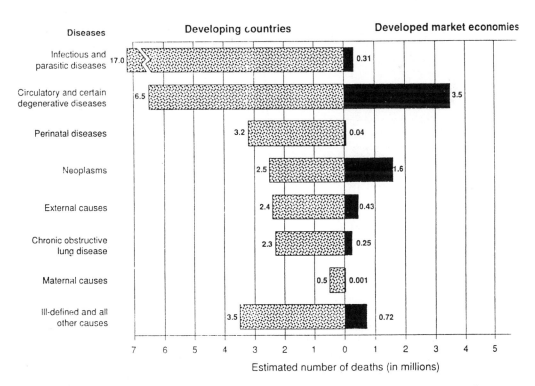

Figure 1.1. Estimated distribution of total deaths from major diseases around developing countries and developed market economies. Source: WHO (1992).

Table 1.2. Estimated Causes of Death in Developing Countries for Children Under 5 Years, 1990

Causes of death	Percentage
Acute respiratory infection (ARI)	27.6
ARI-measles	3.7
ARI-pertussis	2.0
(ARI-mostly pneumonia)	
Pertussis	0.8
Measles	1.7
Diarrhea	23.3
Diarrhea measles	1.4
Malaria	6.2
Birth asphyxia	6.7
Neonatal tetanus	4.3
Congenital anomalies	3.5
Birth trauma	3.3
Prematurity	3.3
Neonatal sepsis and meningitis	2.3
Tuberculosis	2.3
Accidents	1.6
All other causes	6.0

Source: WHO (1992).

Note: Since 1985 the number of deaths due to ARI has decreased; neonatal tetanus has dropped; neonatal sepsis and meningitis have increased; measles and pertussis deaths have decreased; neonatal and perinatal deaths have increased slightly, to 30 percent from 27 percent; vaccine-preventable deaths have decreased from 27 percent to 16 percent.

natal diarrhea and umbilical infections, septicemia, or tetanus neonatorum, as well as birth trauma, low birthweight, and immaturity. In infancy, respiratory tract infections usually head the list, followed by diarrheal disease, nutritional marasmus, and, later, malaria (Table 1.2).

It is the toddler, however, or pre-school child who bears the brunt of the killing diseases. Almost everywhere in less technically developed regions, the "big three" of early childhood morbidity and mortality are pneumonia, diarrheal disease, and protein calorie malnutrition. Children with tuberculosis, whooping cough, measles, intestinal helminths, malaria, accidents (especially burns), and anemia crowd hospital wards. In some areas, there is a seasonal incidence of conditions, for example, summer diarrhea, and winter burns. Large numbers of young children are brought to outpatient and health centers for treatment of less lethal condi-

tions, particularly eye disorders (xerophthalmia, conjunctivitis, trachoma), skin diseases (scabies, ringworm, impetigo), and chronic ear infections.

Women bear the heaviest burden of disease and death. They are most vulnerable in pregnancy, when the commonest causes of maternal morbidity and mortality are hemorrhage, sepsis, toxemia, abortions, obstructed labor, and ruptured uterus.

As well as these universally common diseases, other conditions, such as meningitis in early childhood, tetanus, and intestinal infections, pose important diagnostic or therapeutic problems in urban hospitals, as do widespread diseases with considerable risk of later severe residua, such as hepatitis, leprosy, xerophthalmia, and conjunctivitis leading to blindness. The newly recognized scourge of AIDS has special impact on and significance for mothers and children.

Certain regional forms of disease may require special consideration as, for example, the malignant lymphoma found in parts of Africa, cirrhosis of the liver seen in children in parts of India, lead poisoning in inner-city slums, and genetic problems such as sickle cell disorders. Moreover, beneath the bulk of infective and nutritional disorders lie unrecognized many of the metabolic and genetic conditions that so much preoccupy health workers in Europe and North America.

Most of these devastating conditions that strike mothers and children disproportionately can be prevented by health education, health supervision, medical treatment, fertility control, and immunization. Whether they are prevented ultimately hinges on greater social and economic equity.

Molding Factors

The developing regions of the world have common characteristics, irrespective of geographic location (Table 1.3), that perpetuate preventable mother and child

Table 1.3. Some Common Characteristics of Less Technologically Developed Countries

General
  Poverty
  Monoculture agriculture of cash crops
  Declining food production (per capita)
  Inequitable distribution of income, land, and resources
  High illiteracy
  Non-Western culture
  Dependence on imports (oil, consumer goods)
Demographics
  Mainly rural
  Increasing urban influx
  High young-child population
  Rapid population increase
Health statistics
  High morbidity and mortality (especially among mothers and young children)
  Repetitive pattern of preventable diseases
  Highly prevalent malnutrition
Health services
  Rural neglect
  Urban concentration
  Hospital dominated
  Physician centered
  Technology based
  Costly

health (MCH) problems. These conditions were commonplace in European and North American pediatrics in the past. Kwashiorkor called "flour-feeding disease" by Czerny) was undoubtedly common among ill-fed foundlings in nineteenth-century Europe. Malaria posed a problem in large areas of the United States and was vividly described by Dickens in *Martin Chuzzlewit*. In the 1870s a high percentage of children in "poor law schools" in Britain were found to have trachoma, and in 1877, the two major causes of outpatient attendance at the Children's Hospital in Sheffield were diarrhea and worms. The infant mortality rate in Western Europe at the beginning of the twentieth century was high (McDermott 1966).

The conditions among children in developing countries today and in urban ghettos throughout the world are similar to those documented in Sir Thomas Phayre's *The Boke of Children*, describing conditions in England in the 1540s, and in Rosen von Rosenstein's *Diseases in Children*, describing Sweden in the eighteenth century. Indeed, the earlier books document these conditions better than some recent books on tropical medicine, which give more attention to the minutiae of the mosquito's form than to MCH problems. The preoccupation with microscopic minutia and lack of surveillance has increased parasitic infection prevalence and allowed vectors for their transmittal to flourish in tropical regions. (These parasitic infestations include schistosomiasis, guinea worm, and malaria.)

Briefly, there are four molding factors that contribute to the picture of maternal and child ill health in less technologically developed areas today:

1. The level of progress, measured by standards of general and technical education, economic prosperity, public hygiene and available health services, and the equity of distribution.
2. Cultural influences.
3. Geographic-climatic factors.
4. Genetic variation.

FACTORS IN THE DEVELOPMENT OF MCH SERVICES

Planners of MCH services designed to deal with the numerous problems affecting health must consider numerous complicated and overlapping factors. Ten are of particular importance.

Health Priorities

The services planned must be focused on the dominant health problems of the area. The diseases to be prevented must be those that are the most common and the most serious.

Newly arrived or ill-experienced health care workers must realize that not everything can be done. Rather, the limited resources available must be concentrated on the most widespread health problems in the community. In most tropical regions, for example, little emphasis can be given to congenital heart disease or to the attainment of theoretically desirable intakes of calcium, when tuberculosis and general malnutrition are highly prevalent. Moreover, the services that are provided must be geared to groups, families, or individuals at risk and with the "priority diseases."

Simple vital statistics—for example, illness rates in mothers and children—can be helpful in pinpointing where health efforts are needed the most. This information—some of it perhaps biased but useful nevertheless—can come from hospitals, health centers, and dispensaries. These data may give valuable indications of the main local diseases, although such common factors as bed capacity, difficulties with multiple diagnoses, local communications, the degree of rapport with the people, and cultural concepts about the treatability of disease have to be taken into account. More data are needed, however. Attempts must be made to motivate governments and individuals to appreciate the need for registration of births and deaths. (Major advances in this field will come about only when the value of such registration is recognized—for example, when proof is mandatory for admission to school or for the claiming of a pension.)

Community-based studies are also necessary. In some parts of the world, these have been carried out by means of field prevalence surveys (Jelliffe and Jelliffe 1989). These surveys have some disadvantages; for example, they are made only at one season of the year and thus cannot detect short-term episodes of ill health. On the other hand, they can be used to assess the problems in rural or urban areas, gauge to some extent the various ecological circumstances that contribute to a particular pattern of ill

health, focus attention on issues, involve the community, and serve as training exercises for health professionals such as medical students and nurses.

Longitudinal studies permit an understanding of the dynamic interplay of community factors and the incidence of major and minor episodes of health over an extended period (Mata 1978). Special studies, however, are costly, time-consuming, and complicated to organize and supervise. Much may be accomplished even without these studies if staff working in MCH services collect information and keep simple registers in the course of their work. Properly supervised village workers in Papua, New Guinea, with less than a full primary education and at least two weeks training in recording and/or simple administration of questionnaires, have collected accurate demographic and morbidity data classified by age, sex, and area (Hetzel 1978) (Fig. 1.2). The trust and confidence of mutual respect permits such observations of the real dynamics of the community. In large, diverse countries with minimal communications, the collection of data is harder to accomplish.

Although much information is needed to assess health problems, usually sufficient data are available locally, without special surveys, to be able to make a well-informed assessment of the major problems; the lack of precise information must not hold up the initiation of plans and programs. Data obtained by every means in the future must constantly be fed back to modify the plans that have been put into operation.

Health Economics

The availability of funds is usually one of three principal limiting factors in the development of adequate MCH services (Abel-Smith 1967; Cook 1968; Kaprio 1965; Taylor and Hall 1968). (The others are trained staff, and flexibility and imagination.) Although money alone will

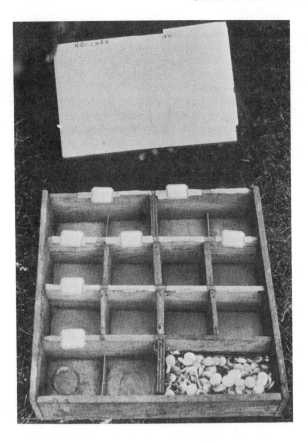

Figure 1.2. Counters used by illiterate community health workers for morbidity data collection, Papua New Guinea. Source: Radford (1978).

not ensure good health, it is generally agreed that in the least technologically developed countries, the extreme poverty of the population and the low level of gross national product (GNP) together with inequitable distribution of resources, is the overriding constraint. Health must compete with other pressing developmental needs for public resources (Gish 1975). Rapid population growth is also adding to the problem at a devastating rate.

Both national revenues and per capita income in developing countries are usually very small indeed, and there is a correlation between low GNP and high infant mortality. Ironically, the richest 20 percent of the world's population receives 83 percent of the total world's income, while the poorest 20 percent receives only 1.4 percent (Fig. 1.3) (UNDP 1992). Expenditures for health, however, have been rising rapidly over the last few decades in both industrialized and developing countries, but this has not included preventive care or unserved rural areas.

Analysis of health care costs indicates they are exploding. In the world as a whole in 1990 the public and private expenditure on health was $1,700 billion or 8% of the world product. High-income countries spent almost 90% of this amount, averaging $1,500 per person per year. In contrast, developing countries spent $170 billion (4% of their GNP), averaging $41 per person per year—less than a thirtieth spent by rich countries. (World Bank Report 1993). The average Indian gets about one-hundredth as much health care as a Briton, though the latter, typically living in a sanitized environment, falls ill less often and less severely. Generally the poorer the country, the poorer is the health coverage. In Bang-

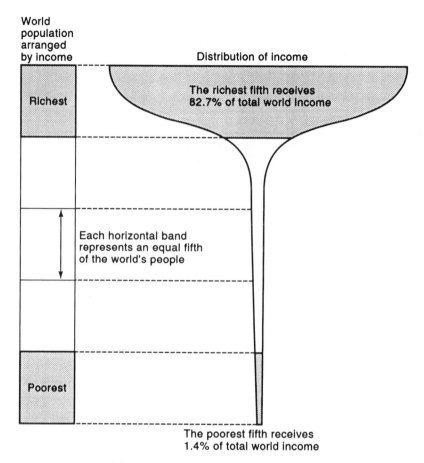

World
population
arranged
by income

Distribution of income

Richest

The richest fifth receives
82.7% of total world income

Each horizontal band
represents an equal fifth
of the world's people

Poorest

The poorest fifth receives
1.4% of total world income

Figure 1.3. Global distribution of income. Source: UNDP (1992).

ladesh, Ethiopia, Indonesia, and Zaire, annual public health expenditures are only $1 per capita. Expenditure is considered one of the socioeconomic indicators (Table 1.4) (UNDP 1992; WHO 1992).

Since recurrent expenditures are concentrated in urban areas, where hospitals and specialized staff are located, it may be concluded that the resources available to operate health services for the rural population are very limited. In the poorest group of countries, the average is substantially less than $1 per capita. In Zimbabwe, for example, Ushewokunze (1980) found that the three large specialist hospitals absorbed half of the total

national budget for health to serve at most 600,000 out of a population of 7 million. The curative emphasis was also evident: only 11 percent of the health budget was allocated to preventive services. Medical resources are generally unequally distributed (Fig. 1.4), with the sickest and the poorest receiving the least services from the least trained.

A substantial increase in public resources for health in poor countries is usually possible only if there is a shift from other sectors. Nevertheless, Sri Lanka, Kerala State in India, and the People's Republic of China have attained a life expectancy close to the level of that of the industrialized world with income

Table 1.4. Health and Socioeconomic Indicators

	Least developed countries	Developing countries	Developed countries
Total population (millions)	4,196	—	1,224
Infant mortality rate (per 1,000 live births)	120	70	18
Life expectancy (years)	51	63	76
Low-birthweight infants (under 2500 g)	75	88	95
Population with access to safe water (%)	50	70	100
Adult literacy (%)	40	65	98
Population per doctor	17,000	2,700	520
Population per nurse	6,500	1,500	220
GNP per capita (U.S. $)	301	684	19,542
Government health expenditure as percentage of GNP	1	2	4
Under-5 mortality rate (per 1,000 live births)	200	120	20

Sources: WHO (1981, 1992); UNDP (1992).

levels in the range of those of the least developed countries. The achievements may be explained in part by the public priority given to literacy, food, health, and sanitation and by special social and political organizations.

For countries with the least resources, the critical issue is the mobilization of the population in the struggle to improve their status. The percentage of the national budget allotted to different aspects of "development"—education, agriculture, communications, industrialization, and health services—can vary, although generally the health services receive a pittance and the military expenditures the lion's share (Table 1.5). The health care situation has become more serious because of the impact of worldwide recession, national debt, and economic adjustment policies that often include a restriction of social services, including those concerned with health. The decreased health care budget has had especially profound effects in Africa (Lancet 1990; WHO 1992) but is evident even in America, where health care has not been a right but a privilege.

Within MCH services, the money available must be balanced in the spending on staff, buildings, equipment, vaccines, drugs, transport, and possibly supplementary foods. Drugs alone can take up to 40 percent or more of the national health budget. In an effort to contain costs, several countries have streamlined drug inventories to include only essential drugs, and some have even begun to produce drugs locally. On the whole, money tends to be spent on visible parts of the system that are politically important, such as buildings, whereas a trained and adequately mobile staff, provided with simple but serviceable equipment, drugs, and vaccines, should take priority. And often, funding is unbalanced, with urban-based hospitals receiving 50 to 60 percent of the national health budget while primary care struggles with shortages of basic supplies (Gilson 1991).

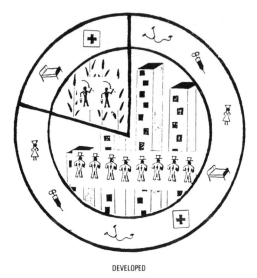

DEVELOPED

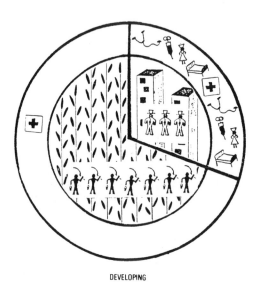

DEVELOPING

Figure 1.4. Distribution of resources. In developed countries where only 20 percent of the population is rural, resources are more equitably distributed. However, in the developing countries where the majority (90 percent) live in rural areas, resources are concentrated in the urban areas for the elite minority.

The economic superiority of preventive health measures, as opposed to the continuous and inconclusive financial drain of exclusively curative services, has been abundantly proved and will be a major and recurrent theme in later chapters. Prevention occurs at three levels: prevention of occurrence, prevention of progression, and rehabilitation or modification of disability. The economics and mechanics of sustained preventive measures also require consideration and often may be substantially greater than is at first apparent (Medovy 1968).

Health administrators must aim at maintaining a rational balance among the different branches of the health services according to immediate national needs and the long-term objectives. Additionally, they must ensure that even generous international assistance is used wisely and not for unjustifiable, inappropriate, unsustainable programs.

Financial considerations have to be built into all aspects of the health services. The difference in cost of a fraction of a cent between one drug and another may be of great importance if it is widely used, as iron tablets are in the preventive treatment of iron-deficiency anemia among the many millions of women and children in India.

The Mother-Child Relationship

In 1969 a World Health Organization (WHO) Expert Committee report found much higher rates of mother and child mortality and morbidity in developing areas, mainly the result of poor nutrition, widespread infection, and hazardous and excessive reproduction associated with inadequate medical care, supervision, and treatment. There has been little change in the report's basic findings. Less than 20 percent of people in technologically underdeveloped countries have access to health care and less than 30 percent have deliveries supervised by trained personnel (WHO 1992; UNICEF 1990).

The need to appreciate the link between women and their children in any part of the world has been emphasized by the very label *MCH*. In less developed areas, this biological and logistical link is

Table 1.5. Defense and Social Expenditures in Selected Countries

Countries	GNP per capita (U.S. $)	Percentage of Central Government Expenditures		
		Defense	Education	Health
India	340	19	3	2
Egypt	640	20	12	3
Ecuador	1,020	12	25	7
Korea Republic	4,400	27	19	2
Costa Rica	1,780	3	13	17
United States	20,910	25	2	13
Netherlands	15,920	5	12	11
France	17,820	6	8	21

Source: UNICEF (1992).

Note: The data were collected between 1986 and 1990.

not only important but vital, and imperative for health and survival (Jelliffe 1967).

The nutrition of women in pregnancy is reflected in the birthweight and maturity of their infants and also by fetal stores of iron, vitamins, and other nutrients needed in early infancy (ICN 1992). Even more important is the need for a lively, vigorous, lactating mother to feed, caress, carry, and care for the infant during this period. Bottle feeding may be virtually a sentence of death in the least developed countries or poverty areas.

This close relationship between mother and child (Fig. 1.5) in the early months has to be considered in the planning of MCH services. When children, particularly breastfed infants and preschoolers, must be hospitalized, provision must be made to admit their mothers as well. The need for accommodation and facilities for mothers, such as those for washing and feeding, is applicable in any unit for low-birthweight neonates. Mothers must stay with their children in hospitals not only to give emotional support and to assist in caring for their babies but also because if the family is not given necessary health education, young patients are unlikely to survive after discharge from hospital. In Mozambique the working mother is considered the "agent of change" and admitted with her child, with no loss of pay.

The nutritional strain of reproduction on the mother requires emphasis. Females may be in a constant state of nutritional drain from girlhood through early teenage marriage, until their premature death from exhaustion in their thirties. The seriousness of this "maternal depletion syndrome" may be roughly assessed by enumerating a section of the popula-

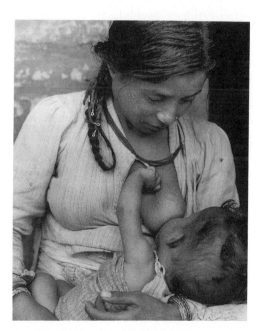

Figure 1.5. Mother–child relationship. A close relationship between mother and infant in the first few years is critical for the child's mental, physical, and social development. UNICEF photograph by Ling, Nepal.

tion by sex into age groups of 0 to 14, 15 to 19, 20 to 44 years, and over 44.

Children are dependent on the mother's nutrition and health. Recently emphasis has shifted toward the importance of nutrition in adolescents, particularly with disorders that have become more prevalent because of the slimming cults of industrialized countries. Antenatal clinics in developing regions need to emphasize maternal nutrition and general health during the life cycle of women, especially relating to childbearing, rather than concentrate exclusively on the mechanical aspects of obstetrics.

Adaptation

This is probably the most important principle in introducing meaningful health services into a developing country (Bryant 1969; Chapman 1968; Horwitz 1968; Titmuss 1962), and it is especially so with regard to MCH. The main difficulty is in introducing scientifically guided methods in difficult circumstances—those characterized by little money, few and often inadequately trained staff, poor communications, large-scale health problems, and a non-Western cultural background. Essentially, this entails adapting the implementation and practice of universal scientific principles to suit local circumstances and constraints.

To introduce a neonatal resuscitation unit into an unsophisticated area is basically an unsound decision but a relatively simple one; to institute appropriate and effective MCH services requires endless consideration and adaptation. *An orthodox type of well-baby clinic entirely focused on preventive pediatrics is an absurdity in an area in which young children are almost continually sick and there are no private practitioners or pediatric departments in the few existing hospitals.*

In Europe and North America, hospitals developed, followed by clinics more or less exclusively concerned with the prevention of disease in children. In developing regions of the world, differentiation into pediatric outpatient departments for the sick and welfare clinics for the protection of comparatively well babies is neither practical nor realistic. It is increasingly realized that clinics for young children or families that offer a blend of preventive and curative work are needed. The proportion in this mix of preventive and curative will vary depending on the particular circumstances, but it must always contain as much diagnosis and treatment as necessary and as much preventive emphasis as practical. Treatment has to be available because it is commonly needed for large numbers of sick children, it instills confidence in the parents, it may prevent more serious developments and hospitalizations, and it ensures continuity of health care within the family. At the same time as much preventive work as possible must always be carried out, including immunization and health education, in homes, clinics, health centers, and hospitals.

Another form of adaptation that is often necessary concerns staff function (Rutstein 1967). Too frequently it is assumed, mistakenly, that staff must be the same everywhere in the world. Yet minor operations and diagnostic procedures, for example, can be carried out by specially instructed medical assistants, and in some countries certain diagnoses, drug treatment, and intravenous fluids can be handled by nurses. The determining factor may be a question of economics. In rural areas of the United States, for example, midwives carry out deliveries (legally or illegally, depending on the state). But in some urban areas where obstetricians abound, midwives are severely restricted or even barred. Nevertheless, maximum use must be made of people selected from, and belonging to, the population—even those without formal education and training. Various grades of unorthodox auxiliaries such as birth attendants are important and ideal for many tasks, provided they are trained, supervised, provided with opportunities for referral, and involved in continuing in-service training. Trainees are often readily available from among the large reserve of discontented, semieducated, young people.

A new program in Mozambique has trained twenty surgical assistants for 36 months in essential obstetric functions. These mid-level health workers have learned to carry out a cesarean section, hysterectomy, dilatation and curretage, tubal ligation, removal of an ectopic pregnancy, and repair of a ruptured uterus. They now make these lifesaving treatments available in rural areas where there is no general physician available. The program has been evaluated as successful and is to be expanded (Safe Motherhood News 1993).

The importance of home care and home visiting must be stressed. It is useless for the most skilled staff to give advice unless they know and appreciate conditions in the homes. For the past century, Western medicine has become more and more firmly based in institutions. It is possible now for doctors and nurses to complete their training without ever having seen the inside of a community home and without any attempt to correlate diseases with the environment that may produce them. Yet only a well-organized system of home visiting will ensure continuity of care, practical advice, and the extension of services to those most in need. Time and transportation must be provided for staff home visits. Sometimes providing bus or taxi fares is cheaper than buying and maintaining vehicles. Bicycles or boats have also been used.

In countries with widely scattered populations and few villages, health policy has to be adapted to suit this dispersal of people. For example, widespread home visiting, though desirable, may be time-consuming, expensive, and impossible in the rainy season. Under these circumstances, carefully thought-out priorities of home visits have to be arrived at, based on the distance of the home from the center and the nature of local at-risk groups. For example, families may be visited when children are weaned from the breast or if malnutrition has been noted in the family. In some situations "mothers at risk" (about to give birth) will have to be housed in the dispensary or "maternity houses" or health centers if they live too far away from a health center or if rainy weather or mountainous terrain cuts them off.

Adaptation is also required with regard to health education as, for example, with suggested improvements in infant feeding. Education must be related to the principal nutritional problems of the women as well as the children in the area, to indigenous cultural concepts of food and sickness, and, as far as possible, to the actual and felt needs of the parents. A classic example of adaptation that does not reflect the needs of the community is the exhortations of health personnel that mothers should feed their babies certain foods from the early weeks of life. In many developing countries mothers are told, for example, to feed their infants orange juice despite the facts that infantile scurvy has not been seen in the community, oranges are unobtainable, fruit juice prepared in the village would be a source of intestinal infection, or the use of "cold" fruit for young children might have not been culturally acceptable.

Adaptation of modern technology has to be made imaginatively—for example, providing health education to a community via the transistor radio. Family care should have continuing supervision and support and use simple field measures.

Public Opinion and Political Will

As much as possible, planning of MCH services has to be in line with public opinion of priority problems. This means accounting for the politically guided national policy of the country concerned, in which the emphasis will almost always be on curative services in their more classical forms or, alternatively, on mass methods for disease control.

An apparent conflict between what MCH planners consider as a community's preventive "needs" and its stated curative "wants" may arise, although the discrepancy may not be as great as it may seem at first. Curative services are, indeed, required, but they should have preventive functions built in from their inception. The distinction between preventive and curative activities is an anachronism, especially in areas with limited resources.

It is important to ensure that politicians, senior administrators, and all other public leaders are aware of the problems as they appear to health workers and communities, as well as the basic economic soundness and the practicality of MCH programs. Cross-cultural misconceptions may be potent molders of public opinion. For example, the idea that infant malnutrition (or indeed growth and health) is related in any way to the foods eaten by the mother may be very difficult for the people to believe if the condition is considered locally to result from "heat" from the pregnant mother. Blood taking and autopsies may be viewed with understandable suspicion if undertaken in a community where magical and mystical forces are considered responsible for disease and other misfortunes. The use of dried skim milk in bags labeled "sterilized" has been known to lead to much confusion and has even been misinterpreted as a sinister form of genocide.

Among less educated segments of all non-Western communities, public opinion about ill health, treatment, and healers operates at various levels. Modern medicines may be sought for the cure of some illnesses, but at the same time, indigenous methods may be employed to discover, ward off, or placate the nonhuman forces that may have been considered responsible for the illness. Dramatic demonstrations of a cure in a particular illness cause modern medical methods to be sought, as when injections of penicillin were introduced for the treatment of yaws. By contrast, in many parts of the tropics, culturally conditioned psychological illnesses have largely remained, and quite rightly so, in the sphere of the indigenous healer. He appreciates the local "causes," and the patient has confidence in his dramatic methods, which often include divination and herbal and magical remedies. In one area in Malawi, the hospital refers "mental" cases to the indigenous healers, who have been trained to recognize cases requiring hospital referral.

The effectiveness of health care should not be oversold to the population. For some diseases, there are no rapid and specific cures, no effective means of immunization or protection. Ignorance, apathy, and fatalism cannot be eradicated with a residual spray. Education is a gradual process. All over the world, the public has heard all too often the imminent solution of medical problems. Even the most conservative newspapers and television programs constantly announce "breakthroughs" in the control of a disease, when there is only a mere hint of a possible new approach. The overselling of taxol for the "cure" of ovarian cancer in the United States is a classic example (Granai 1992).

Organ transplants garner large amounts of public interest, but they are performed at great expense in money, time, and attention. Unfortunately, such research and specialization are the fields that desperately needed medical personnel see as carrying status and promotion.

Until recently, it was assumed that teaching hospitals were medical palaces; anything else was despicable and considered second-rate or "mud-hut" medicine. Yet developments all over the world clearly show that adaptive services, aimed at identifying and helping those most at risk, providing basic services, and training and supervising auxiliaries are vital, universal needs. Scientific research and specialization are obviously essential, but when an immoderate degree of money and attention is given to them and relatively little to generalization and application, then there is an urgent case for reviewing the purpose of medicine worldwide (Titmuss 1962).

Available Health Services

It is a fact of life that MCH innovators have to work with what exists. A major aim, therefore, may be to reorient these services by better utilization, coordination, innovative adaptation, and avoidance of overlap. Usually the health staff of all types is limited (Table 1.6 and Fig. 1.6), hospitals are scattered and situated mainly in towns, and limited attempts have been made to organize principally preventive prenatal and so-called MCH clinics. The latter are probably controlled by a number of authorities, central and local governments as well as voluntary bodies. Organization can be improved by making a specific section of the ministry of health (or the equivalent) responsible for coordination of MCH activities, preferably assisted by an advisory committee composed of those working in various fields of MCH and nutrition, education, agriculture, community development, and statistics.

In most developing countries, the majority of the population live in rural areas, so carrying services outward toward the periphery is always a major challenge. The situation in any particular country or region requires individual analysis. For example, traveling with migrant pastoral people may be the only practical answer, although the expense may be prohibitive. Since it is essential to provide regular supervision, another alternative is to train at least one itinerant community health worker to travel with each group. Without outreach, the difficulties for a mother with a newborn baby on her back who is carrying an ailing toddler for many miles to the nearest hospital or center are self-evident. In some cases, flying doctor services seem to be the only way to reach people, but the costs are usually prohibitive.

An advantage of mobile personnel is that this arrangement somewhat helps the constant problem of trying to persuade trained staff to work in remote rural areas. One arrangement is a personnel agreement that two years will be served in rural areas by those training on government bursaries. So far this has not been too successful because of cultural and educational isolation of the staff and their families.

In the Philippines, the Davao Medical School was established to train medical students closer to home and to emphasize community (as opposed to hospital) practice. The *katiwalas* (community health workers) were trained on the same campus with the medical students to foster the teamwork and camaraderie that should exist ideally in a health team (De la Pax

Table 1.6. Health Professionals in Selected Countries

Country	Population (millions)	Population per physician	Population per nurse	Population per hospital bed
Costa Rica	2.74	958	450	—
Hong Kong	5.74	1,075	241	204
Norway	4.22	451	57	67
Sierra Leone	4.04	13,626	1,090	—
Chad	5.54	38,358	3,395	—

Source: World Bank (1991).

Curative services

Region	Doctors (per 10 000 population)	Population per physician
East Africa	0.6	17,480
Central Africa	0.7	15,387
West Africa	0.7	14,965
S.E. Asia	1.5	6,646
S. Central Asia	2.5	4,021
North Africa	4.7	2,151
Southern Africa	4.7	2,135
East Asia	4.8	2,106
S.W. Asia	5.1	1,947
Caribbean	6.6	1,523
Central America	7.0	1,423
South America	10.7	1,128
Oceania	12.3	813
Europe, N. America	17.5	572

Region	Nurses and midwives (per 10 000 population)	Population per nurse or midwife
East Africa	3.8	2,648
Central Africa	6.3	1,595
West Africa	6.6	1,527
S.E. Asia	6.5	1,535
S. Central Asia	2.5	4,031
North Africa	9.4	1,068
Southern Africa	32.4	309
East Asia	10.7	933
S.W. Asia	9.7	1,027
Caribbean	19.1	522
Central America	8.0	1,245
South America	10.9	997
Oceania	66.0	151
Europe, N. America	55.0	194

Region	Hospital beds (per 10 000 population)	Population per bed
East Africa	27.7	847
Central Africa	51.8	383
West Africa	17.9	971
S.E. Asia	21.7	658
S. Central Asia	8.2	3,136
North Africa	23.5	547
Southern Africa	37.9	313
East Asia	58.7	285
S.W. Asia	30.0	564
Caribbean	53.0	260
South America	25.4	484
Central America	48.8	337
Oceania	69.0	192
Europe, N. America	102.0	109

Figure 1.6. Worldwide distribution of curative services. Source: UNICEF (1980).

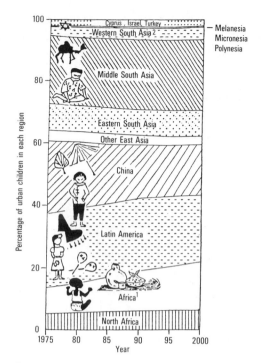

Figure 1.7. Proportion of all urban children in less developed regions, 1975–2000. In Africa and Latin America, the percentage of urban children is rising. Source: Adapted from UN Population Division 1980 estimates.

1983). This example illustrates that training of paramedical personnel can best be carried out regionally in nonurban areas, enabling constant contact with local problems.

One of the largest problems facing the extension of rural health care services is the lack of an infrastructure and a delivery system. Rural problems aside, urban migration is rapidly increasing, and all urban areas suffer from slums that pose the familiar problems of poverty and poor sanitation, plus new ones such as delinquency and family disruption (Fig. 1.7). Urbanization and affluence may bring with them new problems—obesity, dental caries, and so-called chronic diseases of adults, among others. In most developing countries the accessibility to health services is limited and the distribution of services is inequitable, usually concentrated in large, urban centers serving a minority of high-income urban residents.

Training

Suitably trained staff is the top priority for the development of MCH and other family health services everywhere in the world, but especially in less developed areas. Achieving this goal requires political will backed by financial investment. The principal problems are the types of personnel and the level of training feasible and economically supportable with limited financial resources (Fendall 1964).

Training programs must be flexible and constantly improved to deal with long-standing conditions, as well as new problems, such as drug-resistant malaria and AIDS. It is usual for too few highly trained personnel to be available and usual that they are used to occupy key positions as supervisors, coordinators, and catalysts. Equally inevitable, larger numbers of lesser trained staff have to be used for an "interim" period that may actually last years or even decades. All over the world, auxiliaries with limited general education and technical training have major responsibilities in health services. Many countries have developed their own training manuals and programs for local needs.

Training must be flexible but also practical and directly related to the particular country rather than an attempt to copy a model from elsewhere. Midwives and traditional birth attendants need instruction not only in matters of pregnancy and childbirth but also in nutrition and the supervision of young children and mothers, for in many countries the running of clinics for infants and preschool children will be their responsibility. Similarly, if medical assistants are expected to carry out certain types of surgery or if nurses are expected to issue a range of medicines, suitable instruction must be included in their courses, and health professionals must be taught how to teach and supervise supportively. For all groups, functional practicality must be the dominant theme, with an eye to future developments.

Health workers should be encouraged to make use of MCH facilities for their own families and should be taught how to promote their own and their children's well-being. Mass immunizations, oral rehydration, environmental sanitation, pest control, and food distribution are of little use unless individuals also understand and exemplify a better way of living. Basic knowledge of MCH should be included in the training of health professionals, workers in community development, agricultural extension, home economics, social work, and women's clubs, together with administrators. Workers in MCH must understand how the roles and activities of each group affect MCH and how to work together.

Research

Research is vital if health services are to be both reliable and adaptable to the rapidly changing circumstances of modern times.

Students and staff must appreciate that research does not necessarily require much equipment. Simple methods can produce valuable results provided they are carefully planned and guided by modern statistical principles. For example, the collection of accurate data concerning users of hospitals, outpatient departments, and health centers is necessary for planning and feedback. Moreover, research should not be exclusively related to laboratory or theoretical work but should also gather data on attitudes, behavior, and responses to education. At larger centers, such as medical schools, both major forms of research are required: applied or operational, and basic or academic. It is difficult to tell which research will be of practical value. Laboratory research on virus culture ultimately led to the development of measles vaccine, which has had a great effect on child health throughout the world.

With the large-scale problems that face MCH workers in developing regions today, it is necessary to give emphasis to the investigation of problems of an immediate nature, that is, operational research. In delivering services, MCH workers need to be aware of the incidence, prevalence, and impact of an area-specific disease, as well as means of control.

Social Assistance

Many areas suffer from abject poverty of material resources, education, and enterprise. The instinct to rush in with financial social assistance, welfare, and supplementary feeding is often justified in times of emergency but must be carefully considered when conditions are long-standing. A community that has been neglected and exploited may be further demoralized by ill-considered "welfare" of this sort.

It is usually more helpful to show people how to help themselves than to provide for them. It was Plutarch who said, "The real destroyer of the liberties of any people is he who spreads among them bounties, donations and largesse." Of course, the helpless and the disadvantaged must not be abandoned. It is easy enough to give injections to an unsophisticated population, to a social drop-out, or to a problem family. It is also easy to give material help rather than to teach self-help. Patience, persistence, and continuing support are required to teach people how to feed children, to use clean water, and to trust their own resources rather than witchcraft or the welfare state.

Public assistance is not a panacea for all afflictions. How much damage can be done by any but the most carefully considered and continuous type of assistance is a subject about which little is known. To give comfort without humiliation is one of the most complicated of problems—even to give comfort without demoralization. Health workers have the opportunity to identify local resources for people at risk and to develop appropriate community-based support.

Volunteer workers have blazed the trail in medical care, education, and agriculture, and they will continue to provide invaluable help and inspiration. But the entire community must take some responsibility. The care of the helpless and disadvantaged is an important branch of statecraft. Social assistance with funds and food should generally be short-term to develop permanent solutions.

Coordination

Probably no other word (except perhaps *evaluation*) is used as frequently as *coordination* and yet is practiced so infrequently. A general absence of coordination among programs may be the result of tunnel vision training, personal departmental rivalries, or restrictive funding mechanisms and areas of influence, but it is also related to the fact that with so many tasks and so few staff, it is usually difficult to find the time to practice coordination.

Coordination is required for overall planning at health centers. Health staff and other extension workers must learn to work together so they know and appreciate each other's jobs, skills, and limitations. More broadly, a coordinated comprehensive program must evolve as a major component of an overall plan for national development in the form of primary health care (PHC). Instead of providing single-service programs, health planners should integrate services in the interest of efficiency and cost.

In the early 1980s the revolutionary concept that health care is a right, not a privilege, became accepted worldwide. The 1978 joint UNICEF/WHO conference on PHC at Alma Ata in the former Soviet Union had laid down the principles of PHC and set an ambitious goal to achieve

Health for All by the Year 2000. PHC as defined at the Alma Ata conference (WHO 1978) encompassed addressing the main health problems in the community and providing appropriate promotive, preventive, curative, and rehabilitative services. Because these services evolve from and reflect the economic conditions and social values of each country and its communities, they vary by country and community but include at least eight basic elements (WHO 1978):

1. Food supply and proper nutrition.
2. Health education.
3. Provision of essential drugs.
4. Immunization.
5. Maternal and child care.
6. Treatment of common diseases and injuries.
7. Adequate supply of safe water and basic sanitation.
8. Communicable disease control.

In addition to these eight elements, PHC requires action on a wider range of factors crucial for good health, including control of environmental pollution and protection of natural resources. PHC services are needed in the workplace to promote safe work practices and protect workers from the effects of dangerous substances in agriculture and industry. Good housing is a key element in achieving and maintaining health, particularly for vulnerable groups. The status of women is important; women often care for their family's health while neglecting their own health. Their special health needs have to be identified and protected. Public awareness of health and how it relates to daily life must be promoted in the education system, through the mass media, and by training health workers. Finally, PHC must be available, accessible, and affordable.

For the PHC objectives to be achieved, the following prerequisites are essential:

1. Active participation by the community, implying that the local community would exercise some control and authority over the contents and management of the program, as well as responsibility for implementation.
2. A socially relevant strategy adapted to the local context, implying that Western medicine would be shaped to augment rather than replace traditional health systems.
3. Involvement of other sectors—education, housing, water, sanitation, and agriculture—and women's groups to promote general development.
4. A program of health services and health promotion largely operated by paramedical personnel.
5. Use of simple but effective technologies.

In many countries such as Thailand and Botswana, PHC has been effective in strengthening national health systems, and nongovernmental organizations have developed innovative small-scale PHC projects. PHC can work, but it is difficult and complex to implement because of the interaction of social, economic, managerial, and epidemiological factors (AHRTAG 1991). In Thailand, PHC has been augmented with a basic minimum needs strategy, in which the following components are considered the basic minimum needs (Chanawongse et al. 1988):

1. Adequate food intake of good quality and safety.
2. Good housing conditions.
3. Full employment of working-age people.
4. Essential basic services (health and education).
5. Safety in daily life.
6. Maintenance of good culture and habits.
7. Adequate supply of daily income-generating work.
8. Family planning.
9. Community participation and obedience of the law.

In the 1990s, PHC is facing serious challenges. Its lack of dramatic success has led to a call for a new approach, with PHC to be replaced by alternative solutions. UNICEF has moved to vertical strategies in GOBI (growth monitoring, oral rehydration, breastfeeding, and immunizations). Its main thrust now is toward child survival activities, with immunizations heading the list. An attempt has been made to add family spacing and female literacy to the action plan, and maternal health, too, has been included. But without the development of a health infrastructure, the effects of these actions will not drastically alter mortality or improve the quality of life of the poorest of the poor.

FUTURE DEVELOPMENTS

Battling the immediate problems that face mothers and children in developing regions must occur simultaneously with trying to foresee future trends. Improved statistics are vital for this effort, and their collection should be built into all programs. Historical developments in other parts of the world—for example, the change of patterns of disease in Europe that resulted from the Industrial Revolution and urbanization—may act as indicators.

Changes of major significance to the health of women and children will surely occur. Rapid urbanization is a universal phenomenon, and so is industrialization. Perhaps the latter will increase national prosperity and thus the development of improved health, education, and social services. However, industrialization may be slow, the increased earnings may not reach the majority, and the ensuing changes in life-style and health problems already indicate clearly that this trend can be double-edged.

The transition from a rural, agricultural, mainly subsistence economy, in a well-regulated system of life guided by time-honored social mores, to a detribalized cash economy in mushrooming shantytowns on the "septic fringe" of large cities, has considerable significance for the health of women and children. Without traditional social controls or customary "absorptive mechanisms," the number of abandoned, socially unwanted, and abused children and women is increasing, with all the associated psychological, behavioral, nutritional, and other health problems.

Nutritional patterns are likely to alter among these ill-prepared new townsfolk, and especially among children. Most significant, a decline in breastfeeding is usually found, partly because some mothers may have to work in towns where breastfeeding is taboo by modern convention and successful status-giving bottle feeding is carried out by those in higher socioeconomic groups. The harmful effects of ill-advised and inappropriate advertising of expensive proprietary milk are clear. The widespread lack of knowledge of breastfeeding on the part of health staff adds to the anti-breastfeeding atmosphere.

Lack of finance does not permit adequate milk to be bought. Health care providers should ensure that women who chose not to breastfeed understand fully the financial implications of their decision. Costs are both direct and indirect. Direct costs include the baby milk formula, nipples, and bottles, fuel, and work time. Indirect costs include hospitalization for children who have developed diarrhea or other infections and malnutrition because of contaminated or diluted feeds. An unskilled mother has to spend half her income or more for appropriate substitution of mother's milk (Steenbergen 1986).

It has been estimated that at least $429 million (U.S.) could be saved annually if mothers in the U.S. Department of Agriculture's successful Women, Infants and Children's supplementary feeding program (WIC) would breastfeed for just one month. WIC provides food for pregnant mothers and infants up to 3 years of age. Formula is by far the most expensive item in the package and in the last 6 years its cost has risen over 100 percent. WIC accounts for nearly 40 percent of all infant formula purchased in the United States (IBFAN Africa News 1989).

To feed an infant properly on powdered milk formula requires about 40 kilograms of milk powder. When the percent of wages used to buy 40 kilograms of formula was calculated against the minimum wage in urban areas, it amounted to 18 percent in Botswana, 21 percent in Zimbabwe, 40 percent in Kenya, 108 percent in Sierra Leone, and 246 percent in Nigeria. The cost was influenced by type of formula used (Table 1.7).

The cost of feeding a 3-month old baby infant formula, and the treatment of infantile malnutrition and diarrhea

arising from the ill-effects of formula feeding is staggering in terms of foreign exchange. Forty-seven percent of Pakistani families spend about 40 percent of average monthly earnings (about US $10) to feed infant formula to one child. In Barbados, in 82 percent of the cases studied, a tin of milk that should have lasted four days was made to last between five days and three weeks (Helsing and King 1982).

Purchase of breastmilk substitutes not only affects individual families but has far reaching consequences at the national level. It may mean the loss of high grade food, the need to keep milk cattle or to use part of the foreign exchange to import milkpowder for infant feeding. In Pakistan, for example, the baby milk imports increased from $4 million in 1982–1983 to $8.5 million from 1987–1988 (IBFAN Africa News 1989). The resources needed annually to replace

Table 1.7. Costs of Bottle Feeding

Country	Brand of formula	Cost for a year in local money and dollar	Yearly legal minimum urban wage	Percent of wage used to buy 40 kg of formula	Food that could be bought for that money
Botswana	Lactogen	P 432 (US $216)	P 2400 (US $1200)	18	62 kg meat, 36 kg beans, 208 kg sorghum (*all* of those!)
Zimbabwe	Neslac[a]	Z$379 (US $189)	Z$ 1800 (US $900)	21	124 lt sour milk, 37 kg beans, 207 kg maize meal
Kenya	Nan starter and Lactogen	Ksh 4092 (US $189)	Ksh 8676 (US $404)	47	277 lt fresh cow's milk, 83 kg beans, 181 kg maize meal
Sierra Leone	Lactogen	Le 13,200 (US $203)	Le 12,000 (US $185)	108	220 kg fish, 16.5 kg cassava leaves, 92 kg rice
Ghana	Ostermilk	C 84,000 (US $311)	C 42,500 (US $157)	198	105 kg fish, 126 kg beans, 420 kg maize
Nigeria	SMA	N 3960 (US $558)	N 1500 (US $211)	264	158 kg fish, 137 kg cow peas, 305 kg cassava

Source: IBFAN African News (1989).

[a]Neslac contains cornstarch as an ingredient. Newborns lack the ability to digest starch. However Neslac is labelled for newborns and cheaper than Lactogen, so many Zimbabwean mothers buy it.

breastmilk in Indonesia would be $62 million; in Tanzania, $22 million. Worldwide, $15 billion would be required to feed 120 million infants (BFHI News 1992). In addition, the use of formula leads to waste and environmental pollution. (Radford 1991).

Furthermore, inadequate education and poor home circumstances (perhaps with water obtained from a nearby pond, with one saucepan and with no insect-proof storage space) ensure that homeopathic doses of milk will be fed through a heavily contaminated bottle. The result is an inevitable increase in infectious diarrhea and nutritional marasmus.

"Bottle-feeding disease" was uncommon in Mulago Hospital, Kampala, until the mid-1960s, when it accounted for 5 to 10 percent of pediatric admissions. Even among the comparatively well educated and affluent, bottle feeding and early mixed feeding produces gastrointestinal, nutritional, and allergic problems. It is surely a wry paradox that in a world searching for nutritious foods for young children from such exotic sources as algae and leaves, breastmilk, widely recognized as a major national food resource, should be disappearing from the nutritional scene and be consistently ignored by agronomists (Helsing and King 1982).

The crux of the problem is to prevent this development from spreading, especially among poorer communities. Locally, appropriate modification of advertising is highly desirable, but it is difficult to persuade the persuaders. It is probably optimistic to expect the trend toward bottle feeding to be halted or reversed, unless the trend-setters—mothers (including female health workers and the wives of male health workers) in the Western world and educated mothers of the upper socioeconomic groups in developing regions—practice what the health workers preach. The WHO organization and member countries (except the United States) adopted the International Code of Marketing of Breast Milk Substitutes in an attempt to halt the promotional and marketing practices of infant formula companies and develop programs to encourage and protect breastfeeding (WHO 1981), but codes are not enough. Recent surveys have shown them to have only a limited effect since it is impossible to enforce this voluntary code.

Reorientation of hospital practices and training of health personnel are critical and underway in many countries. A massive effort was initiated in Brazil on all fronts to halt the erosion of breastfeeding, especially through mother support groups such as La Leche League International. Up to 280 mother support groups were developed in the *favellas* (urban shanties). Four aspects of breastfeeding require programs with different stresses and variations according to local conditions (Fig. 1.8).

A number of new breastfeeding programs have shown what Clavano (1981) found in the Philippines when exclusive breastfeeding and rooming in were introduced in the newborn units: a decrease in infant mortality, a decrease in neonatal sepsis, and a decrease in the use of intravenous fluids. These results have reinforced the urgency of changing maternity hospital practices and providing mother support groups. In an attempt to stop the erosion of breastfeeding, UNICEF and WHO have launched a breastfeeding initiative. Through this initiative steps have been taken to end the supply of free and low-cost infant formula to hospitals and maternity facilities globally (UNICEF 1992), and to make hospitals "baby and mother friendly" through the "Ten Steps to Successful Breastfeeding" by which every facility providing maternity services and care for newborn infants should:

1. Have a written breastfeeding policy that is routinely communicated to all health care staff.

Information and Motivation

Mass media
Support groups (La Leche league)

Health Services

Services—
Rooming in
Breastmilk bank
(colostrum for all babies)
|
Training—
Theory
Practice
Sanitation

Working Mothers

Lactation leave
Creches
Nursing pauses
Legislation with enforcement
  mechanisms

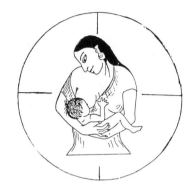

Infant Formula Industry

Legislation (code)
Monitoring

Figure 1.8. Four elements of breastfeeding programs.

3. Inform all pregnant women about the benefits and management of breastfeeding.
4. Help mothers initiate breastfeeding within a half-hour of birth.
5. Show mothers how to breastfeed and how to maintain lactation even if they should be separated from their infants.
6. Give newborn infants no food or drink other than breastmilk, unless medically indicated.
7. Practice rooming in (allowing mothers and infants to remain together) twenty-four hours a day.
8. Encourage breastfeeding on demand.
9. Give no artificial teats or pacifiers to breastfeeding infants.
10. Foster the establishment of breastfeeding support groups and refer mothers to them on discharge from the hospital or clinic.

By December 1992 more than 122 developing countries had acted to end the dangerous practice of distributing low cost and free formula to health care facilities, and 90 developing and 14 indus-trialized countries initiated the process to evaluate and certify hospitals as baby friendly (J. Nelson UNICEF-NGO Liaison Office memo, 1993). Efforts are under way to involve more industrialized countries and to evaluate and certify more baby-friendly health care facilities (UNICEF Guidelines 1992). The ultimate objective is to create a mother- and baby-friendly environment both inside and outside the hospital.

For the newly urbanized population, child feeding patterns may be changed and use of new foods or lack of availability of customary foods may cause nutritional problems. For example, cassava flour may be the most readily available product but may cause protein energy malnutrition because of its low protein content. In addition, berries, leafy vegetables, insects (a source of protein), and other foods gathered in rural areas are unavailable, and as a result the children are at increased risk of micronutrient deficiencies. The establishment of "vegetable clubs" at clinics may solve some problems. To counteract the disadvantages, however, both health and educational services should be concentrated on areas of need and opportunities for maternal education.

Another consideration important today and in the future is the MCH aspects of overpopulation and large, stressful, and ill-spaced families. Apart from the well-known general nutritional and economic effects of population growth expanding in advance of economic development, the cumulative effect of continuous reproduction on Third World mothers is often underappreciated. In poor circumstances, the need for child spacing, as well as family limitation, is an important factor in the prevention of malnutrition.

Family planning in developing regions is fraught with potential misunderstandings, as it is elsewhere, and may be viewed suspiciously as a scheme to diminish the population for sinister, political motives. Motivation is difficult in communities where large families are prestigious evidence of virility and valuable as a work force, as warriors, for bride-price, and for security in old age. Aesthetics, acceptability, economic practicability, and religious sanctions must be taken into consideration in family planning programs. In some parts of the world, traditional child-spacing techniques (by means of exclusive breastfeeding, polygamy, and various customs prohibiting intercourse until a child has reached a certain culturally defined age) may be a useful and an acceptable means of introducing an otherwise foreign concept.

Family planners must recognize that if they are to win the confidence of the community, they should also provide assistance for infertility problems. In some areas, untreated pelvic infections have created a great deal of infertility. The only way to form a strong basis for a family planning program is to ensure that it is safe and will benefit the children and their mothers. It will improve the quality and hence diminish the quantity of population growth.

CONCLUSION

The principal factors in the development of MCH services in developing regions are the problems of vast numbers and minimal resources of all sorts and archaic, unsuitable, and unworkable ideas and methods of organization. To achieve results under these circumstances, it is constantly necessary to reconsider and refine methods that are locally adaptable, practically applicable, of proved and acceptable principles, and geared to the health priorities of the region. The main principles to guide MCH developments can be summarized in three words: *priorities, adaptation,* and *training.*

Efficient fact finding and surveying of needs is necessary everywhere (Backett 1969; Bennett 1979; WHO 1980). The sifting and analysis of data leads to the most effective and logically planned programs. Balanced realism must be employed rather than confused, dissipated efforts covering too broad a spectrum. "Today's needs must sometimes be sacrificed to the interests of tomorrow's children," Fedall (1964) pointed out. The greatest need is often not money but the right attitude. Methods and approaches should not necessarily be hallowed by tradition but should be economical, functional, and realistic.

MCH services can become useful and economic means not only of curing and preventing disease among the most vulnerable but of helping the progress of communities by reaching the majority in need through tailor-made comprehensive services.

REFERENCES

Abel-Smith, B. (1967). *An International Study of Health Expenditure.* Wld. Hlth. Org. Publ. Hlth. Pap., no. 32. World Health Organization, Geneva.

Adenyi-Jones, O. (1956). The importance of child health in developing countries (with special reference to Nigeria). *J. Trop. Pediat.* **2**, 32.

AHRTAG (1991). Goals for primary health care in the 1990's. *Appropriate Health Resources and Technologies Action Group Health Action* **1**, 1.

Babbs, S.; Sanders, D.; and Werner, D. (1993). *Questioning the Solution.* Hesperian Foundation, Palo Alto (in preparation).

Baby Friendly Hospital Initiative News (1992). UNICEF, New York.

Backett, E. M. (1969). Community medicine and the improvement of health services. A model for the university contribution to innovation. *Lancet* **ii**, 39.

Baumslag, N. (1989). *Breastfeeding Passport to Life.* NGO Committee on UNICEF Committee on Nutrition. UNICEF, New York.

Bennett, F. J. (1979). *Community Diagnosis and Health Action: A Manual for Tropical and Rural Areas.* Macmillan, London.

Bryant, J. H. (1969). *Health and the Developing World.* Cornell University Press, Ithaca, NY.

Bull. PAHO (1980). Programs to improve the nutrition of pregnant and lactating women. *Bulletin of Pan American Health Organization* **14**, 22–34.

Caudill, H. M. (1937). *Night Comes to the Cumberlands.* Little, Brown, Boston.

Chanawongse, K., and Singhadej, O. (1988). *Components of Basic Human Needs.* Asean Training Centre for PHC Development, Thailand.

Chapman, J. S. (1968). Problems of medicine in the underdeveloped areas of the United States. *Arch. Environ. Hlth.* **17**, 844.

Clavano, N. (1981). The results of change in hospital practices. A paediatrician's campaign for breast feeding in the Phillipines. *Assignment Children* **55/56**, 139–165.

Cook, R. (1968). The financial cost of malnutrition "Commonwealth Caribbean." *J. Trop. Pediat.* **14**, 60.

Cordier, S. et al. (1991). *Brit. J. Industrial Medicine* **48**, 375–81.

De la Pax, Trinidad (1983). The katiwala approach to training community health workers. *Wld. Hlth. Forum* **4**, 34.

Evans, J. R.; Lashman Hall, K.; and Warford, J. (1981). Health care in the developing world. Problems of scarcity and choice. *New Engl. J. Med.* **305**, 17.

Fendall, N. R. E. (1964). Organization of health services in emerging countries. *Lancet* **ii**, 53.

Gilson, L. (1991). Paying for health care. *AHRTAG Health Action* **1**, 7.

Gish, O. (1975). *Planning the Health Sector.* 2d ed. Croom Helm, London.

Granai, C. D. (1992). Ovarian cancer—Unrealistic expectations. *New Engl. J. Med.* **327**, 197–200.

Harrison, P. (1981). *Inside the Third World.* 2d ed. Penguin Books, Harmondsworth, England.

Helsing, E., and King, F. S. (1982). *Breast-Feeding in Practice.* Oxford University Press, Oxford.

Hetzel, B. S. (1978). *Basic Health Care in Developing Countries: An Epidemiological Perspective.* Oxford University Press, Oxford.

Horwitz, A. (1968). *Balance Sheet of Accomplishments, 1967.* Pan American Health Organization, Washington, D.C.

IBFAN Africa News (1989). Cost of powdered infant formula. Dec., pp. 4–5.

ICN (1992). *Nutrition and Development—A Global Assessment.* International Conference on Nutrition. FAO/WHO, Geneva.

Jelliffe, D. B. (1967). Mother-child interdependence in developing regions. *Matern. Child Care* **3**, 351.

Jelliffe, D. B., and Jelliffe, E. F. P. (1978). *Human Milk in the Modern World.* Oxford University Press, Oxford.

Jelliffe, D. B., and Jelliffe, E. F. P. (1989). *Community Nutritional Assessment.* Oxford University Press, Oxford.

Kaprio, L. A. (1965). The economics of health in relationship to international health activities. *Roy Soc. Hlth. J.* **85**, 395.

King, M. (1990). Health is a sustainable state. *Lancet* **ii**, 664–67.

Lancet (1990). Editorial: Structured adjustment and health in Africa. *Lancet* **335**, 855.

McDermott, W. (1966). Modern medicine and the demographic disease pattern of overly traditional societies: A technologic misfit. In *Environmental Factors Bearing on Education in Developing Countries.* New York.

Mata, L. J. (1978). *The Children of Santa Maria Cauque: A Prospective Field Study of Health and Growth.* MIT Press, Cambridge, Mass.

Medovy, H. (1968). Lapses in prophylaxis: Errors of omission. *J. Pediat.* **73**, 308.

Newman, G. (1906). *Infant Mortality: A Social Problem.* Methuen, London.

PAHO (1970). *Maternal Nutrition and Family*

Planning. Pan American Health Organization Scientific Report, no. 204. Washington, D.C.

Pop. Ref. Bur. (1992). *1992 World Population Data Sheet.* Population Reference Bureau, Washington, D.C.

Pub. Hlth. News (1991). Abstracts on hygiene and communicable diseases. *Public Health News* 66(8), 22.

Radford, A. (1991). *The Ecological Impact of Bottle Feeding.* Baby Milk Action Coalition, Cambridge, U.K.

Radford, A. J. (1978). Village-based health and medical resources. In *Basic Health Care in Developing Countries.* Ed. B. S. Hetzel. Oxford University Press, Oxford.

Rosen, G. (1958). *A History of Public Health.* MD Publications, New York.

Rutstein, D. D. (1967). *The Coming Revolution in Medicine.* Cambridge, Mass.

Sanders, D. (1985). *The Struggle for Health.* Macmillan Education, London.

Safe Motherhood News (1993). Delegating in Mozambique. No. 10, p. 8. (WHO, Geneva.)

Sivard, R. L. (1983). *World Military and Social Expenditures.* World Priorities, Washington, D.C.

Steenbergen, V. W. M., and Kusin, J. A. (1986). *Borstvoeding in de tropen.* Kooninklyk Instituut voor de Tropen, Amsterdam.

Sutedjo, S. M.; Muslichan, S.; and Sudijano (1969). Mortality in infants and children of Indonesian doctors. *Pediat. Indones.* 9, 1.

Sy-Quimsiam, E. B. (1968). The socio-economic aspects of social pediatrics in the Philippines. *Philipp. J. Pediat.* 17, 228.

Taylor, C. E., and Hall, M. F. (1968). Health, population, and economic development. *Science* 157, 651.

Titmuss, R. M. (1962). Medical ethics and social change. *Lancet* ii, 209.

UNDP (1992). *Human Development Report 1992.* United Nations Development Programme, Oxford University Press, New York.

UNICEF (1980). *Assignment Children.* Ed. P. E. Mandl. No. 49/50. UNICEF, Geneva.

UNICEF (1990). *Children and Development in the 1990's: A UNICEF Sourcebook on the Occasion of the World Summit for Children.* United Nations, New York.

UNICEF (1992). *State of the World's Children.* Oxford University Press, New York.

UNICEF Guidelines (1992). Part IV: Ending the Distribution of Free and Low Cost Supplies of Infant Formula to Health Care Facilities: Assisting Government Action and Gaining Industry Committment. October. UNICEF, New York.

Ushewokunze, H. (1980). *Behind and Toward a Health Model for Zimbabwe.* Ministry of Health, Zimbabwe.

World Bank (1981). *World Bank Development Report,* Washington, D.C.

World Bank (1991). *Social Indicators of Development.* World Bank, Johns Hopkins University, Baltimore.

World Development Report (1993). *Investing in Health.* Oxford University Press, New York.

WHO (1969). *Organization and Administration of Maternal and Child Health Services.* World Health Organization Tech. Rep. Ser., no. 428.

WHO (1978). *Primary Health Care, Alma Ata USSR.* World Health Organization, Geneva.

WHO (1980). *Sixth Report on the World Health Situation, 1973–1977.* World Health Organization, Geneva.

WHO (1981). *International Code of Marketing of Breast Milk Substitutes.* World Health Organization, Geneva.

WHO (1987). *World Health Statistics Report.* World Health Organization, Geneva.

WHO (1992). *Implementation of the Global Strategy for Health for All by the Year 2000.* 2d ed. World Health Organization, Geneva.

WHO/UNICEF (1989). *Protecting, Promoting and Supporting Breast-feeding: The Special Role of Maternity Services.* World Health Organization, Geneva.

2

Cultural Factors

*We take our own standards of life so much for granted, that we
simply have no conception that they are not universal.*
C. D. WILLIAMS, 1941

Children everywhere are born into two external worlds. The first is that of physical and geographical surroundings—for example, the dry heat of the arid desert or the ice, snow, and cold of the Arctic. Their second world is that of culture—the interconnected system of customs, ideas, and behavior that has been created for them by their elders and ancestors, mainly through ecological adaptation.

All communities, of all degrees of technological sophistication, urbanization, and industrialization, have evolved their own cultural pattern, which can be defined as a common way of life shared by all members of the group. This includes not only their preferred life goals, their valued ends and sanctioned means, and their attitudes to life and death but also all aspects of everyday life, the relationships between different members of a family, the role of women, customary ways of preparing food (Fig. 2.1), and approved methods of rearing children (Fig. 2.2).

The cultural pattern of a group is based on learned behavior, acquired partly by deliberate instruction on the part of the parents, but mostly absorbed subconsciously by observation of the behavior of relatives and other close members of the community.

All cultures are constantly undergoing change, taking in and absorbing new practices and beliefs when these do not conflict with fundamental tenets, a process described as syncretization (Baumslag 1972). In Lesotho, sexual intercourse is taboo while the woman is breastfeeding, so migrant male workers bring home formula cans to their wives, who can then bottle-feed their babies and have sex.

The process of acculturation begins at birth and is mediated by every contact the infant has with the surrounding world, including the way babies are carried, the role of the parents in child rearing, and the foods that are (or are not) eaten by different groups within the particular community, particularly pregnant and lactating women and infants (Foster 1951; Jelliffe 1964; Williams 1958b). From birth, the frequency and affection of human contacts have a bearing on the progress and development of the infant.

In a similar manner, MCH workers have been molded in their own habits and ideas by their own cultural pattern,

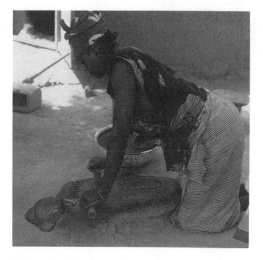

Figure 2.1. Traditional preparation of food. This mother in Mali is pressing out oil from the karitas nut *(beurre de karite)*. If proper attention is paid to hygienic preparation, the oil can be a good source of concentrated calories to augment a weanling's diet. Photograph by Carol Carp.

are intensified when urbanized health workers with no sensitization or cultural preparedness are sent to work in rural areas. Appropriate responses to local problems are often a blend of valuable traditional practices and acceptable modern scientific concepts.

Medical teams are encouraged to seek advice from social anthropologists in order to understand cultural patterns. The collaborative efforts of these two groups can be invaluable. Additionally, health workers who see people and communities in times of crisis can often add to the information collected by anthropologists (Williams 1958a; Pelto 1978). Recently, insights of medical anthropologists and "anthropological medicalists," health professionals who have become sensitive to cultural issues, have been combined (Jelliffe 1992).

Most human beings possess a certain

which, as every culture does, contains both scientifically rational and irrational elements. In fact, it requires considerable insight to realize that the customs and practices of one's own group are neither the only, nor necessarily the best, methods but merely some of the many alternatives possible. It has been said that a fish does not know he swims in water; the lack of cultural awareness of health workers has been related to the fact that social anthropology and other behavioral sciences are still unappreciated as aspects of medical training.

Too many health workers in the past have concentrated on teaching their own ideas rather than on understanding those of other people. Success in the management and prevention of disease depends on recognition of the causes of disease, the resources of the patient, and the cultural pattern and outlook of patients, as both groups and individuals.

Generalizations are dangerous. In every region, there will be some people who are receptive to new ideas, while others cling to ancient practices. The problems

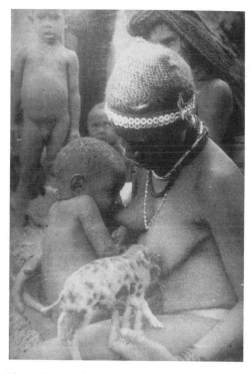

Figure 2.2. Cultural norms vary. In remote rural New Guinea, breastfeeding a piglet alongside an infant is socially acceptable.

amount of common sense based on practical observation as well as local mores. When health professionals in Fiji were puzzled by an increasing fear among the islanders about eating fish, a basic traditional food, an investigation revealed that the fear was well founded. The fish were eating a toxin-producing algae, which was passed on to humans (WHO 1982).

Parents are nearly always devoted to their children; when they see their ill child recover before their eyes, they reconsider their attitudes. In Indonesia there used to be a saying, *"Biar mati anak. Jangan mati adat"* ("Let the child, but not the custom die"), but this now is being reversed. We were once told that the devotion to the whitest of white rice in Southeast Asia was impossible to combat. But in the past forty years, beriberi, a major killing condition of young children in particular, has been vastly reduced because of the awareness of the deficiencies of white rice. The majority of people in Malaya and Singapore now use reinforced or undermilled rice and the correct food supplements for pregnant and lactating women and young children. They still enjoy white rice but much of it is now fortified. The infant mortality rate (IMR) in Singapore was 300 per 1,000 live births immediately after the Japanese occupation in World War II; it fell to 100 in 1950 and 23 in 1968. With social and economic improvements and the extension of health services, it dropped to 6.7 by 1992 (Pop. Ref. Bur. 1992). There has been no vast expenditure in MCH but a steady development of essential services.

In Jamaica, between 1935 and 1960, the propaganda against some herbal teas (such as Senecio and Crotalaria) practically eliminated the incidence of venoocclusive disease of the liver (Asprey 1953; Bras et al. 1954). In spite of the fact that no more than 50 percent of babies were ever taken to a health center, the mothers stopped giving their children the disease-causing teas.

Social anthropologists are apt to ignore how much of human behavior is a response to fear and to a high death rate in children. Show people what they can do for themselves to protect themselves, their families, and their community, and give them confidence that their children will survive, and their attitudes and receptivity to health education will change.

Ill health, whether episodic or chronic, has an effect on behavior and activity. An ancient Chinese philosopher said, "All my problems are associated with my body. If I have no body, I have no problems." Not all of us can speak with much assurance about incorporeal existence, but anyone who has suffered from hunger and hardship, and sickness and deprivation, must have some sympathy. Concern with bodily ills and functions gives medical and other health workers an enormous advantage in understanding, and possibly ameliorating, adverse conditions and their mental and cultural effects (BMJ 1970).

Social anthropologists were trained to observe and to deduce, but now they are also engaged in attempting to change behavior. Health workers, on the other hand, are not a contemplative body of people. They are not there merely for the negative function of controlling disease but for the positive function of helping to create a better use of resources and a better life, best achieved through teamwork.

A mother may tell you that her child is sick because a witch looked at him or a thunderbolt fell on him. But physical signs are of universal significance and all babies speak the same language. Although the mother knows something is wrong, she may not be aware of the cause. Some of the information that health workers desire will not easily be ascertained. Some ideas and beliefs may be forthcoming only after prolonged familiarity with the fieldworker, when with goodwill and the ability to help, confidence is established. Cicely Williams worked in Accra with patients for nearly three years before the local name of *kwa-shiorkor* was mentioned. To utter the word was supposed to be unlucky (Williams 1963). At that time, the disease of protein malnutrition and its symptoms, both acute and chronic, were entirely unknown to "scientific" medicine.

Health workers are in a privileged position. They are given precious opportunities for listening and observing (limited only by time and vast pressures of work). They can often collect examples of treatment, both successful and unsuccessful. Some herbalists in Ghana have been known to treat diseases such as tetanus neonatorum and meningitis successfully (Read 1966; Tanner 1959). Their use of sedatives in certain psychiatric cases is outstanding. But their concept of disease and of treatment can be harmful. The importance of cultural considerations was demonstrated by the work of Dr. Lambo in Nigeria (Lambo 1963). In Mali, studies among the Dogon and the Tuareg showed that in rural areas, mental disturbances fell into one of two categories: either *que-que* ("madness," or antisocial behavior) or *tibi-suogo* (epilepsy). Both types of disturbances were treated with various combinations of herbs and spiritual rituals. An interesting finding from one study is that depressive symptoms, neuroses, and conditions regarded as psychosomatic appeared mostly in patients from urban areas and were best cared for by modern psychiatry, while culturally defined disturbances were most effectively treated by traditional healers (Coppo 1983).

CULTURAL PATTERNS RELEVANT TO MCH

Many cultural patterns affect the organization and implementation of MCH programs. Here we look at five general principles and in succeeding chapters cite various examples of cultural concepts and practices.

Patterns of Household Authority

The family members who purchase and cook the food are those at whom nutrition education must be directed. If the father purchases the food, he is the target. If the mother authorizes the food purchases and cooks, then she especially is the one who should be educated. A large number of households—40 percent or more—are directed by women. In such instances, the mother's mother on the farm, a child, or a neighbor often looks after the infants while the mother works. In rural India the husband's mother is often the director of the mothers' and children's conduct and practice.

Proverbs in many cultures reflect many social values. Some even legitimize violence against women; in Turkey it is said, "Roses bloom where a husband hits" and "One who does not beat his daughters beats himself." Violence against women is ingrained in many cultures and considered a family matter instead of a gender crime. Increasingly, however, it is being recognized as a serious cause of health problems in women (Baumslag 1989).

Child-Rearing Practices

The duration of breastfeeding, time of weaning, and types of foods considered suitable for children depend to a large extent on the cultural milieu. Generally women have a low status and are subservient from infancy (Fig. 2.3). They are fed least and last and are expected to suffer in silence. In India, for example, it was found that females used health facilities less often than males. Their self-image interferes with their utilization of health services.

In all societies, rites of passage represent the transition from one status to another. At each stage, rituals are performed and customs observed. Each year millions of girls have circumcisions, which

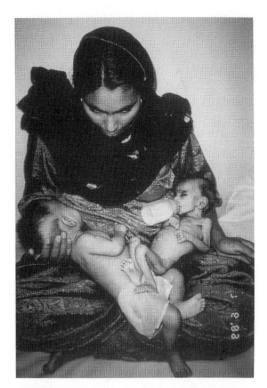

Figure 2.3. Gender preference in feeding twins. Twins: healthy breastfed male (left); marasmic bottle-fed female (right). Courtesy Prof. Khwaja Abbas, Pakistan Institute of Medical Sciences, Islamabad, Pakistan, UNICEF.

lead to serious health problems (Hosken 1982).

In many parts of Latin America, children remain unnamed until they are a year old because of the high infant mortality rate. Infants there are not taken outside until they are a few weeks old for fear of evil spirits or the elements, and so they cannot be brought to a clinic if ill. Home visits are essential in these situations.

In Mongolia and Afghanistan infants are still swaddled and some people believe that this is to prevent touching of genitalia. Swaddled infants in Turkey have a higher incidence of upper respiratory tract infections than unswaddled ones (Yurdakok et al. 1990).

All of these practices have an impact on the health of the community and af-

fect the resources available. Food restrictions in particular abound.

In every culture, there is a wide range of superstitions and fads. The following examples are important to a greater or lesser extent in the field of child health among different socioeconomic groups in Britain: rigid attitudes to toilet training and scheduled feeding, the use of proprietary "colic-water" medicines, and the belief that fish is a specific "brain food" for infants. In the United States, old wives' tales warn that continuous nursing when pregnant will result in deformity of the new infant or poisoning of the older child (Walters 1975). Mothers in Italy believe, as mothers do elsewhere, that eating white foods such as pasta and white wine, improves the production of breast milk (La Leche 1987)—a classic example of "sympathetic magic" ideology (like produces like).

Marriage and Childbirth

Marriage occurs at an early age in most developing countries, usually at 14 to 16 years, increasing the risk of early and prolonged childbearing. Marriages are usually arranged, and fertility is prized. In many cultures, initiation ceremonies are performed, and girls are prepared at puberty for marriage, taught about men, medicaments, taboos, and their own roles. In some societies, there are secret women's groups, as in the Mende tribe in Sierra Leone, where headwomen act as midwives. Some groups have special mothers' villages, where the mother and infant stay for a year.

The range of customs and rituals is amazing. The evil eye or witchcraft is much feared by many women; for this reason, tribes like the Zaramo disregard pregnancy until the seventh month, when the ceremonial presentation of the "sambo cloth" takes place. Such customs may mean a delay in attendance at the antenatal clinic until pregnancy is far advanced (Ebrahim 1979). In many Muslim countries, women are prohibited from going to clinics if male health workers will be examining them.

Fertility generally is highly prized and women who are infertile are abandoned. In some parts of Africa, as many as 40 percent of women are infertile, in contrast to the developed countries, where only 2 to 4 percent are. Many customs are directed against infertility; for example, egg eating in pregnancy is taboo in some societies, for it is believed to result in sterility or abortion. Among the Zulus if a caesarean section is performed, the scar marks the woman as an outcast. Symphysiotomy, a more socially acceptable procedure, has to be performed instead; it has a lower operative risk but a higher danger of urinary tract infections as the women are often immobilized for as long as nine days.

Food Ideology

The food system is of particular importance and direct relevance to MCH (Fig. 2.4) (Jelliffe 1982b). Ingrained practices are difficult to change. In some cultures, deficient dietary intake is not considered a cause of protein energy malnutrition (PEM), which is blamed instead on the mother's alleged infidelity.

From a general nutritional point of view, it is worth noting that the universal, but scientifically irrational, prejudice in Britain against protein-rich frogs, snails, dogs, and insects is so great that even during the period of maximal food shortage during World War II, no suggestion was made that these might be employed for the supplementary feeding of children, despite the fact that these items form customary, much relished, and nutritious foods in other parts of the world. It is important to recognize the cultural absurdities in one's own culture and to prevent their unwitting and harmful export in ill-advised health education.

The most widespread staples ("cultural superfoods") are cereal grains, such as rice, maize, millet, and wheat. Where low-protein foods such as cassava or plantain are the staples, they are often used as weaning foods, with nothing

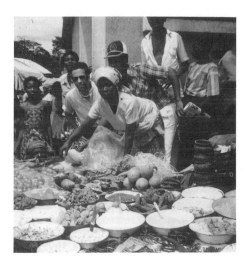
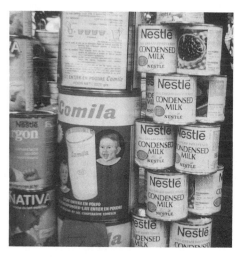

Figure 2.4. Food ideology. Speaking to the people and visiting local markets and shops will give clues as to which foods are available and how they are used. Medicines are often sold alongside food, and some foods are also used as medicines. Both photographs (N. Baumslag) are from a market in Zaire.

added. Not surprisingly, kwashiorkor is more prevalent in populations that subsist on these staples.

Many cultures have their own body image, which includes ideas concerning the workings of the body and its physiology and may be totally different from scientific facts (Brownlee 1978). These ideas may be systematized, as with the ancient Hindu classification of body physiology into *doshas* ("humors"), especially "hot" and "cold." Similar "hot" and "cold" classifications are be found in many parts of the world. The importance of these classifications is that both foods and illnesses are categorized in this way, so that the diet permitted may be of considerable influence in both health and disease, in relation to its supposed influence on the body. For example, in Bengal diarrhea is classified as a "hot" disease, and, to the village mother, it is plainly dangerous to feed her child with sugar and honey because these are "hot" foods, but barley water is "cold" and therefore considered appropriate.

Sympathetic magic foods—in Gujarat, India, the convoluted walnut is considered a brain food—and physiological foods—special items for particular periods—are well recognized and include foods to be consumed, or more often avoided, in pregnancy or early childhood (Vermury and Levine 1978).

Indigenous Health Services

Long before Western-type medicine was introduced in developing countries, a wide range of indigenous practitioners provided the bulk of the primary care and still do (Brotmacher 1935; Jelliffe and Bennett 1960; Mead 1928; Read 1948; Williams 1970). These practitioners include herbalists, bone setters, medicine men (some of whom are concerned with magic and spirits and casting spells), and "lay" midwives, called traditional birth attendants (TBAs). (A WHO-coined term,

TBA is used to describe a wide variety of women assisting with childbirth, from the very experienced to untrained women who help out occasionally.) In many countries, more than 80 percent of deliveries are still supervised by TBAs (Mangay-Maglacas and Pizurki 1981).

In traditional societies, health is regarded as a state of internal and external balance or equilibrium, including balances of opposing forces, such as the Latin American "hot" and "cold" and the Chinese yin and yang. Positive health is identified as the blending of physical, mental, and spiritual welfare (Bannerman 1982). In these cultures, childbirth is considered a social event, whereas in the West it is treated as a hospitalized disease state. (Until recently the American government regarded pregnancy as a period of incapacitation and gave federal employees "incapacity leave." Passage of the Family Leave Act (Feb. 1993) has made it possible for parents to take 12 weeks unpaid leave for childbirth, or care of a sick child, spouse, or parent.)

The WHO has developed several initiatives in the form of a three-pronged approach to increase the utilization of useful and important areas of traditional medicine (Bannerman 1982). The first is to identify drugs used by traditional practitioners that are effective and could replace imported drugs. In some countries, drug purchases consume 40 percent or more of the health budget, leaving little money for anything else. China has effectively dealt with this problem by incorporating into its health care system the use of traditional herbs and treatments. Myanmar, India, Mexico, Nigeria, and Thailand, among others, are researching the effectiveness of traditional remedies for use in health care (Akerele 1983). Problems occur with identifying chemically active ingredients in variable herbal mixtures. Nevertheless, the scientific value of this approach is emphasized by the recent recognition of the effectiveness of *artemisinin,* an ancient Chinese herbal mixture, in the treatment of resistant malaria.

Second, where few people are reached by Western-type medicine, local healers and lay midwives provide the bulk of the primary health care. These workers are now recognized as an important channel for getting services to those most in need (Figs. 2.5 and 2.6). However, where infant and maternal mortality rates are high, maternity services are predominantly provided by unsupervised lay midwives. Certainly they perform an invaluable service, but they often do so in unsanitary environments, and some of their practices leave a lot to be desired. For example the use of oxytocin-like herbal concoctions to hasten labor can result in obstructed labor and other complications, and the insertion of vaginal plugs during pregnancy can introduce infection. Such unhygienic practices emphasize the need for education. The hard-working TBAs are an underutilized source of available, low-cost services, and retraining them to interfere less and to provide hygienic services (especially care of the cord) and timely referrals has been undertaken in many countries, including Sierra Leone, Malawi, Philippines, Nepal, and Honduras (Mangay-Maglacas and Pizurki 1981).

Economics plays a significant role in the use of lay midwives throughout the world. In Arizona, lay midwives have won the legal right to perform deliveries because of the shortage of obstetricians in their area (Yankauer 1983). But in other parts of the United States where there is a high density of obstetricians, midwives are not allowed to function independently (Yankauer 1983). A study in the Sudan found that as the number of trained lay midwives to population increased from 4.3 percent to 6.9 percent, maternal mortality decreased from 23.8 per 1,000 live births to 12.4 percent per 1,000 live births (Bayoumi 1976). In Malawi it was shown to be fifty-nine times

more expensive to train and equip a state-enrolled midwife than a TBA (Bullough 1983). Retraining efforts do not consistently make an impact for several reasons. While TBAs have kits that contain scissors, cord dressing, and other necessary items, they do not always use them. Unsanitary conditions and limited major services for referral also have to be addressed before any improvements in mortality statistics appear. A new problem is that when TBAs are retrained and given certificates, they raise the price of their services.

Third, the importance of traditional medicine is now recognized. Several African medical schools include aspects of traditional medicine in their curricula. Although fundamental differences in concepts of life, health, and disease underlie the philosophy on which the traditional system is founded (Table 2.1), the integration of carefully selected Western and indigenous medical practices can improve health practices.

CULTURAL VARIATION AND MCH WORK

I would rather know something about the man who has the disease, than about the disease the man has.
DR. CALEB PARRY, 1770

Contacts between health personnel and patients or the public may be considered cultural interactions, and conflict may arise when cultures are widely divergent (Jelliffe 1982*b*). The local culture pattern is of great importance to MCH workers anywhere in the world (Jelliffe 1967; Jelliffe and Bennett 1960) for the following reasons:

1. It leads to an understanding of cultural factors that may underlie disease patterns in the community. For example, a high incidence of tetanus among newborns in parts of India may

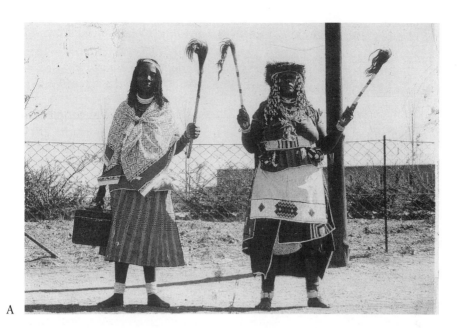

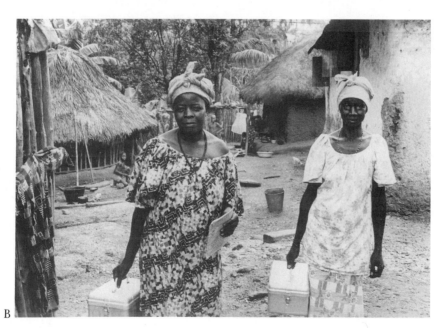

Figure 2.5. (A) A lay midwife with her apprentice. Traditional birth attendants and traditional healers provide the bulk of primary health services in rural areas and urban ghettos. Photograph by N. Baumslag. (B) Retrained traditional birth attendants (Sierra Leone) carrying midwifery kits for their primary care rounds. The cost for retraining is estimated at about $110 per worker. UNICEF photograph by Jette Meng.

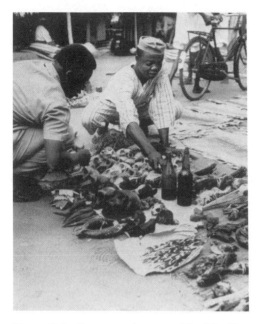

Figure 2.6. Custom, culture, and health. Traditional herbalists sell remedies in the local market and treat common diseases. WHO photograph by P. Almasy.

be related to the use of cow dung, a product of the holy cow, as a cord dressing.

2. It gives insight into people's values and knowledge of and attitudes to health and disease. The relevance may be considerable for the child health worker, if, for example, an infant is not regarded as truly born until after a certain ceremony or a certain age; his or her death before this is not considered of much importance (Mead 1930; Parrinder 1949).

3. It suggests how to ensure the best cooperation with the community, participation in, and appreciation of health work carried out by personnel trained in foreign medicine. Most MCH work in developing countries presents cross-cultural problems to some extent, whether the work is carried out by foreigners or by scientifically trained local people, who may have become cut off from village customs and be-

havior. Conflict is most likely to arise in health education; unless careful thought is given to cultural concepts, the ideas of the scientific health educator may find no common ground with those of local people. Health education is most likely to be successful if it is integrated into the local cultural framework (Williams 1958*b*).

4. It enables scientific medicine to become enriched by new ideas, methods, and techniques. A variety of indigenous herbal drugs await scientific recognition, and the often seemingly bizarre techniques employed in practical psychotherapy by various nonscientific healers in different parts of the world require study and possible incorporation into modern medicine. In the field of child rearing, cross-cultural studies of the numerous different methods employed in other cultures can give information of value to the world as a whole. An outstanding example is the variety of practices traditionally used in breast feeding.

CLASSIFICATION OF CUSTOMS

MCH workers will find the following approach to the problems of an unfamiliar culture a useful guide:

1. Investigate as far as possible the relevant indigenous methods and practices. This study can be initiated by reading the socioanthropological literature and by talking to local residents, both foreign and indigenous (with due allowance for cultural bias by either of these groups of informants). Investigation is usually based ultimately on personal inquiry and observation of behavior (Paul 1955; Pelto and Pelto 1978). The advice of a social anthropologist working among the particular group can be quite helpful, provided that he or she realizes

Table 2.1. Comparisons Between Traditional and Western Health Care Providers

	Traditional	Western
Definition	Long-standing: includes ancient practices and beliefs; culturally ingrained	Relatively new techniques and treatments not known to the population
Method of treatment	Varied; may include herbal, spiritual, and mystical approaches	Technological, drug, and surgery oriented
Approach	Holistic, concerned with body and mind; preventive concerned with wellness; culture and science integrated; spiritual and mystical	Organ centered and disease oriented; curative; science and culture separated; germs and bacteria
Rapport	Good; begins by telling patient what is wrong; may use divination to do this	Begins by asking questions; uses instruments and laboratory tests; relies on measurements
Culture	Familiar	Unfamiliar
Type of care	Continuous, with follow-up rites of passage; pregnancy, not delivery, is the main event	Fragmented; crisis or event specific (e.g., delivery only)
Acceptance	Universal	Selected interventions accepted (e.g., injections for infectious disease or immunizations)
Coverage	Extensive	Limited
Services	Wide range; e.g., TBAs wash clothes, prepare food and herbal remedies, advise on child care and feeding, give massage during pregnancy and delivery	Limited to advice
Type of practice	Often generalist, solo	Specialist, team
Payment	In kind; payment when patient improves; relatively cheap, local resources	In cash; before treatment; costly drugs and procedures
Advantages	Comfort to many, culturally accepted	Saves lives surgically and with immunizations

Sources: Adapted from Bannerman (1982); Mangay-Magaclas and Pizurki (1981).

what information is of special importance to the MCH worker.

Action ultimately has to be taken on information based on a reasonable period of investigation; nevertheless, observation should be continued, with subsequent reappraisals made, since the complexity of motivation behind even apparently simple practices may be considerable.

2. Objectively analyze the effects of these methods and practices on the physical and psychological health of both child and mother on the basis of current scientific knowledge, but bear in mind the realities of the local environment, including climate, geography, economic factors, and agricultural practices (Jelliffe and Jelliffe 1964; Williams 1963).

Cultural practices can be divided into four categories:

1. *Beneficial:* Customs that appear to benefit the health and nutrition of children and women, although they may be very different from Western practices—for example prolonged breastfeeding in an African village, or the vigorous Hindu mouthwash after meals in the prevention of dental caries. Beneficial customs should be incorporated into health education.

2. *Harmless:* No obvious beneficial or detrimental effect as far as the health of the mother or child is concerned. Examples include not cutting the hair until the child can talk (in Jamaica) or thickly outlining the eyes with black kajal to keep off the "evil eye" (in Bengal). This latter practice is harmless if the kajal is clean and not being also used by others with sore eyes. Although practices in this category may be bizarre to the culturally ethnocentric, they are best respected but should not be included as topics in health education. On the other hand, galactogogues (milk-producing) foods and drinks exist in many cultures, and although little researched, mothers swear by them and they may be useful for health education (Table 2.2).

3. *Uncertain value:* Sometimes customs are difficult to classify as either beneficial or harmful—for example, the use by pregnant Baganda women of *emumbwa,* a mixture of possibly mineral-containing clay and chopped herbs. Without analysis of the mixture, it is impossible to be certain of its value as a source of minerals or a danger. In many cultures, pregnant women crave and eat clay or starch known as geophagia, a form of pica. This behavior may be prompted by iron-deficiency anemia. With customs in this uncertain group, further observation and investigation are required before they are included in health education.

4. *Harmful customs:* Customs such as failing to give fish, a good source of protein, to young children (rural Malaysia), using pepper enemas (West Africa) (Fig. 2.7), placing a cow dung dressing on the umbilical stump (India), forced hand feeding (Nigeria), sedating infants with opium (India), circumcising females (Sudan), restricting diet extremely in pregnancy (Burma), and failing to ligate the umbilical cord (parts of Uganda) may be deleterious to health (Ismail 1982; Gelfand 1981). Harmful practices are, of course, found in all cultures, including those of the Western world. A sympathetic appreciation of cultural relativity is a prerequisite of success for work outside one's own community or within it.

Table 2.2. Galactogogues: An Explanation

Mothers continents apart have, and still are, using herbs, teas, soups, and foods for increasing their milk supply. These galactogogues may improve the mother's diet and fluid content, or they may reduce anxiety and encourage the let-down reflex. The medical literature abounds in treatments to ensure a sufficient milk supply.

Some of the galactogogues from Nepal have been analyzed chemically, and the calcium content has been found to be high. The exact significance is not known, but it may be important for the contraction of the milk duct muscles. The velvet bean drink contains high iron, zinc, and copper and may act as a hematinic. Although most of these remedies have not been scientifically tested, the women who use them considered them important supplements.

Galactogogues used vary throughout the world. Following is a list of some of them:

India:	Ginger, jaggery, powdered earthworms.
Pakistan:	Cumin, lassi cottonseeds, goat's stomach.
Mexico:	Gruels made from legumes, groundnuts, chickpeas, sesame, cottonseed, abyinth.
Tunisia:	Herb teas called "ververine" made from fennelreek, coriander seeds, barley, and cous-cous.
United States:	Thistle tea with comfrey and fennel.
China:	Soups made of pigs' legs, tailbones, or fishtails and boiled with ginger or cooked with beans and peanuts; eggs; chicken soup made from adult roosters.
Nepal:	Juana seed, fennel, dill, carraway, gendrik.
Guatemala:	Ixbut tea from leaves of the *Euphorbia lancifolia* plant.
Honduras:	Velvet bean cocoa drink.

Table 2.3. Approaches to Categories of Cultural Practice

	Beneficial	Neutral	Uncertain	Harmful	
Approach	Incorporate (positively, prominently)	Ignore or unobtrusively incorporate	Observe and categorize later	Integration	Dissuasion (conviction)
Examples	*Doula* (female assistant at child-birth: India and most cultures): rest and good diet in puerperium (Chinese in Malaysia); prolonged breastfeeding (most traditional cultures); weaning food vegetable oil with rice (Myanmar)	Avoidance of "twin" bananas in pregnancy (East Africa); symbolism of color (yellow = danger/ill health), used in weight charts (Indonesia)	Cosmetic outlining of eyes: *Kajal* (carbon and oil), harmless; lead compound, harmful, maternal prechewing of foods for infant, beneficial	Restriction of items for sick young child (hot/cold incompatibility)—use alternative food with hot/cold compatibility	Nutrition rehabilitation concept (mother's preparing foods and feeding)—observation important

Source: Jelliffe (1982*b*).

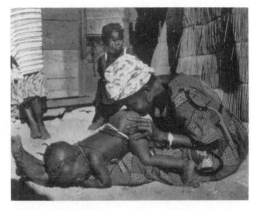

Figure 2.7. Examine local health practices. Harmful practices are found in all cultures, including so-called Western cultures. Home-administered pepper-water enemas used in West Africa are harmful and should be discouraged.

Health workers who know the culture and classify the cultural practices can improve the services and identify conditions prevalent in the community (Table 2.3). In Zimbabwe, traditional healers are being involved in AIDS education and spiritual support (Women's AIDS Support Network 1990).

Health workers need to preserve the beneficial cultural practices and beliefs and try to modify the harmful practices by health education or by cultural inte-

gration. The ill effects of a particular custom can be modified while retaining the essence of the culturally accepted practice. For example, in Bengal, cow's milk, which is classified as "hot," should not be given to children recovering from diarrhea, whereas "cold" buttermilk should be. Through this awareness, an increased protein intake can be achieved within the cultural framework of the Bengali village.

The fact that the observance of tradition and rituals, even if they are apparently unnecessary or irrational, helps people to identify with their family or community is a cardinal factor in social development and stability. It may be that many of the "overdeveloped" countries are now suffering from "withdrawal" from such observances.

REFERENCES

Akerele, O. (1983). Which way for traditional medicine? *Wld. Hlth.*, June 4, 3–4.

Asprey, G. F., and Thornton, P. (1953). Medicinal plants of Jamaica. *W. Indian Med. J.* **2**, 28.

Bannerman, R. H. O. (1982). Integrating traditional and modern health systems. In *Ad-*

vances in *International Maternal and Child Health*, vol. 2, Ed. D. B. Jelliffe and E. F. P. Jelliffe. Oxford University Press, Oxford.

Baumslag, N. (1972). *Family Care*. Williams and Wilkins, Baltimore.

Baumslag, N., and Vogel, L. (1989). *Violence Against Women: A Global Problem*. Proceedings of a workshop at PAHO, May 22, WIPHN, Bethesda, Md.

Bayoumi, A. (1976). The training and activity of village midwives. *Trop. Doct.* **13**, 118.

Beasher, S.; Beasher, T.; and Cook, R. (1983). Traditional practices in women in the eastern Mediterranean region: Recent developments. In *Advances in International Maternal and Child Health*, 3:63. Oxford University Press.

BMJ (1970). Editorial: Mothers of premature babies. *Brit. Med. J.* **2**, 556.

Bras, G.; Jelliffe, D. B.; and Stuart, K. L. (1954). Veno-occlusive disease of liver with non-portal type cirrhosis, occurring in Jamaica. *Arch. Path.* **57**, 285.

Brotmacher, L. (1935). Medical practice among the Somalis. *Bull. Hist. Med.* **29**, 197

Brownlee, A. T. (1978). Traditional and modern health systems. In *Community Culture and Care: A Cross-Cultural Guide for Health Workers*. C. V. Mosby, St. Louis.

Bullough, C. H. W. (1983). Editorial: Traditional birth attendants. *Trop. Doct.* **13**, 49.

Coppo, P. (1983). Traditional psychiatry in Mali. *Wld. Hlth.*, June 10–12.

Ebrahim, G. J. (1979). *Care of the Newborn in Developing Countries*. Macmillan, London.

Foster, G. M. (1951). A Cross-Cultural Analysis of a Technical Aid Program. (Mimeo. Smithsonian Institution, Washington, D.C.

Gelfand, M. (1981). African customs in relation to preventive medicine. *Cent. Afr. J. Med.* **27**, 1.

Hosken, F. P. (1982). Female circumcision in the world today: A global view. In *Traditional Practices Affecting the Health of Women and Children*. WHO/EMRO Technical Publication, 2 (2). WHO, Regional Office for the Eastern Mediterranean, Alexandria.

Ismail, E. A. (1982). Female circumcision— physical and mental complications. In *Traditional Practices Affecting the Health of Women and Children*. WHO/EMRO Technical Publication 2 (2). WHO, Regional Office for the Eastern Mediterranean, Alexandria.

Jelliffe, D. B. (1956). Cultural variation and the practical pediatrician. *J. Pediat.* **49**, 661.

Jelliffe, D. B. (1957). Social culture and nutrition. Cultural blocks and protein malnutrition in early childhood in rural West Bengal. *Pediatrics* **20**, 128.

Jelliffe, D. B. (1962). Culture, social change and infant feeding. Current trends in tropical regions. *Am. J. Clin. Nutr.* **10**, 19.

Jelliffe, D. B. (1964). Report of the forty seventh Ross Conference on paediatric research. *Int. Child Hlth.* **52**.

Jelliffe, D. B. (1967). Parallel food classification in developing and industrialized countries. *Am. J. Clin. Nutr.* **20**, 279.

Jelliffe, D. B. (1982*a*). Cultural aspects of nutrition. *Prac. Pediat.* **6**, 1.

Jelliffe, D. B., and Bennett, F. J. (1960). Indigenous medical systems and child health. *J. Pediat.* **57**, 248.

Jelliffe, D. B., and Bennett, F. J. (1961). Cultural and anthropological factors in infant and maternal nutrition. *Fed. Proc.* **20** (Suppl. 7), 185.

Jelliffe, D. B., and Bennett, F. J. (1962). Worldwide care of the mother and newborn child. *Clin. Obstet. Gynaec.* **5**, 64.

Jelliffe, D. B., and Jelliffe, E. F. P. (1982*b*). Culture in primary child health care. In *Advances in International Maternal and Child Health*, 2:53. Ed. D. B. Jelliffe, and E. F. P. Jelliffe. Oxford University Press, Oxford.

Jelliffe, D. B., and Jelliffe, E. F. P. (1992). Medical Anthropology and Anthropological Medicalists: Complementary Partners (in press).

Jelliffe, E. F. P., and Jelliffe, D. B. (1964). Children in ancient Polynesian Hawaii. *Clin. Pediat.* **3**, 604.

La Leche League International (1987). *The Womanly Art of Breast Feeding*. 4th ed. La Leche League International, Franklin Park, Ill.

Lambo, T. A. (1963). *African Traditional Beliefs: Concepts of Health and Medical Practice*. Ibadan, Nigeria.

Mangay-Maglacas, M., and Pizurki, H. (1981). *The Traditional Birth Attendants in Seven Countries: Case Studies in Utilization and Training*. Wld. Hlth. Org. Publ. Hlth. Pap., no. 75. World Health Organization, Geneva.

Mead, M. (1928). *Coming of Age in Samoa: A Psychological Study of Primitive Youth for*

Western Civilization. Blue Ribbon Books, New York.

Mead, M. (1930). *Growing Up in New Guinea*. Peter Smith, Magnolia, Mass.

Parrinder, G. (1949). *West African Religion*. Epworth Press, London.

Paul, B. D. (1955). *Health, Culture and Community*. Russell Sage Foundation, New York.

Pelto, P. J., and Pelto, G. H. (1978). *Anthropological Research: The Structure of Inquiry*. Cambridge University Press, Cambridge.

Pop. Ref. Bur. (1992). *1992 World Population Data Sheet*. Population Reference Bureau, Washington, D.C.

Read, M. (1948). Attitudes towards health and disease among preliterate peoples. *Hlth. Educ. J.* 6, 166.

Read, M. (1966). *Culture, Health and Disease*. Tavistock Publications, London.

Tanner, R. E. S. (1959). Sukuma leachcraft: An analysis of their medical and surgical system. *E. Afr. Med. J.* 36, 199.

Van Der Hoeven, J. A. (1958). Taboos for pregnant women, lactating mothers and infants on the North Coast of Netherlands New-Guinea. *Trop. Geogr. Med.* 10, 71.

Vermury, M., and Levine, H. (1978). *Project on Beliefs and Practices That Affect Food Habits in Developing Countries*. CARE, New York.

Walters, M. (1975). The folklore of breast feeding. *Bull. N.Y. Acad. Med.* **51**, 870.

Williams, C. D. (1938). Child health in the Gold Coast. *Lancet,* i, 97.

Williams, C. D. (1958a). Milroy lecture: Social medicine in developing countries. *Lancet,* i, 863, 919.

Williams, C. D. (1958b). Social aspects of nutrition. In *Matrix of Medicine*. Ed. N. Malleson. Pitman Press, London.

Williams, C. D. (1963). The story of kwashiorkor. *Courier* **13**, 361.

Williams, C. D. (1970). Witch doctors. *Pediatrics* **46**, 448.

Women's AIDS Support. Network (1990). Women's AIDS Support Network. *WIPHN News* **8**, 13.

WHO (1982). *World Health Statistics*. World Health Organization, Geneva.

WHO (1983). Newsbriefs: Fear of feeding on fish. *Wld. Hlth.,* June 31, 31.

Yankauer, A. (1983). The valley of the shadow of birth. *Am. J. Pub. Hlth.* **73**, 635.

Yurdakok, K.; Yazuz, T.; and Taylor, C. E. (1990). Swaddling and acute respiratory infections. *Am. J. Pub. Hlth.* **80**(7), 873–875.

3

Historical Developments

*Human history becomes more and more a race between
education and catastrophe.*
H. G. WELLS

There have been great improvements in health and medical care in this century and it is in the field of mother and child health that progress has been most noticeable. In most ancient societies, less than 50 percent of the babies born alive survived to maturity, and in nineteenth-century Europe, the figures were not much better. Modern medicine has learned not only how to cure many diseases; it has discovered that the vast majority of children's disorders are preventable. In technically advanced countries, the survival rates is over 97 percent. In less developed countries, over 50 percent of total deaths are of children under the age of 5, and the average life span is about 35 years. In scientifically advanced countries, only 5 percent of the total mortality occurs among the under 5s, and the average life span is over 70 years.

Before the advent of scientific medicine, it was taken for granted that a large proportion of children born alive would die in childhood, and therefore parents felt it necessary to have many children in the hope that some would survive. In 1900, no one in England dreamed that by 1960 the infant mortality rate would be reduced from 150 to 20 or that the 1- to 4 year-old mortality rate would plummet from 20 to 0.6. In 1991 infant mortality had dropped to 7 per 1,000 live births and the under five mortality to 9 (UNICEF 1993).

The ancients took it so much for granted that children would die in large numbers that few of them paid much attention to childhood diseases. Some traditional societies still do not give a child a name until he or she is some months old, because they regard the child's hold on life as so insecure that he or she is not considered a fully established person.

Hippocrates (c. 460–375 B.C.) recognized that children need special attention and noted that the conditions most commonly found in small babies were thrush, vomiting, cough, sleeplessness, terrors, inflammation of the navel, and discharging ears. He stated that fevers, convulsions, and diarrhea were common during teething; later, asthma, stones, roundworms, and skin diseases would occur. The works of other authors of this time—Aristotle, Celsus, and Pliny—also contain references to children.

Galen (c. A.D. 130–200), whose ideas dominated medicine for the following one thousand years, wrote about child care. He emphasized the need for cleanliness, and recommended salting and swaddling, which are still practiced in many lands. The bladder stones he mentioned may be associated with the diarrhea and dehydration that were common, and still are, in some regions.

In the later days of the Roman Empire, infanticide was practiced among both the wealthy, because children were a nuisance, and among the poor, because they were an expense.

The first book on pediatrics in the English language was *The Boke of Chyldren* by Sir Thomas Phayre, published in 1545 and popular for many years. "Here to doo them good that have the most nede, that is to say, chyldren." He listed a number of conditions (which are symptoms rather than diagnoses), "for most commonly the tender age of children is chiefly vexed and grieved with the diseases following: . . . stiffness of the limbs, watering eyes, scabbiness or itch, canker of the mouth (noma), streytness of the wind, feebleness of the stomach and vomiting, cramp, colick and rumbling of the guts, flux of the belly, worms, failing of the skin, stone, fevers, consumption, leanness, lice and goggle eyes (squint)." This list represents an accurate picture of many of the diseases common today in developing countries. In fact, children there are damaged most not by the so-called tropical diseases but by those that stem from the educational and socioeconomic status of their parents.

Over the next two centuries, little progress in child health was made, although many authors referred to the care of children in their writing and teaching in a number of countries. Europe at this time was fraught with political, ideological, and economic upheavals, and it was still taken for granted that life was likely to be "short, nasty, and brutish."

But amid these years of ignorance and inconclusiveness, there appeared, between 1709 and 1789, two brothers, John and George Armstrong, who qualified in medicine in Edinburgh and then went to London (Maloney 1954). They made some money in private practice, but their main interest was to set up a dispensary in Soho, London, for "sick children of the poor." They were not only extraordinarily successful in caring for these children but also found time to compare their results with the general average. In 1767 in London, there were 16,042 baptisms and 8,229 deaths in children under 2 years of age—a 50 percent mortality. In their dispensary, the Armstrongs counted 140 children under their care, of whom only 6 had died. Altogether in eleven years, they treated and supervised 11,000 children, and pauperized themselves in the process. Although their work was admired by some, it never achieved adequate appreciation or support. Their work died with them—a major tragedy, because the dispensary was run on sound lines:

I have not confined myself to the therapeutic or curative part of physic only; I have also extended my care to the prophylactic branch, or that which concerns the prevention of disease. . . . I always inquire into the diet of the children and give particular instruction about it, not only while they are ill, but also after they are recovered (Maloney 1954).

Remarkably, the Armstrongs appear to have reduced child mortality at their dispensary in the first two years of life from about 50 percent to less than 5 percent, and this without thermometers, a second-hand on their watches, antibiotics, or immunization, and practically nothing in the way of hospital care. They could rely only on what Florence Nightingale regarded as the essentials: good food, cleanliness, and fresh air. Another two hundred years were to elapse before the need for comprehensive care and supervision was again recognized, together with the importance of environmental hygiene and nutrition.

Monastic medicine (food and shelter for the sick provided by the church) had been practiced in many countries and continued to be so. But throughout Europe as a whole, the function of the hospital as a place for treatment rather than a place of refuge developed only with the advent of scientific medicine and the demand for special equipment and techniques. In England, for example, Christ's Hospital (1537) and the Foundling Hospital (1741) were endowed primarily for homeless and neglected children.

The Industrial Revolution (c. 1760–1840) created new problems in child care and in urbanization, just as is now the case in many developing countries (Jelliffe 1970). Medical treatment for sick children was rudimentary. When the Great Ormond Street Hospital for Sick Children was founded in 1852, it refused admission to children under the age of 2 years, because nearly all of them died when placed in institutions. Manchester started a Children's Hospital in 1829 and Edinburgh in 1837.

The eighteenth and nineteenth centuries were a time of rapid scientific progress, particularly in medicine. The need for vital and health statistics was recognized, and from that time, figures gradually became more accurate. In 1789, Jenner discovered vaccination against smallpox, and in the middle of the nineteenth century Pasteur introduced bacteriology and Lister antiseptic surgery. Anesthetics were first used. Florence Nightingale made sweeping reforms in nursing and midwifery and started to train health visitors. Control of a cholera epidemic in London (even before the recognition of the cholera bacillus) led to widespread improvements in water supply and sewage disposal. The training of doctors was extensively reformed, and

specialists in surgery, medicine, and midwifery were beginning to establish their expert technology. The efforts of Lord Shaftesbury led to greatly increased opportunities for education of the masses. Labor laws and factory acts were introduced to improve working and living conditions, and to prevent exploitation of children. Care of the helpless became not only a religious virtue but a humane and economic necessity.

Yet in spite of these discoveries and advances and the establishment of children's hospitals, it was found that the infant mortality rate in England in 1899 had reached an all-time high—163 per 1,000 live births (Newman 1906), higher, in fact, than the 149 recorded in 1843. Nevertheless, there was a stirring of interest in the fate of children in Europe and in America. The United States and Germany were the first countries to develop pediatrics as a specialty, although individual doctors such as Phayre in England and Nils Rosen von Rosenstein of Sweden (1706–1773) had previously concentrated on child care. George Frederick Still (Still 1965) was appointed to a specialist post in the diseases of children at King's College Hospital in London in 1906. However, it was another twenty years before other similar appointments were made in England. Before the twentieth century, medical students and nurses had little or no special training in child health.

There were other indications of this interest, especially the Gouttes de Lait and the Consultations des Nourissons started by Dufour and Budin in France, the "milk stations" in New York, and the "infant welfare centers" and "schools for mothers" in Scotland and England. These centers, established by volunteers, were designed not only to treat the sick but to visit homes and teach parents how to improve the day-to-day care of their children—an activity that previously had been mainly ignored by the doctors in practice and still more by the hospitals.

The movement toward establishing centers for treatment and supervision of babies spread rapidly. In the twenty years between 1890 and 1910, hundreds were organized by voluntary agencies in Europe and America. Even in Jamaica, the first center was set up as long ago as 1912. The doctors were usually assisted by a number of voluntary workers, who had little specialized knowledge of child care but common sense and goodwill.

The infant welfare centers were a resounding success. Even an untrained voluntary worker visiting homes was a valuable agent of progress. Between 1899 and 1921, the infant mortality rate in England dropped from 160 to 83. Early in the twentieth century, local government authorities began to take over the infant welfare centers and also to train health visitors and district nurses. Between 1913 and 1917, a hundred child welfare centers were established in London alone, and trained health visitors were replacing and assisting voluntary workers. The success of these centers was such that the hospitals and general practitioners began to feel that they were being supplanted. Local government authorities therefore decreed that these centers were to undertake "preventive" work, with "curative" medicine left to general practitioners and hospitals. Thus, through a historical accident, there was introduced into modern medicine the false and disastrous idea that preventive and curative medicine can be separated in the care of individuals.

Since the early part of this century, child health has shown marked improvement. In the United Kingdom, the infant mortality rate was reduced from 150 per 1,000 in 1900 to 55 in 1940. This was due to in part to improvement in environmental hygiene, education, and economics, but certainly "as much to an advance in the mother's skill, as to the newer methods of medical treatment" (Spence et al. 1954). The health visitors and midwives were mainly responsible for teaching these skills. Naturally, improved standards of education have made mothers easier to teach. Since 1940, the progress in medication and surgery, in biochemistry and immunizations (especially for diphtheria, measles, and whooping cough), and the continuing education of parents have played a major role in decreasing the infant mortality rate in the United Kingdom to 7.9 in 1992 (Pop. Ref. Bur. 1992).

Improvements in health result in reduced mortality and morbidity. They also result in a changed pattern of disease (Table 3.1). As diseases are prevented, the attention of pediatricians in highly developed countries is increasingly concentrated on rare and largely nonpreventable conditions, particularly congenital abnormalities and metabolic disorders. Behavior disorders of children and their parents may occupy a great deal of the time and energy of pediatric specialists in private practice. The anomaly is obvious: the healthier people are, the more medical attention they demand. And the more doctors and nurses who are trained for the developing countries (that desperately need medical care), the greater tendency for them to take better-paid jobs in relatively healthy and "overdeveloped" regions of the world, resulting in "brain drain."

HISTORY AND PREVENTIVE MEDICINE

Through the historical accidents that led to the separation of curative and preventive pediatrics in Europe and North America, the idea has grown that preventive or "social" pediatrics is an upstart, low-status subject and different from "pediatrics proper." This separation occurs in no other specialty. Obstetricians accept that it is part of their duty to train students of medicine and midwifery in the supervision of normal pregnancy, as well as in the management of its disorders. Other specialties are equally respon-

Table 3.1. Proportional Infant Mortality in the United States

	1900	1954	1979	1989
Death rate per 1,000 live births	150	26	13	—
Causes of deaths (percentages)				
Infective and parasitic diseases	8	1	2	1
Diarrhea and enteritis	25	3	1	0
Pneumonia and influenza	15	7	3	3
Congenital malformations	6	13	20	21
Certain diseases in early infancy	35	52	51	47
All other causes	12	17	25	38

Sources: NCHS (1982, 1992 [for 1989]).

sible for various aspects of their subject, including prevention in the community.

Traditional medicine is similar. Even where sickness is usually ascribed to enemies or to witchcraft, the traditional healer advises his clients to wear a lizard's jawbone or a blue bead around the neck in order to prevent disease but is prepared to treat the illness too. The ancient Chinese are said to have paid their doctors only while they were in good health; in some parts of Africa, the midwife is given a fruit tree when the baby is born, and she is entitled to the produce as long as the child remains alive. Both are useful incentives toward preventive medicine.

Hippocrates undoubtedly advocated preventive or social medicine. He stated: "Physicians' studies should include a consideration of what is beneficial in a patient's regimen while he is yet in health." Moreover, in the fourteenth century, Chaucer's Doctor of Physic was praised because

He kept his patients wondrously and well
In all hours by his magic natural.

General practitioners used to be family doctors. They were aware of family stresses and physical disorders; knew all about the condition of the drains and the temperament of the grandmother; and gave treatment and advice without being aware that curative and preventive medicine could be separated. There are still such practitioners and they work closely with public health or district nurses and midwives. Recently, there have been countless efforts to emphasize social medicine—to correlate diseases with the factors that produce them, and not only with their bacteriology and biochemistry—but the training of students is still mainly confined to scientific institutions and to a procession of specializations, many of which are impersonal and episodic and result in irrational and ineffective medical or health care.

The progress of child health is slowly moving toward a more integrated approach. Pediatrics is still sometimes regarded as a subspecialty, and in some universities there may be little reference to the subject, clinical or social, in the final examinations. Nevertheless, some teaching hospitals now have centers where students can observe normal and convalescent children and learn to appreciate the need for continuing care and supervision. Some pediatric departments have health nurses attached to them; students can visit in the homes; mothers can stay in the hospital with their children, and good follow-up is maintained. Two classical linked studies, "A Thousand Families in Newcastle upon Tyne" and "Growing Up in Newcastle upon Tyne," are the best examples of how much may be learned through continuing observation (Miller et al. 1960; Spence et al. 1954). Most universities now have training and elective periods when students may work with family practitioners and in peripheral areas, including internships in developing countries.

The word *prevent* comes from the Latin *praevenire*—"to go in front, to anticipate, to protect." It was thus not originally a purely negative concept. Preventive or social medicine is not a recent, upstart specialty. It is an ancient, indispensable function of medicine, which is temporarily in eclipse because of concentration on specialist institutional medicine.

CHILD HEALTH IN DEVELOPING COUNTRIES

A traditional society that lacks scientific explanations and rational guides to conduct lives in fear. Children and marriage, crops and houses are all menaced by hazards that are imperfectly understood and universally dreaded. The forces that govern them have to be propitiated by rituals and by certain forms of homage or sacrifice. The fatalism and apathy that are often found in communities with high child mortality and morbidity are gradually eroded when people find that they can avoid many of the dangers that threaten their children and their homes. Health care can produce better survival and efficiency, and it can help to liberate the spirit.

The early impact of scientific medicine on tropical and subtropical areas was confined to the care of expatriate personnel and then to the control of major epidemic diseases that menaced the whole population, including laborers in some major enterprises. Gradually, local populations began to appreciate the advantages of scientific medicine and demanded treatment. The Indian Medical Service, for example, was a semimilitary organization, while the establishment of the Colonial Medical Service was an attempt to ensure that scientific medicine

would no longer be a luxury for the well-to-do and the educated but available to everyone who believed they could be benefited. The major preoccupations continued to be control of epidemics and medical care for government servants. Few women and children seemed to claim the attention of such organizations. Instead, the hospitals established by religious missions were among the first to attract mothers and children and to provide facilities for them.

Statistics on disease control programs, with which tropical medicine is still largely concerned (Williams 1957), must always be checked against carefully compiled vital statistics. Otherwise, much money and personnel might be expended on controlling disease while a large proportion of other diseases are not being dealt with. Some disease control programs have temporarily saved lives, which are then lost to starvation. Preventing diseases that are not amenable to mass control methods may depend on changing personal and domestic activities and attitudes. Where disease control programs are balanced by good personal medicine, particularly in maternal and child health, people begin to have confidence in the survival of their children and can look to the future. Then, and then only, will they make use of family planning and have only the number of children whom they can expect to bring up properly.

In Singapore, pediatric wards were opened in 1933 under Dr. Hari Das. In India, the first departments of pediatrics were established by Dr. R. K. Chaudhuri (in Calcutta), by Dr. G. Goelho (in Bombay), by Dr. S. T. Achar (in Madras) between 1940 and 1950. Other universities soon began to follow suit. But in most tropical universities and medical schools, a department of pediatrics was deemed necessary only years after other specializations were established. In 1954, a conference on malnutrition in African mothers, infants, and young children was held in the Gambia, West Africa. Of the six pediatricians attending, only one held a post in Africa. There were no obstetricians at the meeting (Williams 1957). It is only within the last 40 years that serious attention has been given to MCH as an essential factor of tropical medicine.

When the WHO was established in 1948, its four priorities were proclaimed to be malaria, tuberculosis, MCH, and venereal disease. An expert committee advised that each medical headquarters should include a deputy director of maternal and child health. It was believed that there was no need to build up a large, separate department, but that by this means it would be possible to direct the organization so that the care of mothers and children, the most vulnerable members of the population, could be coordinated by obstetricians and pediatricians, nurses and midwives, nutritionists and health educators. Now MCH is part of family health in the WHO structure, which includes nutrition, family planning, and health education.

There are signs that the medical profession is beginning to realize the importance of preventive care for women and children in particular and that health care cannot function effectively in isolation. In the 1978 WHO/UNICEF Joint Conference on Primary Health Care at Alma Ata, the then revolutionary concept that health care is a right and that everyone is entitled to basic health care was endorsed. The representatives from over 130 countries around the world agreed that maternal and child care is an essential component of a primary health care system (Primary Health Care 1978), with primary health care identified as "the key to achieving an acceptable level of health throughout the world." A major thrust was that primary health care must involve the community at all levels. However, the ambitious goal to attain Health for All (HFA) by the Year 2000 has met with many problems, among them lack of political will, limited resources, and the attractiveness of vertical programs for donors.

In an attempt to lessen the gap between the haves and have-nots, there has been a major effort on several fronts to promote child survival by providing immunizations against the six immunizable diseases and oral rehydration to prevent diarrheal dehydration deaths. However, "selective health care" measures make use of targeted technical interventions that can rapidly—but perhaps only temporarily—reduce mortality, but they do not address the basic causes of undernutrition and poor health. The basic causes are rooted in the economy and society and are unlikely to be amenable to short-term selective health care interventions. It is becoming increasingly recognized that these programs may have the effect of delaying the development of the material and human infrastructure necessary to begin to address the fundamental causes of childhood ill health. Certainly there is a need for such important and effective components of PHC such as immunizations, oral rehydration, breastfeeding and acute respiratory infection (ARI) prevention. The PHC approach should also incorporate long-term goals of equipping communities to improve not only their survival but also their health, nutrition, and quality of life through social and economic development (Sanders and Davies 1988).

Only through concerted, coordinated, comprehensive programs in the future will the continued waste of child life be avoided and a positive contribution made toward the health and prosperity of people as a whole.

REFERENCES

Jelliffe, D. B., and Jelliffe, E. F. P. (1970). The urban avalanche and child nutrition. *J. Am. Diet. Assoc.* 57, 111.

Maloney, W. J. (1954). *George and John Armstrong of Castleton, Two Eighteenth*

Century Medical Pioneers. Livingstone, Edinburgh.

Miller, F. J. W.; Court, S. D. M.; Walton, W. S.; and Knox, E. G. (1960). *Growing Up in Newcastle upon Tyne*. Oxford University Press, London.

NCHS (1982). Advance report of final mortality statistics, 1979. *Monthly Vital Statistics Report* **31** (6), supplement.

NCHS (1992). *Monthly Vital Statistics Report* **40** (8), supplement 2.

Newman, G. (1906). *Infant Mortality: A Social Problem*. Methuen, London.

Pop. Ref. Bur. (1983). *World Population Data Sheet*. Population Reference Bureau, Washington, D.C.

Pop. Ref. Bur. (1992). *World Population Data Sheet*. Population Reference Bureau, Washington, D.C.

Primary Health Care (1978). *A Joint Report of the Director-General of WHO and the Executive Director of UNICEF*. International Conference on Primary Health Care, Alma Ata, September 6–12.

Sanders D., and Carver R. (1988). *The Struggle for Health*. Macmillan, London.

Sanders, D., and Davies, R. (1988). Economic adjustment and current trends in child survival: The case of Zimbabwe. *Hlth. Pol. Plng.* 3(3), 195–204.

Spence, J. C.; Walton, W. X.; Miller, F. J. W.; and Court, S. D. M. (1954). *A Thousand Families in Newcastle upon Tyne*. Oxford University Press, London.

Still, G. F. (1965). *History of Paediatrics*. 2d ed. Dawsons of Pall Mall, London.

UNICEF (1993). *State of the World's Children*. Oxford University Press, London.

Williams, C. D. (1957). World nutrition. *Roy. Soc. Hlth. J.* 77, 447.

4

The Reasons for Mother and Child Health Services

*There is the serious phenomenon of the man of science who
sticks to the facts of his own scientific discipline, but sees no
connection at all between what he does in science and the
posture he adopts towards life and the world.*
BERNARD DELFGAAUW, 1961

*Whatever may be its value as a science, and whatever the social
and financial preferment that attend it, medicine is still a major
vehicle of compassion, of charity in its true sense.*
MAURICE KING, 1966

The World Health Organization became fully established in 1948 as a specialized agency of the United Nations. The first General Assembly had decided that not only should there be conferences, expert councils for advice, and publications in the area of health (in the tradition of the Health Department of the defunct League of Nations), but that active programs should be undertaken. The priorities were specified in the following order:

Malaria.

Tuberculosis.

Maternal and child health (MCH).

Venereal disease (later expanded to include all forms of treponematosis).

Although maternal and child health was included in a list of diseases, for the first time the care of mothers and children was placed high on a list of priorities.

Whatever the label—community medicine, comprehensive care, family health, social medicine, social pediatrics, primary health care—women and young children require the most attention for medical care and supervision. Furthermore, it is increasingly realized that social pediatrics must be an integral part of pediatrics as a whole.

At the 1978 WHO-UNICEF International Conference on Primary Health Care at Alma Ata, a comprehensive strategy to achieve "health for all" (HFA) was identified (WHO 1978). Maternal and child care was seen as one of the essential components of primary health care, which included other preventive and curative services, such as the promotion of proper nutrition and safe water, immunizations, health education, and the treatment of common diseases and injuries undertaken with and through community participation. The importance of health care to mothers and children was affirmed later in UNICEF's annual report, *The State of the World's Children 1982–92.* It emphasized the potential of simple, available technologies in countering high infant and young child mortality in developing countries. The combined approach was given the acronym *GOBI-FFF,* for "growth changes, oral rehydration, breastfeeding, immunizations, feeding (mother and weanling), family planning, and female education" (Grant 1985). Child survival programs were first initiated by the U.S. Agency for International Development (AID) in 1985 to reach the poorest of the poor in the world (estimated to be 950 million) and to decrease child deaths through programs promoting immunization, breastfeeding and child feeding, prevention and treatment of acute respiratory infections, oral rehydration therapy, child spacing, and initiatives to lower the rate of maternal mortality in childbirth. Although the results have been encouraging, 13 million children still die each year from largely preventable causes. UNICEF, working with others, developed the Convention on the Rights of the Child, which was ratified by world leaders at the World Summit for Children in 1990. The following goals were agreed upon (UNICEF 1991):

Reduction of 1990 under-5 child mortality rates by one-third or to a level of 70 per 1,000 live births, whichever is the greater reduction.

Reduction of 1990 maternal mortality rates by half.

Reduction of severe and moderate malnutrition among under-5 children by half of 1990 levels.

Universal access to safe drinking water and to sanitary means of excreta disposal.

Universal access to basic education and completion of primary education by at least 80 percent of primary school-age children.

Reduction of adult illiteracy rate to at least half its 1990 level (the appropriate age group to be determined in each country), with emphasis on female literacy.

Protection of children in especially difficult circumstances, particularly in situations of armed conflict.

However, unless there is a continuity of services and curative medicine practiced with prevention and full community participation, the interventions will not improve the health situation over the long term.

MCH services differ in scope and organization from country to country. Services may be split up among a number of agencies or even neglected. It is preferable for MCH services to be guided by a unified authority to ensure that the mothers and children concerned, and all aspects of their care, receive adequate consideration in all sectors. Far too often in the past, MCH services have been regarded as fancy trimmings to a health service whose only serious functions were to stamp out major communicable diseases and to provide hospital accommodation for grave disorders. This orientation has tended to continue, with an overemphasis on oral rehydration, immunizations, and treatment of acute respiratory infections with relative neglect of the other aspects of MCH.

Following are some of the important reasons for the priority given to mothers and children (Baumslag 1980; Williams 1964; WHO 1978–1983, WHO 1980).

1. *Children are the future of the nation or community.* This is not a sentimental or a nationalistic statement but a simple fact; a community's survival value rests with its children.

2. *Women and children form the ma-*

jority of the population. This is particularly true in the less developed areas. Where the life span is short, the population is mainly made up of the younger age groups. For instance, whereas in the United Kingdom in 1983 children under age 15 formed about 20 percent of the population, in India, Mexico, and Uganda, they may form as much as 45 to 50 percent of the total, and mothers and children together may make up two-thirds of the population (Pop. Ref. Bur. 1992).

3. *The health of mothers and infants is interrelated.* The majority of conditions women suffer during pregnancy and delivery that increase the risk to them of death or severe morbidity also have an adverse effect on the fetuses or the newborns (WHO 1991) (Table 4.1). Infants born of mothers with moderate to severe toxemia have been shown to have as much as four times greater risk of cerebral palsy, mental retardation, or impaired school performance (Taylor et al. 1985). The mother-infant dyad in pregnancy and the neonatal period is now receiving more attention and resources.

4. *Mothers and children are particularly vulnerable to disease.* The health progress of a country can be gauged by the proportion of deaths that fall into the various age groups. Less developed countries may have up to 20 percent of their total deaths in children under 5 years of age, and there are even higher percentages of maternal mortality, which inevitably have an adverse effect on the health of children. The significance of maternal

Table 4.1. Pathology Affecting the Mother-Infant Dyad

Nearly always maternal only	Maternal-infant shared problem	Newborn problem largely
Postpartum hemorrhage	Obstructed labor	Asphyxia
Puerperal sepsis	Hypertension	Neonatal tetanus
Chronic diseases (e.g., cancer, lupus, sickle cell anemia, maternal hemoglobinopathies)	Anemia	Ophthalmia neonatorum
	Syphilis	Hypothermia
	Gonorrhea	Sepsis and pneumonia
	HIV and other sexually transmitted diseases	Hypoglycemia
	Malaria	Herpes simplex
	Hepatitis A	Neonatal jaundice
	Amnionitis	Rubella
	Malnutrition	Toxoplasmosis
	Multiple gestation	Cytomegalovirus
	Substance abuse	Hepatitis B
	Gestational diabetes	Rhesus incompatibility
	Environmental xenobiotics	Certain drugs
	Emotional disorders	

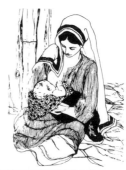

Source: WHO (1991).

Table 4.2. Proportional Mortality, Sweden, 1751–1987

	Deaths under age 5 years (%)	Deaths over age 65 years (%)
1751–1761	36	25
1851–1860	27	33
1891–1900	17	47
1941–1950	5	71
1951–1960	3	74
1961–1970	2	73
1985	1	82
1987	0.8	82

Source: UNDP (1992).

mortality is often not appreciated. In contrast, Sweden, which has devoted social services to child care and provides basic services for its population, has drastically reduced its under-5 mortality rate (Table 4.2).

5. *Most of the diseases that cause mortality and morbidity in children and those associated with pregnancy are preventable.* In countries with low levels of maternal and child mortality and morbidity, these diseases are now being prevented by various methods of prevention. The major epidemic diseases need no survey to make them apparent; an epidemic of measles or cholera is all too evident and can be controlled by vigorous isolation, treatment of patients, and wholesale immunizations. However, in order to prevent recurrences, there must be long-term programs, including health education, improvement in environmental sanitation and economics, and regular supervision (Fig. 4.1). In the case of AIDS, preventive measures involving behavioral changes and protection of blood supply through screening and sterilization of needles and equipment can go a long way toward disease containment.

Other diseases—for example, malaria and whooping cough—may call for more investigation and necessitate different methods of attack. The measures taken often depend on community action, but they also may depend on individual care.

For example, with malaria, care should include the use of mosquito nets, the prevention of mosquito breeding, and the regular provision of suppressive and therapeutic drugs. For whooping cough, care must be taken to obtain good nursing and early preventive inoculation for the protection of young babies. Adequate facilities for treatment will reduce the transmission of these diseases, and adequate health supervision will teach parents how to nurse their children when they are sick at home, depending on the availability of health care, provided by home visits and other professional services.

Control of diseases such as diarrhea, intestinal worms, malnutrition, skin diseases, and most forms of sepsis depends not only on community action but also on the attitudes, education, and diligence of the parents. In some countries, public health measures failed to control epidemics such as schistosomiasis in spite of much effort and much money; in China, a concerted community effort has made the difference. Schistosomiasis depends not only on eradicating the parasite and the water snail but also on toilet facilities and toilet technique.

Although community efforts in housing, sanitation, and public health education are of some value, the ultimate solution rests with the education and responsibility of individuals—with respect given to them and their children. The question, "If preventable, why not prevented?" requires careful and honest examination before it can be answered. Diarrheal diseases and some intestinal parasites are often related not only to the protected and available water supply but to cultural concepts and to the attention of individuals to washing their hands, collecting water in a clean bucket, and drinking out of a clean cup. Young children must be protected in the home.

Malnutrition in some parts of the world probably results not only from the short-

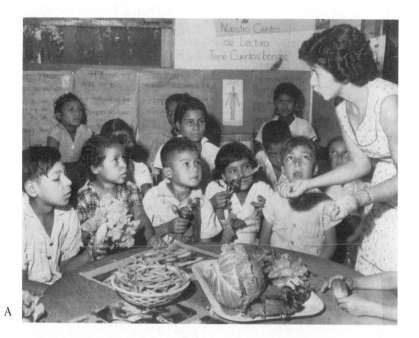

A

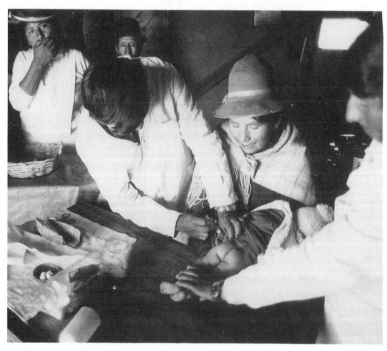

B

Figure 4.1. Direct, low-cost methods of education and treatment. (A) Nutrition education in a Latin American school. Photograph by UNICEF. (B) Immunization in Peru. Photograph by UNICEF. (C: *facing page*) First aid in India. Photograph by A. S. Kochar, WHO.

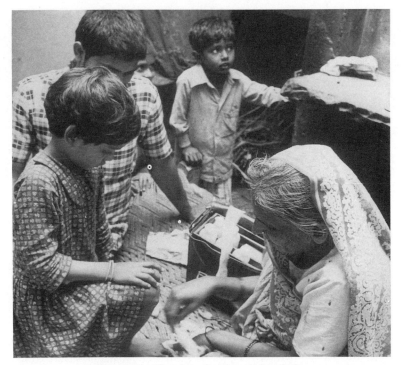

C

Figure 4.1 (Continued). First Aid in India.

age of foodstuffs but also from the failure of individuals to select, prepare, and give available foods to children at the right ages and in the right way. Again, culture as well as economics plays a part.

6. *MCH services provide an appealing and appreciated introduction to appropriate aspects of Western medicine.* The health of a community ultimately depends on the ability of individuals to understand and apply knowledge from the biological and social sciences with respect to their own well-being and on their responsibility to make use of this knowledge. Both health staff and the public must learn how to correlate diseases with the factors producing them. MCH services provide an admirable approach. Everyone is, or should be, interested in the health and well-being of their children. Children respond dramatically to sound pediatrics. When MCH services start with good treatment facilities, parents can see their children recovering under their eyes, particularly when child and mother are together in a hospital

(Fig. 4.2). They can watch the child continuing to flourish instead of dying young, or inevitably becoming a pot-bellied and ill-nourished toddler. MCH services do not merely control diseases; they ensure progress in a community.

A well-organized and consistent MCH program can provide an acceptable and appealing introduction to health and well-being, even if this means changes in behavior. It can spearhead the initiation and adaptation of health services as a whole and of educational and economic progress (Williams 1956).

7. *The incidence of lives damaged by physical, mental, and social burdens can be reduced.* The human race long ago recognized that the impulse to protect the helpless and the weak is one of its most valuable attributes. Through preventive measures, MCH services can reduce the incidence of mental and physical disability and provide special services for disabled children so that their lives can be normalized and they are as independent as possible. These services can provide

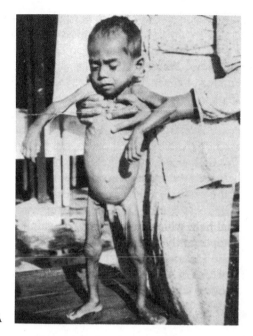
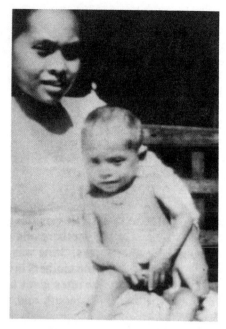

A　　　　　　　　　　　　　　　　　　　　　　　　　　　B

Figure 4.2. Involving mothers. (A) A rejected Malay child, age 2 years, weighed 9 pounds. The mother had run away but was later found and persuaded to stay and help care for the child. (B) After six weeks of treatment and the mother's involvement, the same child weighed 17 pounds.

counseling as well as respite care and family assistance.

8. *Women and children represent the least powerful members of society. Without special consideration, their needs are neither considered nor understood.* In many of the less developed countries, the provision for children in hospitals and health centers is inadequate and grossly out of proportion with the number who desperately need these services. It is recognized that the breadwinner is most essential to family well-being, but this does not justify a situation where wards and outpatient departments are sometimes overcrowded with adults often with minor complaints, while there is little accommodation for sick children.

In many countries, women have little or no part in the formation of policies, domestic or community, and because of this lack of representation, they are often neglected or even overlooked. MCH services need not be elaborate, and they do not need to be separated from other aspects of a health service. But women must receive the necessary consideration in hospitals and health centers and at home.

In some countries, perhaps for the sake of national prestige, investments are made in elaborate and impressive hospitals or equipment. Yet the general health of the population would benefit far more from the training of more auxiliary health nurses or better facilities for the supervision of midwives.

9. *Certain mental, physical, and economic characteristics are found to be typical of areas where there are high child mortality rates.*

Mental. People who live in poverty become apathetic and fatalistic. If they do not understand the causes of death in children, they attribute all deaths to the malevolence of their enemies, to the work of witches, to their own sins, or to transgression of customs. MCH curative and preventive work can do much to correct this apathy and fatalism. Some diseases, such as pneumonia and scabies, can be cured dramatically and readily. The obvious cause and effect gives parents confidence in the health worker's ability.

Physical. In regions where there is a high maternal and child mortality rate, there is illness, malnutrition, and shortage of amenities. The physical effort and calories that go into the making of a child are often wasted. The fact that many children die forces parents to have as many other children as they can in the hope that at least some will survive. This sequence of events leads to physical exhaustion and a high maternal mortality and morbidity.

Economic. In the more developed countries, the life span is approximately 70 years or more. This gives forty to fifty years of productive and independent existence, and many of the aged are able to look after themselves financially and domestically. In countries where the average life span is only 35 years, the productive period is much shorter, and productivity is reduced by chronic illness or the permanent scars of diseases in childhood. Half the population may consist of children below the age of 15. This short and inefficient working life, and the high proportion of dependents, has a serious effect on the whole economic picture. The needs of the family are seldom recognized by those who advocate birth control as an enterprise distinct from other aspects of health work. Family planning services must be integrated with other health services to maximize their effectiveness.

MCH services in the community have certain requirements, which are simultaneously opportunities:

1. *Attention to special problems of nutrition.* Malnutrition is now recognized as a widespread disorder of children and one of the greatest health hazards, particularly in the developing world. How much malnutrition is primary (due to inadequate diet) or secondary (due to factors other than the food itself) can be determined only by careful clinical observation and consistent supervision. Usually malnutrition is due to multiple causes, including dietary inadequacy (for various reasons) and infections. It is useless to campaign primarily for increased food production unless the malnutrition is directly due to food shortage. Moreover, it is useless to expect that increased supplies of food will benefit malnourished children unless there is a skilled and conscientious service for the use of food within the family. Most of the areas where malnutrition exists have no such facilities. Information from a MCH service is one of the best ways of ascertaining the malnourished state of mothers and children.

The gradual establishment of a MCH service aware of the particular needs and resources of a community is a useful step toward the wise distribution of available food, both inside and outside the family, and for the best utilization of food.

2. *Adaptation to local needs.* Some areas of medicine that have developed in scientifically advanced countries, such as radiology, surgery, and biochemistry, must be equipped to reproduce as nearly as possible those conditions under which they were designed to work. But although the basic requirements will be the same, improvisation and modification may be called for. In the field of maternal and child health, adaptation is essential if the work is to be either efficient or successful. Moreover, health workers will find that there are many subjects—for instance, the type and incidence of behavior problems, the management of lactation, the stages of child development and the factors that influence it, the mother-child relationship, and the treatment of certain disorders—about which so-called scientific medicine has much to learn from traditional medicine. Many aspects cannot be appreciated in short-term surveys but need prolonged and careful observation.

Failure to accept the need for adaptation may lead to vast expenditure on institutions, equipment, and personnel with very little in the way of results. Worse, discouragement may inhibit further development of the MCH services. For example, units for premature infants may be needed. These units are complex and expensive in most of Europe and North America and require sophisticated electronic apparatus and biochemical monitoring. Different units must be devised for these infants in areas with different climates, no electricity, and the need for the presence of the infant's lactating mother (Jelliffe 1967). "Demonstration centers" (model training centers) have been instituted by well-meaning international and other organizations, but they have sometimes been so unrelated to the local conditions that their work has been ineffective and has left very little impression.

Doctors insufficiently trained in local diseases can be damaging to the image of scientific medicine. For example, a child may have died of kwashiorkor because the doctor believed that the rash was caused by scalds. Indeed, large numbers of children have died because the doctors did not appreciate the dangers of substituting a bottle for breastfeeding. Many other patients have gone blind or died because the doctor did not recognize xerophthalmia.

In one hospital in Central Africa, the supervising nurse came from a temperate climate. She had worked in that hospital for six years and was a capable and devoted worker. For the patients' food, she sent to a farm some one hundred miles away, at great trouble and expense, for cabbages, leeks, and carrots for the daily diet. But the cook did not want to put these vegetables into the stew, and the patients did not want to eat them. Yet within a quarter of a mile of the hospital, a market sold an abundance of sweet potatoes, tomatoes, eggplant, peas, beans, groundnuts, several sorts of spinach, melons, oranges, pumpkins, bananas, and other no less excellent and thoroughly acceptable foodstuffs.

Only by establishing locally relevant MCH services can both staff and patients ensure that investigation, understanding, and continuing adaptation can be developed.

3. *Provision of comprehensive community-based care that will ensure the efficiency of the hospital services.* A doctor or nurse could deduce from crowded wards and outpatient departments that most people in the community bring their children for treatment. But research might show that a considerable proportion of the children die within a few weeks of being discharged from the hospital and many others have died without ever having been to a hospital or a doctor. Or a nutritionist taking a history may learn that an underweight baby was breastfed for three months and then was introduced to orange juice, milk powder, cereal, and banana. The diagnosis might be protein energy malnutrition, and the mother may be advised to supplement the child's diet. The health worker, however, may be unaware that the child spends several hours a day sitting or crawling around in an insanitary yard. The child may be putting assorted objects in his mouth and may suffer from recurrent attacks of diarrhea or even be infested with worms (Fig. 4.3).

Too often, a nutrition department has its own area of influence, a health education department another, the community health center another, and a "women's society" yet another, and none of them has much to do with a grossly overcrowded and understaffed child health clinics. Parents with two or three children between the ages of 6 and 14 may benefit greatly from guidance and support and ideally should not be excluded from any care and advice that an MCH center can provide. But it is the mother with her first pregnancy or first baby, with a newly weaned child, or with a child with a chronic disorder or mental or physical

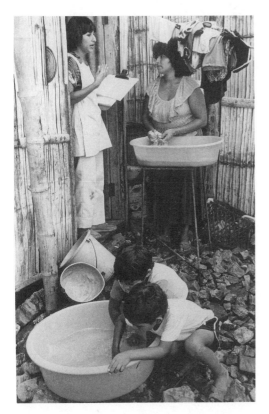

Figure 4.3. A PHC worker discusses ways to provide basic hygienic measures with a mother in a slum in Guayaquil, Ecuador. UNICEF photo by Bernard Pierre Wolff.

abnormality who needs concentrated and continuing guidance and care. To identify mothers and children at risk is a vital function in the development of rational MCH service with limited resources.

A number of areas in the world are plagued with the problems of population explosion. Comprehensive family care will provide parents in these areas with help and knowledge and will encourage them not to have more children than they can look after properly. Health workers will also encourage parents to use this knowledge consistently and help to ensure the stability of the family (Titmuss and Abel-Smith 1961) and they will try to ensure that all services are integrated.

4. *Optimum utilization of health personnel.* MCH services are a good training ground for all health personnel. Doctors and nurses can observe the natural history of disease and not merely a static, textbook presentation. "Growth and development" become associated with all the multifarious factors that affect them and are not merely visions of immutable concrete escalation. Doctors and nurses can learn how to identify cases at risk and how to provide the necessary care and support. It is becoming increasingly recognized that all countries must devise their own methods of training auxiliary staff. Auxiliary health workers can receive much of their most valuable training in the context of MCH services, and the doctors and nurses can learn how to provide the most effective training and supervision.

The reasons for an emphasis on MCH services are many and various. One of the chief reasons is that they should serve to coordinate some of the efforts now being made to improve living conditions—to weigh the imponderable, to reach the unreachable, and to teach the unteachable, as well as to give assistance and advice to those who are striving against serious odds. Continuity of care and comprehensive care will develop the ideal of family service.

REFERENCES

Baumslag, N. (1980). *Mothers and Children—Nutrition and Health Care in Kenya, Zimbabwe, Mozambique and Botswana.* Ford Foundation, New York.

Delfgaauw, B. (1961). *Teilhard de Chardin.* Baarn, Wereldvenster.

Ebbrahim, G. J. (1991). Adjustment with a human face: Is it feasible? *J. Trop. Pediat.* 37, 3.

Grant, J. P. (1985). *The State of the World's Children.* Oxford University Press for UNICEF, New York.

Jelliffe, D. B. (1967). Prematurity. In *Obstetrics and Gynecology in the Tropics and Developing Countries.* Ed. J. B. Lawson and D. D. Stewart. Edward Arnold, London.

King, M. (1966). *Medical Care in Developing Countries*. Oxford University Press, Nairobi.

Pop. Ref. Bur. (1992). *World Population Data Sheet*. Population Reference Bureau, Washington, D.C.

Taylor, D. J.; Davidson, J.; Howie, P. W.; and Drillien, C. M. (1985). Do pregnancy complications contribute to neurological development of disability? *Lancet* i, 713–716

Titmuss, R., and Abel-Smith, B. (1961). *Social Policies and Population Growth in Mauritius*. London.

UN (1989). *UN Demographic Yearbook 1989*. United Nations, New York.

UNDP (1992). *Human Development Report*. United Nations Development Programme. Oxford University Press, New York.

UNICEF (1991). *1991 Annual Report, United Nations Children's Fund*. UNICEF House, New York.

Williams, C. D. (1956). Maternal and child health in Kumasi in 1935. *J. Trop. Pediatr.* 2, 141.

Williams, C. D. (1964). Maternal and child health services in developing countries. *Lancet* i, 345.

WHO (1978). *Primary Health Care*. World Health Organization, Geneva.

WHO (1978–1983). *Sixth General Programme of Work Covering the Specific Period 1978–1983*. Global Medium Term Programme for Family Health, FHE/79.4. World Health Organization, Geneva.

WHO (1980). *Towards a Better Future: Maternal and Child Health*. World Health Organization, Geneva.

WHO (1991). *Child Health and Development: Health of the Newborn*. World Health Organization, Geneva.

5

Population Problems

Much has been written on the subject of overpopulation. By the year 2025, the world population is projected to be about 8.5 billion. Two-thirds (5.3 billion) will live in the developing world, where abject poverty and misery abound, food and water are scarce, housing is inadequate, and public community services are lacking or rudimentary (WHO 1992). Funneling resources of food, land, and money to those most in need is the challenge.

The focus on the very real problem of population explosion has led to a neglect of the main problem of inequitable distribution. World food supplies are produced globally but inequitably distributed, for economic and political reasons (Lappe 1977).

Despite recent reports of slowing birthrates in some countries, a doubling of population is expected by the year 2000 for a number of reasons: a declining mortality rate, a high fertility rate, a low marriage age in technologically developing countries, young populations (over 45 percent of the population is under 15 years of age in the least developed countries), and a rapidly growing number of women entering childbearing age. (The population doubling time will vary from the low figure of 41 years in the underdeveloped countries, excluding China, to a figure of 148 years in the technologically developed countries.) However, new diseases such as AIDS, war, and natural disasters could cause a decrease in population.

Many areas in the world, including Southeast Asia, Africa, and south and central America, have populations that are expanding so rapidly that their progress toward technological development is delayed (Fig. 5.1). Expanding health, education, and other social services are continually outstripped. Some observers claim that if the world population continues to increase at its current rate, there will be standing room only by the year 2700. Additionally, overlarge families with too closely spaced children have been shown to have an increase in low-birthweight infants and a higher prevalence of malnutrition in both mothers and children (Rosa and Thurshen 1970).

Most countries are in a state of demographic transition, with a falling death rate and a high fertility rate. In Latin America and Mexico, in spite of eco-

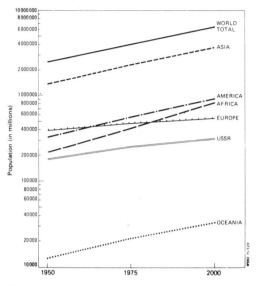

Figure 5.1. Population increase by continent or macro-region, 1950–2000. Source: WHO (1980*a*).

Table 5.1. Number of Women (in millions) of Childbearing Age (15 to 45)

	1950	1975	2000[a]
Developed countries	203	247	286
Developing countries	350	601	1,120

Source: WHO (1980*a*).

[a]Estimated.

ricultural technology gives some grounds for encouragement. Appropriate technology, small loans, and other incentives to assist traditional subsistence farmers to increase the family's food production is vital. However, an unsolved problem of increasing magnitude is posed by the urban avalanche of rural agriculturalists moving to city shantytowns (Fig. 5.2), where they experience the "worst of both [urban and rural] worlds" (Garner 1991).

nomic development, fertility has remained high (PAHO 1990). In several African countries where fertility rates have declined very little and mortality has slowed, the population growth rate is at its peak. In Kenya, for example, the population growth rate was 4 percent a year. Calculations have shown that if the total fertility rate were reduced from 8 to 4 by the year 2000, there would be 28 percent fewer primary schoolchildren to educate (World Bank 1981) (1990 population growth rate in Kenya dropped to 3.6 percent).

MCH services must be based on projections of the number of women of childbearing age (women aged between 15 and 45 years) (Table 5.1). Estimates of the age and sex structure of the population are crucial because the disease spectrum and health care needs vary with age and sex, educational levels, attitudes, psychological capabilities, occupation, income, and consumption patterns.

How far the world's economic and nutritional resources are capable of further development is open to conjecture, although the application of modern ag-

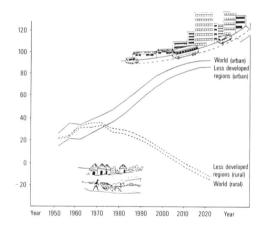

Figure 5.2. Average annual increment in urban and rural population for the world and less developed regions, 1950–2025. In twenty years or less, half of the world's population will live in urban areas in search of amenities and opportunities. In the expanding megacities of the developing world, the major increase will be in the slums and shantytowns, which are growing at twice the rate of cities as a whole. In 1987 it was estimated that slum and shantytown dwellers represented between 30 and 60 percent of the urban population. Sources: Population Crisis Committee (1991); UN Economic and Social Council (1982).

Clearly, the rapid increase in population is a serious problem in most areas of the world (although in underpopulated areas, an increase in population may bring no immediate hardship), it is equally obvious that there are only two ways of combating this increase: high mortality and low fertility. In the past, it was high mortality that acted as a damper. It is necessary to examine the reasons for a high mortality and how the rate has been diminished.

THE MORTALITY RATE

Vital statistics are the least accurate—and often nonexistent—in the areas and at the times when mortality is highest, especially since some governments give lower indicators of poor health and higher-than-actual figures for good indicators. But in every society in all parts of the world, the uneducated poor living in unsanitary environments show high mortality and morbidity rates. These rates are especially high in children, but the adults also have a short average life span.

Several processes counteract high mortality rates: peace (law and order), health and education, and economic progress. The three processes are in fact interdependent, for none of them can succeed without the other. Matters such as food production and conservation are closely associated with health and education, and with economics—in fact, food economics. Peace and freedom from civil unrest, however, are of the first importance in reducing mortality rates and also in increasing birthrates. Second, improvement of health, nutrition, and education services will lower mortality rates (Fig. 5.3) (Zeitlin et al. 1982).

Health measures will save many lives, but if they are merely imposed on a passive population, they will increase the birthrate. If, on the other hand, health measures are accompanied by education, health education, and responsible coop-

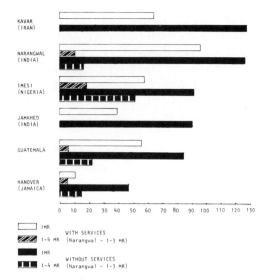

Figure 5.3. Mortality rates in infants and children. Mortality rates (infant and child) in six integrated MCH nutrition programs, were lower in populations receiving services compared to those in the same area without services. Source: Zeitlin et al. (1982).

eration, the birthrate will tend to fall. The third factor, economic progress, will also reduce mortality, provided it benefits all sectors of the population. Because economic progress is impossible without health and education services, it should eventually tend to solve problems of overpopulation.

Let us look at examples of these three processes in different countries.

The Effect of Law and Order on Population Size: India

After the fall of the Mogul empire in the mid-eighteenth century, the Indian subcontinent was in a state of chronic war and disorder, and health services were nonexistent. During British rule, between 1800 and 1950, the population more than doubled. This increase may have been due, to some extent, to the control of epidemic diseases as some segments of the population came in contact with modern medicine, but it is likely that the establishment of law and order, which implies improved transport and organized services during these years, had a more profound effect on population increase than medical care and disease control (PAHO 1970; Population Council 1968; Rosa 1967).

The Effect of Transport and Food Production on Infant Mortality: The Netherlands

Accurate figures are rarely available in the less developed countries, but the effect of war and disorder can be examined in countries where statistics exist. In the Netherlands, during World War II, infant mortality rose from 37 in 1940 to 78 in 1945. By 1964, it was reduced to 14.8. Toward the end of the war, there was a severe famine. The average food intake in October 1944 was approximately 1600 calories; it was only 1300 calories by April 1945 (Fig. 5.4) (NCHS 1968; Stein et al. 1975). Immediately before the German surrender, the food intake was as low as 500 to 600 calories per capita per day (Stein et al. 1975) and the infant mortality rate (IMR) increased to 80/1,000. After the war, with the reestablishment of transportation, food production, and services, infant mortality dropped markedly. In 1983, it was 8.6 per 1,000 live births, one of the lowest of the world, and by 1992 it was just 6.2 (Pop. Ref. Bur. 1992).

The Effect of War, Education, Industry, and Economics on Infant Mortality and the Death Rate: Italy

Italian statistics give a vivid picture of the rise in infant mortality and the decrease in the birthrate that result from war (Fig. 5.5). Families were disrupted, and that alone brought a big reduction in birth rate.

Italy, a Roman Catholic country, has never had an official campaign for family

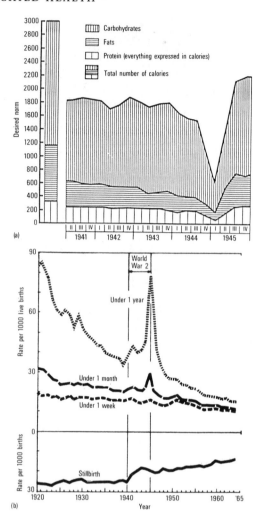

Figure 5.4. Availability of food and infant mortality: (A) average quarterly distribution of food rations in calories, protein, fats, and carbohydrates; and (b) stillbirth rate and infant mortality in the western Netherlands, 1941–1945. Source: Stein et al. (1975).

planning. Moreover, apart from malaria control in certain areas, there have been few campaigns for the control of major epidemic disease that are comparable with those conducted in some developing countries. Analysis of the figures by region shows that in the north, which has more education, industry, economic advance, and better health services, the improvement in infant mortality and the

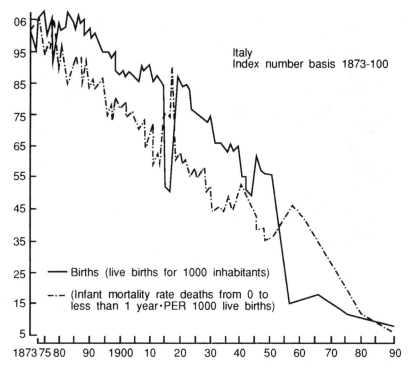

Figure 5.5. Infant mortality and birthrate in Italy, 1873–1990. Sources: UN (1979); WHO (1982); Pop. Ref. Bur. (1992).

decrease in the birthrate have been steadily better than in the south and on the islands. Since World War II, despite the peak in the birthrate that always follows the restoration of peace and family reunions, there has been a steady decline in both the IMR and the birthrate. In 1962 the former stood at 40 and the latter at 19 (about the European average). According to 1992 data the infant mortality rate has dropped to 8.6 and the birthrate to 10 (Pop. Ref. Bur. 1992).

The Effect of War on the Birthrate and Death Rate: The Former Yugoslavia

The effect of two wars on the total population can be seen in the population pyramid for the former Yugoslavia (Fig. 5.6). In World War II, one-tenth of the population was killed, and a large proportion of the adults who died were

among the skilled and professional classes. Wars also limit the number of births because of family disruption. It is likely that the civil war of the 1990s resulting from the collapse of the communist system may show the same pattern as in World War II.

The Effect of Disruption of Family Life on the Birthrate: Scotland

Scotland suffered no enemy occupation and comparatively little in the way of aerial attack during World Wars I and II, but the birthrate fell nevertheless (Fig. 5.7). In 1945 many of the men ages 25 to 35 years were away from their country. Thus, Scotland saw not increased mortality and morbidity as a result of the war but a monumental disruption of family life and, hence, decreased births. When peace was restored and families were reunited, a baby boom followed.

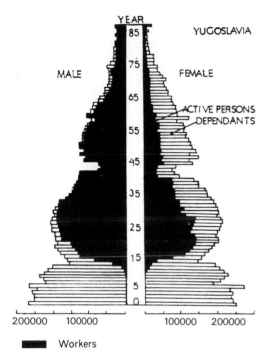

Figure 5.6. Effect of war on the total population of the former Yugoslavia. Source: Federal Statistical Bureau.

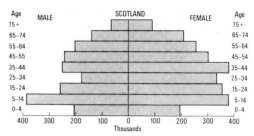

Figure 5.7. Effect of war on total population of Scotland, 1945. Source: Crew (1948).

Because of a decline in fertility since the late 1980s, the Singapore government has started offering incentives for large families in a pronatalist program mainly directed to the "graduate mothers." Parents without a high school education and earning less than $2,750 per year, on the other hand, were offered a $5,000 down payment for an apartment if they were sterilized. This program has since been altered to remove its "superior genes" stigma and is now called the Social Development Unit (SDU). The SDU offers organized sea cruises and computerized matchmaking to promote its pronatalist policy (Lee et al. 1991).

The Effect of a Pronatalist Policy and the Development of Services on Fertility: Singapore

Myanmar (Burma), Malaysia and Singapore, and Indonesia all suffered from harsh enemy occupation during World War II, and in all these areas, the infant mortality rate stood at approximately 300 in 1945. By 1950, resettled conditions and the rule of law were restored in Singapore, and the IMR was 90, but in Myanmar and Indonesia, disturbances still occurred, and the IMR remained at 250 for some time. By 1978 the IMR for Singapore had dropped to 12; but in Indonesia and Myanmar it was still high—91 and 140, respectively (Pop. Ref. Bur. 1980). In 1992 the IMR in Myanmar was 72; in Indonesia, 70; and in Singapore, 6.7. Singapore's infant mortality is lower even than that of the United Kingdom, 7.9 (Pop. Ref. Bur. 1992).

The Effect of War on Infant Mortality: England and Wales

War and civil disorder not only destroy and damage; they result in hardships and deaths among the more vulnerable groups and always cause a reduced birthrate. The effect on the population, however, will vary according to the degree of disruption of amenities. England and Wales in World War II experienced no enemy occupation, although they were hit hard by severe aerial attacks, interruption of food supplies, and industrial reorganization. Nevertheless, there was no actual increase in the death rate among children (Table 5.2) (Frederiksen 1960). This was achieved by detailed and elaborate planning during the war on behalf of the vulnerable groups, including improved nutrition for mothers and infants. After

Table 5.2. Effect of Organized MCH Services in the United Kingdom, 1840–1990

Date	Birth rate	Death rate	Infant mortality rate	Mortality rate of children ages 1–4
1840–1845[a]	32.3	21.4	148	35.0[b]
1851–1855[a]	33.9	22.7	156	35.7[b]
1861–1865[a]	35.1	22.6	151	38.8[b]
1871–1875[a]	35.5	22	153	32.4[b]
1881–1885[a]	33.5	19.4	139	28.0[b]
1891–1895[a]	30.5	18.7	151	25.5[b]
1901–1905[a]	28.2	16	138	20.3[b]
1910–1915[a]	23.9	14.3	110	15.3[b]
1921–1925[a]	19.9	12.1	76	8.5
1931–1935[a]	15	12	62	6.6
1941–1945[a]	17.6	12.8	50	3.5
1946	20.2	12	43	2.1
1948	18	11	34	1.8
1951–1955	15.2	11.7	27	1.1
1960	17.2	11.5	22	0.9
1965	18.3	11.5	20	0.9
1968	17.1	11.8	19	0.8 (1967)
1970	16.3	11.8	18	0.8[c]
1980	13.3	11.8	12	0.5[c]
1990	13.7	11.8	8	0.3

Sources: Office of the High Commission, Malta; Professor D. D. Reid; UN (1979); WHO (1982), World Bank (1991).

[a] Averages.

[b] Calculated.

[c] Derived from average rates of males and females (rates per 1,000 population).

the conclusion of hostilities, the birthrate jumped as a result of the reunion of families.

A society in which the essential services have been thoroughly disorganized suffers infinitely more than one that maintains some semblance of administration and sanitation in times of war and other disturbances. In the latter, the increase in mortality is moderate, even though the birthrate falls. In the former, the population is decreased by both high mortality and low fertility.

The instinct to protect the unfortunate and the defenseless is perhaps the most valuable of all human attributes and the basis of all health education. However it should be noted that the challenge offered by the sick and the handicapped to medicine and science has led to methods of cure and prevention that would never have been discovered if "liquidation of the unfit" had been practiced universally.

Lowering the Mortality Rate

The mass approach. The causes of mortality are often multiple, and an integrated "strategy of struggle" that can be maintained must be woven into the infrastructure of primary health care. There must be community services for water supply, sewage and refuse disposal, food hygiene, pest control, housing, transport, recreation facilities, and occupational health. Health education programs may be carried out through the mass media, although this method is expensive and often not very effective. In times of disaster, these programs can supply shelter and mass feeding. Services of this sort undoubtedly save many lives and are indispensable to good community development, but they need to be balanced by family care and supervision.

The control of communicable disease absorbs a great deal of the attention, personnel, and money available for health work. It is essential that such diseases should be controlled but without developing isolated vertical programs that are in competition with each other. A great deal of money and attention is spent on mass methods—for example, in malaria control. Sri Lanka is often cited as an area where antimalaria programs have resulted in a spectacular reduction of the infant mortality and general death rates. These findings, however, have not been altogether substantiated, and it has been suggested that these rates in both the malarious and nonmalarious areas were similar (Frederiksen 1960) and the reduction in death rates had actually started before malaria control was instituted (Karunaratne 1956).

Mass immunization has eliminated smallpox. Polio and guinea worm (dracunculosis), it is hoped, will be the next. Other endemic and communicable diseases, such as malaria, schistosomiasis, whooping cough, and measles, are more difficult to eradicate because of their more complex etiologies, often superimposed on malnutrition, problems with immunization (when such exists), and in some instances more resistant microorganisms and parasites.

The individual approach. Family medical care and personal, domestic, and community hygiene depend to some extent on the responsibility of individuals. Health depends on the capacity of the people to ensure "cleanliness, good food, and fresh air"—the basic three principles of Florence Nightingale's work. Nightingale should have added a "serene outlook." Health depends more on this capacity than on passive acceptance of immunization. In the same way, there are three factors that prevent the exercise of individual health: ignorance, indifference, and dependence. Patients and parents will readily accept advice on prevention from those who show their ability to cure disease. Unsophisticated people will have confidence in individuals rather than in systems and are often confused—and antagonized—by having to listen to a number of different health workers. When a mother is admitted to a hospital with a sick baby and sees her baby recovering as a result of medical care and diet, she will more readily accept advice on future care and feeding, especially when she herself, while in hospital, has beaten the egg into the porridge.

A balanced approach. Everyone with medical experience in less developed countries knows that almost any form of medical care is met with clamorous interest; the hopelessly overcrowded wards, the vast hordes of outpatients, and the eager groups at home visiting are evidence. But it is the MCH services that can form the spearhead and the continuing weapon of attack on disease and ignorance if they are intelligently adapted to local needs and resources. Food distribution and other mass methods are comparatively more expensive and less effective.

Communities subjected to an unbalanced program dominated by mass methods of disease control, mass immunization, mass distribution of vitamins, milk, and clothing, and the general philosophy of "mass impact" become dependent. In Mauritius (Titmuss and Abel-Smith 1961), social assistance has actually tended to increase the numbers of indigent families; in New Zealand, the Maoris have been affected in the same way. Indeed, many international overseas aid programs have had disappointing results because the donors have not appreciated how much damage can be done by inappropriate giving. In Newcastle-upon-Tyne (Miller et al. 1960), observers found that the three great obstacles to child well-being were deprivation of normal family care, deficiency in physical amenities, and dependence on outside assistance.

Short-term dependence is bound to arise in national emergencies, cataclysms, and certain personal disasters and misfortunes. For long-term planning, however, dependence must be avoided. Unless a health, education, and social assistance program is balanced in its mass and individual approach, whole communities may be physically and mentally pauperized by too much impersonal disease control, food distribution, and assistance. No community can thrive unless it learns how to use these amenities with responsibility at the personal and individual levels.

Tuberculosis, whooping cough, and measles cause large mortality and morbidity among children in developing countries. How much this is due to lack of immunity, how much to poor nursing and medical care, and how much to underlying malnutrition varies with each community and each individual. Health supervision, immunization, and early, economical treatment must form a balanced whole.

In communities where mass disease control programs have been instituted, there may be a considerable saving of life, but unless there is a corresponding attention to individual services, education, and economic progress, the result is a population explosion, with the numbers increasing faster than the social and economic resources. A great deal of money and effort has been spent on mass control of disease in India, but this has not been balanced by other methods of health promotion. The population is now increasing so rapidly that it is considered necessary to spend no less than 3 percent of the total national budget on family planning. The death rate in Sri Lanka (Fig. 5.8) is steadily decreasing among infants and adults, but mass disease control programs have outstripped the individual health programs that are needed for the increasing population. In spite of major efforts to popularize family planning, there is still an excessive birthrate. In Malta, however, the improved health among children and a higher standard of living resulted in a fall in the birthrate and in the infant mortality rate.

In India there are serious complaints of overpopulation. In fact, where the population is healthy, educated, productive, and generally reasonably well-to-do, "overpopulation" is not an immediate obstacle to progress, although this will not be so in the near future if the infrastructure is not properly maintained to avoid sanitary and environmental hazards and development of slums.

Health professionals and other providers of community services can be responsible for health education. Teaching is carried out in communities where the general practitioner and health assistants have overall charge of families. But in the hospital setting, with crowded wards and clinics, specialist staff have no contact with the patient's environment or responsibilities, and doctors and nurses feel they have little time or opportunity to investigate anything beyond the presenting disease.

The supervision and coordination of community services is often complicated by inadequate numbers of staff. In some cases the training curriculum of the health providers is hospital oriented for registered nurses, while that of the "enrolled nurses" (who receive less training) whom they are supposed to supervise is community oriented, resulting in different messages and information. When hospital-trained staff have to work in the community, problems can arise.

Economic progress measured not only by per capita income but by the distribution of wealth, the trend of vital and other statistics, and the use and the potential of a nation's population—is impossible in a country where there is a high death rate and the inevitable short average life span (Beasley et al. 1969). It

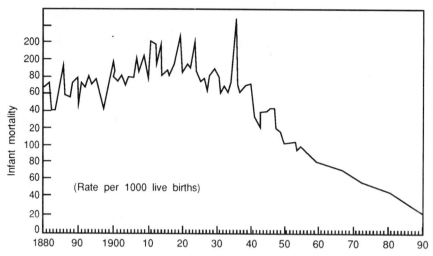

Figure 5.8. Infant mortality rate in Sri Lanka, 1870–1990. Sources: Karunaratne (1956); UN (1979); WHO (1982), Pop. Ref. Bur. (1992).

is rapid in countries with established peace and well-organized social health and education services.

Some of the less developed countries have tried to rush into industrialization, as if this were the answer to their economic problems. But the benefits of industrialization cannot be realized if the workers are kept unhealthy and uneducated and the population has no purchasing power. It is important to encourage housing, transport, land reform, agriculture, agricultural development, and horticultural research into bigger and faster-maturing crops; for without good food, available at affordable prices, good education, and good living conditions, industrial development may be a liability. It may result in a few low-paying jobs that lure the rural population to the cities, creating slums with diseases and crime. Conditions that make for a sound, balanced economy are identical with those that lead to a reduced mortality and morbidity and to a rationalized birthrate.

With Death Control Comes Birth Control

In 1925, Singapore's IMR was over 250 per 1,000, and the birthrate 25 because the population was predominantly male, a result of large numbers of male immigrants from China, Indonesia, and other neighboring islands. In 1928 the MCH services began to operate. In the late 1930s, many women came from these countries to join their husbands, and these two factors raised the birthrate to 40 and lowered the IMR to 150. It was only 90 in the rural areas because the services there were more effective, supervising children up to school age; those of the municipality undertook supervision only during the first year of life. During the Japanese war (December 1941–August 1945) all the MCH services were discontinued. By 1950 family planning services were offered in close cooperation with existing MCH services; the IMR as well as the birthrate fell consistently. In 1980 the IMR was 11.7 and the birthrate 17.1 (Fig. 5.9) (WHO 1982). In 1992 the IMR was 6.7 (lower than 7.9 in the United Kingdom) and the birthrate was 19.

THE FERTILITY RATE

A high mortality cannot be accepted as a solution to population control, but low-

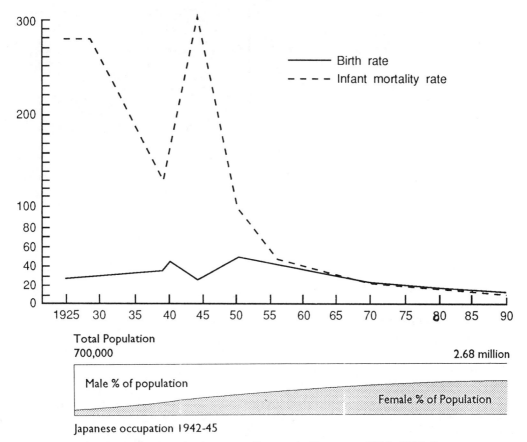

Japanese occupation 1942-45

Figure 5.9. Birthrate and infant mortality rate in Singapore, 1925–1990. Sources: WHO (1982); Pop. Ref. Bur. (1992).

ering fertility can (Table 5.3). One physician has said:

If women could choose to have the number of children they want and no more the number of births would fall by a third in Latin America and Asia and by 17 percent in Af-

rica. Maternal mortality would fall by at least an equivalent proportion. (Sadik 1992)

The reasons that fertility remains high among the more impoverished communities must be examined and not assumed. When a group of uneducated

Table 5.3. Trends in Fertility and Mortality, 1985–1990

	Crude birth rate		Crude death rate		Total fertility rate		Life expectancy for both sexes	
	1985	1990	1985	1990	1985	1990	1985	1990
Developing countries	31.3	30.4	10.2	9.4	4.1	3.8	61.0	62.8
Least developed	45.1	44.3	17.4	15.8	6.3	6.1	48.5	50.7
Eastern Europe	17.8	16.7	10.8	10.4	2.3	2.2	69.5	71.0
Development market economies	14.2	13.8	9.2	9.3	1.8	1.8	74.9	75.8

Source: WHO (1992).

women in Jamaica who lived in an overpopulated area, with high unemployment and a high birthrate were asked why they continued to produce so many children, many of whom they neglected or even abandoned, they gave following answers:

"Having children is fate."

"No women can be healthy unless she has children."

"A woman needs to have children to look after her when she is old."

"If I have no children, everyone will call me a mule."

Where only 50 percent of the children survive to maturity, having numerous children is considered the only way of ensuring the survival of a few. It is not until people find other status symbols and other security than in their fertility, or until they have confidence in the survival of their children, that they become interested in limiting their numbers for the sake of their well-being. Large families may be a response to poverty, not a cause of it.

Before the concept of family planning had become either acceptable or feasible, even the most educated and privileged families looked upon their fertility as a matter that was not within their control, and many women still regard any type of interference with possible pregnancies as immoral. Various types of diseases (particularly pelvic infections) went undiagnosed and untreated, thus exerting some sort of restraint, though a toxic and damaging one, on unrestricted childbearing.

Now, even in seemingly underpopulated countries (such as Romania or some African countries), the advantages of family planning are becoming increasingly apparent. In every country, it appears that when people arrive at a certain stage in education and economic development, families tend to become smaller. The parents have confidence that the children are likely to survive, and they wish

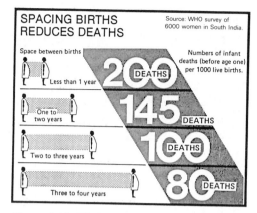

Figure 5.10. Birth spacing and infant mortality, based on a WHO survey of 6000 women in South India. As the pregnancy interval decreases, the risk of infant death increases. Source: Courtesy of UNICEF.

to provide them with good care and education. Studies in Nepal have shown that acceptance and utilization of child spacing increase when there are two or more live sons per family. In every study, it has been proved that the educated classes have fewer children and fewer deaths in almost every age group than the uneducated. Where births are spaced at intervals greater than two years, infant and neonatal mortality is halved (Fig. 5.10) (Omran 1976).

Whatever the methods individual couples choose to limit fertility, it is necessary for them also to consider the problem from the point of view of the children among whom resources (food, clothing), attention, education, and so on must be divided.

Meeting Basic Needs to Improve Health and Nutrition

Countries with a deep concern for their citizens and a willingness to invest a major share of their resources in social welfare have made dramatic improvements in the health and nutrition of their people in a short time. Life expectancy has risen and infant mortality declined in China,

Cuba, Sri Lanka, and Kerala State in India. Social conditions have altered, and health and education services especially have been improved. These changes, rather than the increase in GNP or selective primary care interventions, have been vital to the improvements. With death control has come birth control.

Lowering Fertility: Two Examples

China. China in 1992 had an IMR of 34 and a life expectancy for females of 71 and for males 68 years from birth (Pop. Ref. Bur. 1992), and there has been a rapid reduction in fertility. The birthrate declined from 40 per 1,000 in the mid-1960s to less than 20 per 1,000 in the early 1990s. This lowered birthrate has been achieved through a one-child-per-couple government family planning policy and an extensive health service structure. Health education; obstetric and gynecological services, including abortions and sterilization; and enticing inducements and incentives such as priority education, employment and housing, and free vacations are available to those who comply with the policy. Families with two or more children are penalized and socially ostracized. In addition, late marriage is encouraged (28 years for urban males and 25 years for urban females; 25 years for rural males and 23 years for rural females).

All women are educated at the primary level, and this education has changed attitudes about family size and family planning, which family planning supplies and services are provided, even at the household level, and health education of the individual and masses. For example, family planning posters abound in the railway station where people congregate. China with its low GNP has been able to check population growth rapidly (Fig. 5.11) (Coale 1982; Hux-Xingluan 1982).

Costa Rica. Approaches at the national level vary according to the political sys-

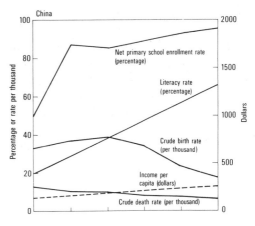

Figure 5.11. Provision of extensive and basic health services has improved health statistics in China. Source: World Bank (1981).

tem of the country. Costa Rica has targeted money and services to the poorest of the poor: increased availability of water, nutrition rehabilitation, education of women, and child spacing. Over a period of thirty years (1960–1990), this effort has resulted in a drop in the total fertility rate from 7.3 to 3.1 and the infant mortality rate from 76 to 17.2 (Bixby 1983; WHO 1980*b*, 1992).

Methods of Limiting Fertility

Most people, including politicians and religious authorities, now agree that responsible people should avoid having more children than can be properly looked after. However, economic and cultural considerations, such as a bride-price, marriage image, and female dowry, continue to be influential. Here we examine some of the main methods for limiting fertility that are available (Wallace et al. 1969; WHO 1965; Hatcher et al 1990).

Infanticide. This was practiced in the distant past in Greece, Rome, China, Mexico, Polynesia, and elsewhere. It is still practiced deliberately or through neglect in some circumstances. But even where it has been defended as a "mercy killing," the majority of people still regard it as an outrage.

In China, where the one-child family planning policy prevails, female infanticide is rising (Women of China 1983); in some areas, there are five times as many male as female infants. Females are the "go-away child"; they do not provide insurance for the aged and do not perpetuate the family name and are thus considered an economic liability. Although legislation has been passed to allow women to stay at home when they marry, cultural practices prevail, and the bride typically goes to live with her husband's parents. Increasing education of girls may lead to the end of this practice. The percentage of girls with primary school education has risen from 57 percent of school-going age in 1960 to 81 in 1990 (World Bank 1991).

In India, amniocentesis is used for selective abortion of female fetuses. Results in one hospital revealed that of 1,500 requests for amniocentesis, 5 percent were for detection of genetic defects, 1 percent to destroy the male fetus, and the remainder to abort the female fetus (Lancet 1983)—and this occurred after legislation had been passed prohibiting female infanticide. On the other hand, when Bhopal victims asked to be provided with amniocentesis to detect birth defects, this test was not allowed (WIPHN News 1991).

Legislation. Legislation deferring the age of marriage, especially where it is customary for the young to marry before they are 16 years old and are physically or mentally full grown, has not been very successful in altering social customs. However, in some countries, higher education seems to be associated with later marriage. To defer the age of marriage, as China does, helps to limit the years of childbearing, reduce the rate of population increase, and make marriages more stable. Unfortunately, it is very difficult to enforce. In many countries there has

been an increase in teenage pregnancies, despite fewer early marriages, due to cultural changes and economic pressure.

The fear of having no children and therefore of indigent old age may be combated by the introduction of old-age pensions (Spengler 1969). Pensions are expensive but may be well worth the money spent and the effort involved. As livelihood is depending more on employment than peasant farming, old-age pensions will be the only way older people can support themselves.

Sterilization. Some countries have legalized sterilization on a voluntary basis. In India an attempt was made to encourage sterilization of both men and women by giving a bonus to those who would submit to surgery, but it became politically unpopular because of coercion and was dropped (Eubank and Wray 1980). Nevertheless, new and faster field surgical procedures such as minilaparotomies for tying fallopian tubes have been developed for mass use in countries such as Thailand, although they are still very expensive. Some countries, moreover, have made sterilization of the "unfit" (e.g., the mentally retarded) obligatory, as was the case in the United States in the 1950s. Some doctors will encourage sterilization where there are already "enough children." But it is not an easy decision for the individuals concerned or for the medical adviser. The mental as well as the physical effects of sterilization have to be considered, particularly in communities where fertility is profoundly respected. Vasectomy and tubectomy are more permanent methods of sterilization, and specialized client counseling is important to avoid regrets and psychological stress later.

Abortion. After World War II, abortions were encouraged and undertaken in some countries, including Japan, in order to control population size rapidly. Abortions are currently widely practiced in countries where other types of fertility control are unobtainable, such as in Latin America. Abortion has also been encouraged in China and was the form of family planning available in the former Soviet Union. But an abortion program is expensive, it is never totally safe, and it may be repugnant to the medical staff taking part. In Zambia, for example, although abortions are legal, Catholic doctors will not perform them. They prefer to employ contraceptive methods rather than to encourage abortions.

The Japanese have succeeded in controlling population growth by a major program of abortion, but they also have an extensive system of health centers and health nurses, and certain cultural factors have helped to implement this program. Many of the pregnancies in Japan spontaneously abort. The causes are genetic, together with infectious, physical, and chemical factors and less well-defined causes related to neurological, emotional, or nutritional factors. Induced abortion, on the other hand, is a deliberate measure to interrupt a pregnancy before the fetus is viable.

Whether legal or not, abortion is probably the most widely used method of fertility regulation. It is estimated that one-fifth to one-third of all pregnancies end in induced abortion. In certain urban areas where abortion is legal, about three abortions for each live birth have been recorded. Two-thirds of the world's population, mostly in Asia, Europe, and North America, live in countries where there are liberal abortion laws and policies, but the remaining one-third live in countries, mainly in Latin America and Africa, where abortion is either illegal or permitted only to protect a woman's life or health.

Regardless of the legal status of abortion in most parts of the world, for the majority of women wanting this procedure, health services are inaccessible (physically or financially) or are not sought, for many reasons (Tietze 1979). And in countries where women have no choice but to resort to illegal abortions,

they are admitted to the hospital if bleeding with a diagnosis of menstrual irregularity or if infected as acute pelvic inflammatory disease. Women worldwide are demanding the right to choose abortion. Legal restrictions have resulted in untold misery, preventable maternal deaths, and unwanted, orphaned, abandoned, and abused children.

Family Planning

Mechanical appliances. These take the form of condoms (including a recently developed female condom), caps, jellies, barrier creams, foams, sponges, and spermicidal tablets. Probably the cheapest method is a piece of sponge rubber soaked in oil and inserted into the vagina. Yet most of these methods are not cheap enough for the underprivileged, none is 100 percent reliable, and all entail some sort of discipline and forethought. They are widely used though not approved by some religious authorities. Intrauterine coils and devices (IUD) made of plastic have also been widely used. Although they are cheap and easy to manage, recent reports have indicated a high rate of side-effects such as salpingitis, tubal occlusion, and tubal pregnancies. Menorrhagia and failure to retain the IUDs have also been reported.

Oral contraceptives. These consist of varying combinations of estrogens and progestogens (WHO 1970; Eubank and Wray 1980; Hatcher et al. 1990). They can have serious side effects, especially interference with lactation and a tendency to thrombosis if the estrogen content is high and in certain women. Therefore, they need careful monitoring. The risk of complications increases in women over 35 years of age and with smoking. No one yet knows all the long-term effects of taking them, but "the pill" is now cheap, available, and popular in many countries.

A lot of controversy surrounds RU

486, a pill that is a competitive antagonist of progesterone and is being used in France and the United Kingdom as a "morning-after pill." It prevents implantation and cause sloughing of the fertilized zygote. This abortifacient has supplanted surgical abortions in many European countries but is not as yet available in the United States or in many developing countries.

Injectable contraceptives. Depo-Provera (methoxyprogesterone) is widely used in technologically developing countries (but not in the United States, where the Federal Drug Administration has blocked its use because it may cause cancer of the cervix). Its advantage is that it is simple to administer (one injection every three months), and it is not a lactation suppressant. However, it is not easily withdrawn and may disturb menstrual periodicity (Population Reports 1975).

Surgical contraception. Tubectomy (tubal ligation) for women and vasectomy for men is the method of choice for families who want no more children. These procedures are done on outpatient basis under local anesthetic.

Hormone implants. Norplant, a new progestin implant, is being hailed as an important and promising development in fertility control. Microcapsules containing the hormone are inserted beneath the skin of the woman's upper arm, and these are gradually absorbed over five years. The sterilization effects are reversible by removal of the implant. The initial cost is quite high, and the implant is not so readily removable. Depression and bleeding have been reported by women's groups as side effects. There is also a danger of misuse of these implants, as well as other provider-dependent contraceptives.

Natural methods. Rhythm methods, withdrawal, and abstinence entail little expense, but they require discipline and calculation and may impose a considerable strain on a marriage. The effectiveness of the rhythm method depends on the regularity of the woman's menstrual cycle. The fact that religious authorities approve of some of these methods indicates that they have little objection to the concept of family limitation, but they do not approve of all the methods to ensure it.

In some cultures sexual abstinence is practiced; the mother does not resume cohabitation until the baby is 1 year old, has cut two teeth, is eating solids, or has passed some other milestone. Abstinence, however, is not easily practiced in a monogamous family.

Prolonged lactation. All over the world lactation is known to act as a contraceptive. Breastfeeding prevents more births than all other methods of contraception put together when it is exclusive (during night and day). In the first six months postpartum, a 98 percent protection from another pregnancy can be expected unless menstruation has resumed (Kennedy 1989). Once menstruation has returned, other forms of contraception are needed. As a general guideline, other measures of family planning are needed six months postpartum, if menstruation returns, or if breastfeeding ceases to be exclusive. The lactation amenorrhea method (LAM) should be incorporated into the overall strategy of family planning (Ebrahim 1991).

Contraceptives should preferably be nonhormonal (e.g., condoms or other barrier methods) since hormones. are excreted in the milk. If (as is usually the case) hormonal preparations are given, oral mini-pills (with low estrogen) should be used because they do not interfere with lactation.

To summarize, there is no method of conception control yet known that is universally acceptable, easy, cheap, and dependable. Methods available to men are limited. Furthermore, many of the effects on women have not been well studied.

There is no doubt that voluntary associations and some government authorities have done much to make people aware of the benefits and the techniques of family planning, and advice is now available to an increasing number of people. But those who would appear to be most in need of limiting their families are the lowest users. Fear, unavailability, prejudice, cost, and lack of awareness are among some of the reasons for low use.

Moreover, the mere provision of facilities for birth control is not enough. In England, the number of family planning clinics has doubled, but births of unwanted babies and the number of abortions have also increased.

Fertility regulation has generally remained a specialized service reserved for a privileged few. There are wide differences in the use of contraceptive methods within and between countries. For example, an estimated 53 percent of sexually active women of reproductive age practiced family planning in the western Pacific region, whereas in West Africa the figure was only 3 percent (WHO 1968). Differences may depend on the availability of fertility control measures to some extent, but in the end, the method chosen will be an individual decision. Only mature consideration will defer immediate satisfaction for the sake of long-term social and economic fulfillment.

Fertility and Infertility

A family planning program should be prepared to give help and advice on a whole range of problems beyond contraception; moreover, a program is often most effective when it emphasizes the benefits to and care of children (WHO 1964; Ebrahim 1991). Families may need advice on infertility, artificial insemination, and adoption. In developed countries, 4 percent of women are infertile; in less developed countries, it may be as high as 40 percent. A comprehensive health service should be aware of these facts. Above all, the services should include counseling for all who need it, young and old. The subject of fertility is not merely a public health problem; it is a deep and intimate concern of individuals and families.

Family planning is often misunderstood. Some politicians may claim that this is a campaign used by one race to eliminate another. A minority group may feel themselves more in jeopardy if their numbers are further reduced, while those who are indifferent to the welfare of their children remain indifferent to the responsibilities of procreation. India alone already has over 8,000 clinics where contraceptives are available free or at subsidized rates to low-income groups. Their programs have only just begun to touch the core of the problem by initiating a downward trend in the birthrate.

Even if they are interested, women are often reluctant to visit a center specifically known for family planning. Often their husbands prevent them from using the services. Integrating family planning into MCH services may make it more acceptable. MCH services may need government approval, cooperation, and funding if they are to offer family planning. Though they become interested in the subject, parents are often inconsistent in their efforts because of lack of education, and visits to the family planning center frequently end in failure. However, there have been notable successes, including programs previously developed in Louisiana in the United States (Beasley et al. 1969).

Rural areas present special problems. People are wrapped up in age-old traditions and habits. Even where there is obvious overpopulation, they still believe that wealth and security rest in numbers of children and numbers of cattle. Moreover, it is difficult to find, train, and maintain workers for isolated areas.

CONCLUSION

Providing the techniques for reducing fertility in women is not enough. Male contraception is also needed. Family planning programs need to be accountable; for example, if oral contraceptives are used, services must provide blood pressure monitoring. Women do not want provider-dependent contraception. They want freedom of choice and control of their bodies. They need education and motivation. Both can be achieved through health and education services that are incorporated in plans for economic development and through MCH services (that ensure education and services for adolescents in particular), adapted to local needs and resources.

Sick, dying, or neglected children are not simply the result of overpopulation. Even in underpopulated wealthy areas, there are neglected, unwanted, and maltreated children. Reducing the population is not in itself an answer to the world's problems. A loaf of bad bread is not made better simply by cutting it in half. The quality of the bread must be improved. If we can improve the quality of the population, the quantity will take care of itself.

In developing areas, progress is slow because so much of the available health resources and staff is spent on disease control campaigns and mass-approaches. maneuvers. Education must include health, and health must include education.

REFERENCES

Baumslag, N., and Ingras, S. (1991). *Report on International Health, Women's Meeting in the Philippines*. WIPHN, Bethesda, Md.

Beasley, J. D.; Frankowski, R. F.; and Hawkins, C. M. (1969). The Orleans parish family planning demonstration program. *Milbank Mem. Fd. Quart.* 47, 225.

Bixby, L. R. (1983). Social and Economic Policies and Their Effects on Mortality: The Costa Rican Case. Paper presented at the Seminar on Social Policy, Health Policy and Mortality Prospects, Institute National d'Etudes Demographiques, Paris.

Catterall, R. D. (1970). Modern contraception

and venereal disease. *Med. Bull.* (Peoria) 4, 4.

Ctr. Pop. Ops. (1992). *Adolescent Fertility in Sub-Saharan Africa*. Center for Population Options, Washington, D.C.

Coale, A. J. (1982). Reassessment of world population trends. *Pop. Bull. UN* 14, 1–16.

Comment (1991). Fertility decline and pronatalist policy in Singapore. *Intl. Fam. Plng. Perspec.* 17(2), 65–71.

Crew, F. A. E. (1948). *Measurements of the Public Health*. Oliver and Boyd, Edinburgh.

Ebrahim, G. J. (1991). The contraceptive effect of breastfeeding—An update. *J. Trop. Pediat.* 37, 210–212.

Eubank, D., and Wray, J. D. (1980). Population and public health. In *Public Health and Preventive Medicine*. 11th ed. Ed. J. M. Last. Appleton Century-Crofts, New York.

Frederiksen, H. (1960). Malaria control and population pressure in Ceylon. *Publ. Hlth. Rep.* (Wash.) 75, 865.

Frederiksen, H. (1961). Determinants and consequences of mortality trends in Ceylon. *Publ. Hlth. Rep.* (Wash.) 76, 659.

Garner, P. (1991). Urbanization: The worst of both worlds. *Brit. Med. J.* 302, 1562.

Hatcher, R. A. et al. (1990). *Contraceptive Technology 1990–1992*. 15th rev. ed. Irvington Publishers, New York.

Hout, M. (1980). The Role of Household Production and Commodity Trade in Latin American Fertility: 1900–1975. Paper presented at the Annual Meeting of the Population Association of America.

Hu-Xing-juan and Zhang Boa-juan (1982). Women's health care. *Am. J. Pub. Hlth.* (Suppl.) 72, 33.

International Planned Parenthood Federation (1970). Oral contraceptives. *Med. Bull.* (Peoria) 4, 1.

Jelliffe, D. B., and Jelliffe, E. F. P. (1970). The urban avalanche and young child nutrition, *J. Am. Diet. Asso.* 57, 111.

J. Trop. Pediat. (1982). Editorial: Contraceptive effect of breast feeding. *J. Trop. Pediat.* 28, ii.

Karunaratne, W. N. (1956). Some population trends in Ceylon (causes and effects). *Ceylon Med. J.* 3, 93.

Kennedy, K. I., and McNeilly, R. R. (1989). Consensus statement on the use of breastfeeding as a family planning method. *Contraception* 39, 477–496.

Lancet (1983). Round the world. India. Misuse of amniocentesis. *Lancet* i, 812.

Lappe, F. M., and Collins, J. (1977). *Food First.* Houghton Mifflin, Boston.

Lee, S. M.; Alvarez, G.; and Palen, J. J. (1991). Fertility deadline and prenatal policy in Singapore. *Intl. Fam. Plng. Perspec.* 17(2), 65–69.

Miller, F. J. W.; Court, S. D. M.; Walton, W. S.; and Knox, E. G. (1960). *Growing Up in Newcastle upon Tyne.* Oxford University Press, London.

NCHS (1968). *Infant Loss in the Netherlands.* National Center for Health Statistics, U.S. Public Health Service, Hyattsville, Md.

Northam, D., and Fisher, J. R. (1982). *Population and Family Planning Programs: A Compendium of Data Through 1981.* 11th ed. Population Council, New York.

Omran, A. R., and Standley, C. C. (1976). *Family Formation Patterns and Health.* World Health Organization, Geneva.

PAHO (1970). *Maternal Nutrition and Family Planning.* Pan American Health Organization Scientific Publication no. 204. Washington, D.C.

Population Council (1968). India: The family planning program since 1965. *Stud. Fam. Plan.* 35, 1.

Population Crisis Committee (1991). *Cities: Life in the World's Largest Metropolitan Areas.* Washington, D.C.

Pop. Ref. Bur. (1980). *World's Women Data Sheet.* Population Reference Bureau, Washington, D.C.

Pop. Ref. Bur. (1992). *World Population Data Sheet.* Population Reference Bureau, Washington, D.C.

Population Reports (1975). *Injectables and Implants.* Series K, no. 1. John Hopkins University, Baltimore.

Rosa, F. W. (1967). Impact of new family planning approaches on rural MCH coverage in developing countries: India's example. *Am. J. Pub. Hlth.* 57, 1327.

Rosa, F. W., and Thurshen, M. (1970). Fetal nutrition. *Bull. Wld. Hlth. Org.* 43, 785.

Sadik, N. (1992). *Safe Motherhood,* no. 7. WHO, Switzerland.

Seiver, D. A. (1975). Recent fertility in Mexico: Measurement and interpretation. *Pop. Stud.* 29, 341.

Spengler, J. J. (1969). Population problem: In search of a solution. *Science* 166, 1234.

Stein, Z.; Susser, J.; Saenger, G.; and Marolla, F. (1975). *Famine and Human Development.* Oxford University Press, London.

Tietze, C. (1979). *Induced Abortion.* 3d ed. Population Council Fact Book. Population Council, New York.

Titmuss, R., and Abel-Smith, B. (1961). *Social Policies and Population Growth in Mauritius.* London.

UN (1979). *Demographic Yearbook.* United Nations, New York.

UN (1982). *Demographic Indicators of Countries.* Department of International Economics and Social Affairs, United Nations, New York.

UN Economic and Social Council (1982). *Urban Basic Services: Reaching Children and Women of the Urban Poor.* Report by the Executive Director, E/ICEF/L.1440. June 7. United Nations, New York.

UNICEF (1992). *The State of the World's Children.* Oxford University Press, London.

Wallace, H. M.; Gold, E. M.; and Dooley, S. (1969). Relationship between family planning and maternal and child health. *Am. J. Pub. Hlth.* 58, 1355.

Wells, F., and Lau, K. S. (1960). Incidence of leukemia in Singapore, and rarity of chronic lymphocytic leukemia in Chinese. *Brit. Med. J.* 1, 759.

WIHPN News (1991). Amniocentesis denied to Bhopal victims. Vol. 9, p. 3. (Women's International Public Health Network, Bethesda, Md.)

Williams, C. D. (1966). Population problems in developing countries. *Trans. Roy Soc. Trop. Med. Hyg.* 60, 23.

Women of China (1983). *Why Female Infanticide Still Exists in China?* China Publications Centre, Bejing.

World Bank (1981). *World Development Report,* 109. World Bank, Washington, D.C.

World Bank (1991). *Social Indicators of Development 1990.* Johns Hopkins University Press, Baltimore.

WHO (1964). *Biology of Human Reproduction.* World Health Organization Tech. Rep. Ser., no. 280. Geneva.

WHO (1965). *Mechanism and Action of Sex Hormones and Analogous Substances.* World Health Organization Tech. Rep. Ser., no. 303. Geneva.

WHO (1968). *IUD: Physiological and Clinical Aspects.* World Health Organization Tech. Rep. Ser., no. 397. Geneva.

WHO (1969). *Developments in Fertility Control*. World Health Organization Tech. Rep. Ser., no. 424. Geneva.

WHO (1970). *Health Aspects of Family Planning*. World Health Organization Tech. Rep. Ser., no. 442. Geneva.

WHO (1980*a*) *Sixth Report on the World Health Situation, 1973–1977*, Part 1: *Global Analysis*. World Health Organization, Geneva.

WHO (1980*b*). *Sixth Report on the World Health Situation, 1973–1977*, Part 2: *Review by Country and Area*. World Health Organization, Geneva.

WHO (1982). *World Health Statistics Annual*. World Health Organization, Geneva.

WHO (1992). *World Health Statistics Annual*. World Health Organization, Geneva.

Zeitlin, M. F.; Wray, J. D.; Stanbury, J. B.; Schlossman, N. P.; Meurer, M. H.; and Weinthal, P. J. (1982). *Nutrition and Population Growth: The Delicate Balance*. Oelgeschlager, Gunn, and Hain, Boston.

6

Women's Health Problems and Status

Eighteen goddess-like daughters are not equal to one son with a hump.

CHINESE PROVERB

WOMEN'S STATUS IN SOCIETY

The mother is the key to the provision of health services for the family, yet she has been both neglected and exploited by health services traditionally geared to serve infants. The *M* in MCH should be the focus because the mother is the central figure who provides the child care, hygiene, nutrition, and even primary health care. Without good mental and physical health care for the mother, child-oriented programs are doomed to failure. Therefore, the *M* in MCH must be emphasized, and appropriate programs and services developed for all women, starting in childhood.

Women comprise 50 percent of the world's population, carry the burden of the world's work hours, receive 10 percent of the world's income, and own less than 1 percent of the world's property (UNICEF 1980). National economic statistics usually omit women's work in the subsistence sector, yet rural women in developing countries account for at least 50 percent of food production. In Bang-

ladesh 90 percent of the female population is engaged in agriculture, and in Africa women do 60 to 80 percent of agricultural work (UNICEF News 1980).

Women are also the most oppressed social group in the male-dominated world (Fig. 6.1). In the less developed world, peasant women are among the least articulate and least heard members of society (Bronstein 1982). Generally development has been measured in terms of social and economic changes affecting the male population. Until recently, social scientists and health planners have shown little interest in the specific needs of women, typically ignoring the factors affecting women's ability to participate fully at social, economic, and political levels. In many countries women are beasts of burden. They work a double day as food and child producers and caretakers. This double-day is the most persistent form of women's oppression, even in the most socially advanced countries, capitalist and socialist (Engle 1983). In these countries women work outside the home, and in one way or another the vast majority are

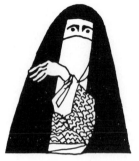

The top social group among women in Third World societies is those who live in total seclusion, often behind the veil, never taking part in outdoor activities. In farming communities, their husbands would typically be well enough off to employ field labour. This pattern of life is typical of Indian upper castes and the Middle East.

The next ranking social group is one in which the women do domestic duties, craft work and occasional poultry raising, but never earn money. Their menfolk do their own ploughing, planting, and agricultural work. This pattern of life is typical of that of most women in Latin America, and the Indian cultivator caste.

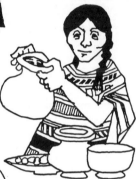

The third group is equivalent to low caste women in an Indian village. They assist their men in the fields, go to market, and at certain times of year do extra paid work. Most women in Asia live like this. In the Philippines, for example, women work 30 hours a week on the family farm, while men work 43 hours.

The fourth and lowest group consists of those women who are expected to support themselves and their families virtually independently. In Asia they regularly seek work as landless labourers, as do India's Untouchables. In Africa, where this is the typical pattern, the woman obtains the right to work a piece of land by marriage and then bears all the responsibility for food production.

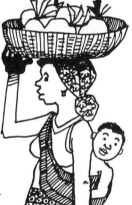

This classification of women's roles is based on research cited in Woman's Role in Economic Development *by Esther Boserup.*

Figure 6.1. Socioeconomic roles of women. Source: UNICEF (1980).

expected to look after children as well, the same demands that mothers in developing countries face.

In most traditional societies, women are viewed as reproductive machines and their fertility is prized. From an early age, they are conditioned to a subservient role, fed last and least, expected to be fertile, but remain chaste until married. This emphasis on chastity takes many forms; the most extreme is female circumcision, which affects millions of girls in Africa and the Middle East. An extreme form of female circumcision is infibulation, in which the external genitalia are excised and the vagina virtually closed. Genital mutilation subjects young girls to extraordinary physical and psychological harm that lasts a lifetime. Complications—hemorrhage, urinary tract infections, sepsis, vesico-vaginal fistulae, difficult childbirth—can cause death (WHO 1992). At the very least, an extensive episiotomy has to be made at each birth. The custom of circumcision is, however, inculcated; its goal is to ensure marriageability of girls. There is no religious sanction for this practice, which has been condemned by African women's groups working toward integration of women in development (Blair 1980).

Females have a low social value. In traditional societies they are discarded if they produce no offspring, rejected or beaten if they produce female offspring, stigmatized if raped, and, in India, rejected (sometimes burned) if they do not bring enough dowry. If their infants fall ill, they are likely to be accused of infidelity. Usually more male infants are born than females, but the ratio eventually evens out. In some countries, like India and China, however, the male-to-female ratio reflects a male preponderance because female mortality is engineered. In China, female infanticide has been on the rise; the male-to-female ratio was found to be five to one in one region. As part of the Chinese population control policy, families are expected to have only one child per couple. Males are preferred because they can work on the farms, look after their elders, and bring their wives and their children home. A girl in China is known as "the go-away child." In spite of legislation that allows girls who marry to stay with their parents, older cultural patterns prevail (Women in China 1982). Female oppression continues, and social and mental servitude is perpetuated in their offspring. In India, amniocentesis is used for selective abortion of female fetuses (Lancet 1983).

Late marriage is an effective means of lowering the birthrate, yet in such countries as Bangladesh, India, Sudan, Yemen, and Nepal, marriages are arranged at an early age. Early marriage not only increases the risk of early and more frequent pregnancies but raises the risks because complications are more frequent in adolescents. Adolescent fertility is a growing problem globally. In some parts of Africa and Latin America, 50 percent of births occur in women less than 20 years old, as do 25 percent of second births and 10 percent of third births (Center for Population Options 1992).

Traditional male domination is perpetuated through female illiteracy. Few resources are expended on the education of females, since their worth is measured primarily in terms of their reproductive function and physical work capacity. Nearly two of every three illiterate people in the world are women. In some countries, for example, Bangladesh, the rate of female illiteracy is as high as 78 percent (Fig. 6.2).

More than 40 percent of young women are still illiterate in Africa and southern and western Asia. Those who obtain minimum literacy skills are not able to maintain them and soon are illiterate again. As these societies develop, the illiterate mothers are confronted by written rules, regulations, labels, and instructions that they can neither read nor understand, and they therefore remain dependent and powerless (Freire 1970). Lack of education for mothers restricts their opportunities to raise the quality of their life and that of their families. Moreover, infant mortality and birthrate decrease when

mothers are educated. In Tanzania, children born to mothers with no education have half the chance of survival compared with children of mothers with five or more years of education. In Kenya, Mosley (1983) found a strong correlation between child mortality and the level of maternal education (Fig. 6.3).

Disruption of the family—migration of males to farms, mines, and cities—leaves women with land they do not own, primitive tools, and helpless dependents. The number of unmarried women is also increasing; it is as high as 50 percent in countries such as Botswana. Consequently, an increasing number of women are household heads: 30 percent in some parts of Latin America, 20 percent in Panama, 28 percent in Cuba, and 31 percent in the United States. Similar estimates have been made for Africa. In Botswana 45 percent of all households are headed by women (UN 1991). Data suggest that where women are household heads, the incidence of malnutrition and infant mortality rates is higher than when men head the household.

When women follow their men to the cities or are forced to earn money in the cities to support the family, the children are often left at home with grandmothers, friends, or other caretakers, including siblings. The caretakers are often unaware of the infant's and toddler's needs and healthy habits. Alternatively, when the mother takes her young children to city slums, they face an uncertain, unhealthy future. Even in the city such common ailments as malaria, anemia, and malnutrition are diagnosed late. In some developing countries, men leave their wives and children in the villages where sanitation and water hygiene are poor and food scarce. Many of these women are divorced or abandoned, and they have little or no support.

Female household heads earn much less than men, and international data show a significant linkage between female family headship and poverty. In Chile, 20

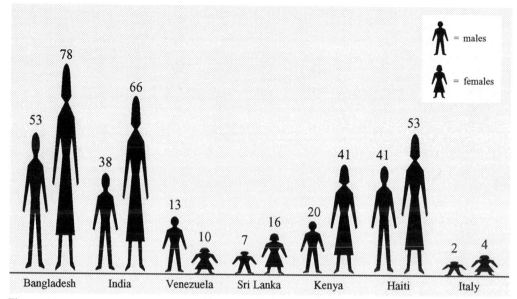

Figure 6.2. Percentage of illiterate adults in selected countries. Illiteracy data are not internationally standardized and are therefore difficult to ascertain accurately. In some countries, literacy is defined as the ability to read and write, while other countries define it as the ability to write one's name. Source: Adapted from UNICEF (1992).

percent of female family heads fall in the lowest income bracket as compared with 10 percent of male family heads. In Brazil, the percentages are 41 percent and 26 percent, respectively (UNICEF 1990a). Although maternal work for wages generally has a positive effect on child survival (Darrow et al., 1981), the stress of wage earning on the single parent has not been determined. For example, working women in Sweden accounted for the entire increase in sick leave during the 1980s and for the rising early retirements in a work environment dictated by men. The fault lies not with women but subordination, double employment, and the way work is organized and allocated (Ekelof 1991).

HEALTH PROBLEMS SPECIFIC TO WOMEN

Too little attention is paid to women's health problems. MCH services are centered mainly on reproductive function and pregnancy outcomes.

Maternal Mortality

Information on women's health and nutritional status is sparse, but the little available on maternal mortality is disturbing. There are more than 700 million women of reproductive age (15 to 49 years) in the developing world. Half a million of these women die every year, from largely preventable conditions caused by complications of pregnancy, abortion, and childbirth, leaving at least 1 million motherless infants. (Despite the high abortion rate in Latin America, the total maternal mortality there is lower than in Africa or Asia.) According to a 1991 WHO report, the maternal death rate has been constant since 1983. The majority of these deaths were in Southern Asia by virtue of the high numbers of births in this area. In some countries in Africa, like Somalia, women may be one hundred

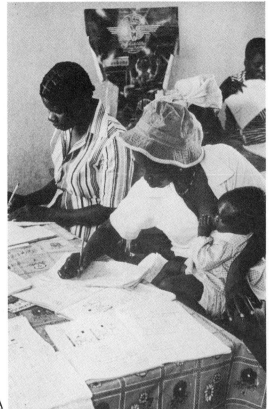

CORRELATION OF CHILD MORTALITY BY LEVEL OF MATERNAL EDUCATION
WITH LEVEL OF POVERTY IN 6 RURAL PROVINCES
KENYA - 1979

A

B

Figure 6.3. Education of mothers is associated with lower child mortality. (A) Education of mothers in Botswana. Photo M. Kahn Gaberone. (B) Increasing poverty has a greater impact on mortality levels for women with the least education, as can be seen from the graph of child mortality in different regions of Kenya. Two factors, maternal education and level of household poverty, were identified in this Kenyan study. Source: Mosley (1983).

times more at risk for dying in childbirth than women in Western Europe. The overall world maternal mortality risk has dropped by 5 percent, but this has been counteracted by a 7 percent increase in total number of births.

It must be realized that the accuracy of statistics depends on the information system. China's improved data collection, for example, has resulted in higher levels than previously reported.

In countries with well-developed health care where the maternal mortality rate is documented, the rate is one-hundredth or even one-thousandth that of developing countries (WHO 1982). Age-specific rates may vary and are important for targeting those most in need. For adolescent mothers in Bangladesh, the rate was 1,770 per 100,000 live births (WHO 1980c). It is estimated that 20 percent of women in the world are pregnant before they are 20 years of age. At any one time in the developing world, one-sixth of women of childbearing age are pregnant, whereas only 1 in 17 is pregnant in the developed world. (Pop. Ref. Bur. 1980).

Within-country variations can be striking. In Malaysia, the highest maternal mortality rate in one district was eighteen times that of the lowest-ranking district. Urban-rural differences are common. In Afghanistan, the maternal mortality rate was 700 per 100,000 live births in rural areas; the urban rate was almost half that of the rural. Such differences demonstrate the inequality of services. Berkeley (1979) compared national mortality rates in Scotland with those in the Kilimanjaro region of Tanzania and found that the rates showed a tenfold difference, probably reflecting the hygienic standard of the services, as well as the nutritional status of the mothers (Table 6.1). In addition, in Kilimanjaro, there was a very high frequency of ruptured uteri, very uncommon in countries where obstetrical care is adequate.

In almost every country, maternal complications are among the five leading causes of death in women of childbearing age. In most of Africa and South and East Asia, which have the highest maternal mortality rate, underreporting of deaths for a variety of reasons may be as high as 50 percent. In some areas, maternal death is a reportable complication but described differently to avoid problems (Campbell and Graham 1991). In some parts of the Philippines, for example, a required registration fee acts as a reporting deterrent. Even in the United States,

official statistics on maternal mortality underestimate the incidence by 20 to 30 percent. In developing countries the inaccuracies are greater. For example, a 1978 report from Egypt showed national maternal deaths to be 82 per 100,000; however, a report from a well-designed study in 1982 showed a figure of 190 per 100,000. Maternal mortality accounts for 25 percent of all deaths in women ages 15 to 45 years in the developing world but only 1 percent of the same age group in the United States.

Maternal mortality is largely preventable. It is attributed directly to the lack of health services before, during, and after delivery (PAHO 1982). The most frequent causes are postpartum hemorrhage (more common in the multiparous mothers), with increased mortality because of existing anemia puerperal sepsis; obstructed labor; and toxemia (Table 6.2). Toxemia accounts for one-fifth to one-fourth of maternal deaths, frequently affecting mothers at both extremes of the parity spectrum: adolescents and high-parity malnourished "maternally depleted" women (Baumslag et al. 1981).

Table 6.1. Causes of Maternal Deaths

	Scotland 1972–1975	Kilimanjaro 1971–1977
Total births	294,519	24,292
Maternal deaths	92	80
Obstetric (selected causes)	50	45
Abortion	12	4
Ectopic	6	4
Hemorrhage	7	6
Ruptured uterus	1	10
Sepsis	5	7
Associated (selected causes)	42	35
Enterocolitis	0	12
Epilepsy	4	0
Maternal mortality rate per 100,000	32	329

Source: Berkeley, (1979).

Note: Although the proportion of deaths from puerperal causes is similar (54 percent and 56 percent), there is a tenfold difference in maternal mortality rates. Mortality rates are limited in their usefulness because they refer only to diseases that cause death and give no direct information on the occurrence and severity of nonfatal diseases.

Table 6.2. Estimated Cause-Specific Maternal Mortality Rates (MMR) in Selected Countries (per 100,000 live births)

Country	MMR	Hemorrhage	Infection	Toxemia	Abortion	Uterine rupture/ obstructed labor	Other
United States	15	2	1	3	1	0.5	9
Cuba	31	2	6	4	5	—	15
Jamaica	108	25	10	33	11	3	—
Zambia	118	20	18	24	20	—	36
Tanzania	378	67	58	13	63	24	153
Indonesia	718	329	75	34	49	—	231

Source: Herz and Measham (1990).

Note: Barbara Kwast (1985) found in Ethiopia that half of the mothers who died in childbirth had unwanted pregnancies.

Antenatal screening for albuminuria, edema, and hypertension can identify those at risk. Another significant contributor to maternal mortality is illegal abortion, which is not reported even when it is a cause of death. (Sepsis is often found in these cases, and the cause of death is described as pelvic inflammatory disease.) Although two-thirds of countries have liberal abortion laws and policies, health services are inaccessible for the majority of women wanting a legal abortion (Tietz 1979). Induced abortions are the first or second cause of maternal mortality in much of Latin America, and are responsible for more than half of maternal mortality in Trinidad and Tobago (PAHO 1990).

Although the life span of women is biologically longer than that of men, in some developing countries, life expectancy at birth for women is almost the same as or lower than that for men (Fig. 6.4). In the industrial world, where nutrition and public health standards are high, and medical care widely available, the reverse is true. In Kerala State in India and in Sri Lanka, where literacy rates are relatively high and social services widely available, women's life expectancy rates are correspondingly high. The female disadvantage ratio measures women's status compared with men in their own society. It is based on life expectancy and literacy rates and provides a concrete indicator of women's hardships in different parts of the world: lower female disadvantage scores are associated with higher birthrates. Improved services for mothers at and after delivery could reduce the incidence of maternal mortality to some extent (WHO 1980c), but raising women's awareness of the need for a more equitable distribution of resources and work load is essential, as well as bringing the clinics near the users and reducing the waiting time at outpatient clinics.

In addition to their community responsibilities and the risks of childbirth, women must contend with hard physical activity, such as water and fuel collection, which may be required right up to the moment they begin labor. In a number of traditional societies, the chores in the puerperium were assumed by family members, and women were given forty days' recovery time. This has changed, as shown by a review of the activity and work during pregnancy and postpartum period in 202 societies. The study showed that most women continued their full work and activities until labor began and after childbirth, limiting their duties for only a short time (Jiminiz 1979), particularly if the woman is the sole breadwinner in the family.

In an attempt to alleviate mothers' work load and improve pregnancy outcome, "lying-in villages" have been established (for example, in Zaire) for women in the last weeks of pregnancy. These women rest and receive supplements of rice and

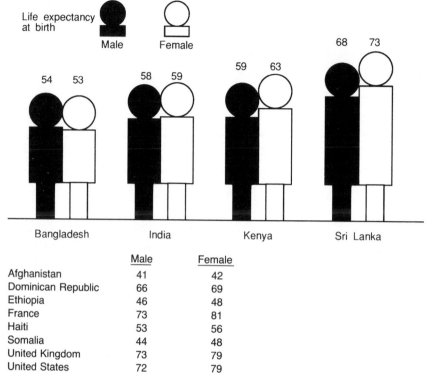

Figure 6.4. Life expectancy at birth, selected countries. Source: Pop. Ref. Bur. (1992).

	Male	Female
Afghanistan	41	42
Dominican Republic	66	69
Ethiopia	46	48
France	73	81
Haiti	53	56
Somalia	44	48
United Kingdom	73	79
United States	72	79

palm oil. The reported stillbirth rate for these women was 1.9 percent compared with 4.2 percent for women who were not in the lying-in village. Unfortunately, the health of the women was not studied.

Infection

A vicious cycle of infection and malnutrition is prevalent among poor women in developing countries. Moreover, a high rate of infection may increase nutritional needs during pregnancy and is an important factor in maternal health. In Guatemala, Leonardo Mata found that a large percentage of pregnant women had at least one attack of diarrhea, dysentery, or an acute respiratory disease, such as pneumonia or bronchitis (Mata 1980) (Table 6.3).

The observed rate for infectious disease is probably underestimated, espe-cially since rural mothers are accustomed to disease throughout their lives and do not complain or report symptoms unless they are severe. Findings of high serum immunoglobulin levels tend to corroborate the high rate of ongoing infection. In Zimbabwe, for example, infection is a major cause of maternal mortality (Brown 1981).

The most common sources of infection in women are those related to the unsanitary conditions of childbirth (puerperal sepsis). Other sources are urinary tract infections, unrecognized amnionitis, and sexually transmitted diseases (STD), a growing problem for which there are usually no diagnostic or treatment services (Germaine et al. 1992). These conditions also affect newborn infants. Infections may be acquired through inappropriate care or poor hygiene during the menstrual period, childbirth, or abortion and

Table 6.3. Percentage of Pregnant Women with Infectious Diseases

	Trimester			
	First	Second	Third	Total
Upper respiratory diseases (including bronchitis, pneumonia)	21	31	36	88
Diarrhea, dysentery	6	6	9	21
Cystitis, pyelonephritis	2	2	1	5

Source: Modified from Mata (1980).

may result in pelvic inflammatory disease (PID), ectopic pregnancy, and infertility. In the developed world infertility affects 2 to 4 percent of women compared to as many as 40 percent in parts of Africa (WHO 1980*a*). Although infertility constitutes a major health problem, infertility services are generally not available.

Infective hepatitis, pulmonary tuberculosis, amebiasis, hookworm, and schistosomiasis are widespread in developing countries, particularly in malnourished women, and contribute to high mortality rates. Malaria is a particularly debilitating disease. During pregnancy, women lose part of their acquired immunity to it, and malarial attacks are more severe. Apart from maternal mortality, malaria of the placenta is associated with low-birthweight infants and miscarriage. Suitably trained and well-informed staff, necessary laboratory facilities, and drugs for treatment would cure many of these infections.

HIV Infection and AIDS

Human immunodeficiency virus (HIV) is the causative agent for AIDS (acquired immunodeficiency syndrome). This virus has a preference for lymphocytes, which help to produce antibodies. The loss of lymphocytes leads to a lowered body defense system, characterized by secondary infections such as tuberculosis, candidiasis and other fungal diseases, and Kaposi's sarcoma. AIDS represents the later stages of the HIV infection.

Several modes of HIV transmission have been identified. Sexual intercourse, both homosexual and heterosexual, is the main mode of transmission through contamination with infected semen, open wounds, and "sores" exposed to blood or body fluids. The other major route of infection is by the use of contaminated needles among drug abusers or even in unhygienic clinical settings. Of the 8 million persons in the world so infected, 3 million are women (WHO 1991*a*), 80 percent of whom are in developing countries (Fig. 6.5). There are a million or more HIV infections in Asia, most of them in Thailand and India (UNICEF 1992). The Asian caseload could exceed the African caseload within a few years, given the large population and the high incidence of prostitution. Approximately 700,000 HIV-infected births have already occurred. An estimated 10 million cases of HIV are predicted by the turn of the century.

This pandemic could be contained by changes in sexual behavior. Special target groups that have been identified are street children, AIDS orphans, and HIV-infected women. Young girls can be sexually influenced by dependence, coercion, exploitation, or lack of knowledge of the implications of sex. It is not surprising that in some societies young women between the ages of 15 and 19 years are at substantially higher risk of HIV transmission than boys of the same age. Improving the social status of young women in particular, as well as providing advo-

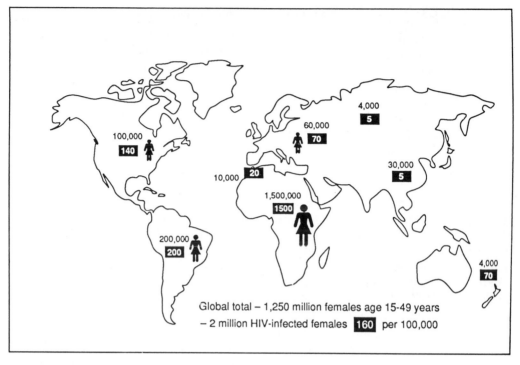

Global total – 1,250 million females age 15-49 years
– 2 million HIV-infected females 160 per 100,000

Figure 6.5. Worldwide estimates of HIV infection in women. WHO estimates that more than 1.5 million African women are infected with HIV. Preventing infection in women is the key to reducing infection in infants. Source: UNICEF (1990).

cacy and education, is of paramount importance.

The diagnosis of AIDS in adults is defined by the existence of at least two major signs and associated with at least two minor signs in the absence of known immunosuppression, such as cancer or severe malnutrition (WHO 1986):

Major Signs

Weight loss: more than 10 percent of body weight.

Chronic diarrhea (lasting more than one month).

Prolonged fever (lasting more than one month, either intermittent or constant).

Minor Signs

Persistent cough (for more than one month).

Generalized pruritic dermatitis.

Recurrent herpes zoster.

Oropharyngeal candidiasis.

Chronic, progressive, and disseminated herpes simplex infection.

Generalized lymphadenopathy.

The presence of generalized Kaposi's sarcoma or cryptocoocal meningitis is sufficient by itself for a diagnosis of AIDS.

In the absence of a vaccine, treatment, or cure, AIDS prevention is dependent primarily on changes in sexual behavior, such as safer sex through use of condoms.

Transplacental transmission of the virus is about 20 percent to 45 percent, though diagnosis of infants is not easy since maternal HIV antibodies are passively transmitted to infant and persist for eighteen months from birth. Nevertheless, diagnosis can be made if other clinical signs and symptoms are evident. Pregnancy has been found to hasten the progress of AIDS, which may lead to premature labor or abortion. Premature infants are at a higher risk than term babies of contracting HIV if their mothers are HIV positive (Peckham 1992). WHO recommends that HIV-positive mothers in developing countries breastfeed since the risk of diarrheal dehydration death is greater for infants than the risk of being infected with HIV through breastfeeding. The Centers for Disease Control (CDC) has just recently added pulmonary tuberculosis, recurrent pneumonia, and cervical cancer to the definition of AIDS (MMWR 1993).

Mental Health

Social status and servile conformity negate women's individuality and persuade them to endure abuse and hardship for the sake of the family, husband, and security. Physical and mental abuse, rape, battery, neglect, starvation, and the threat of murder lead to depression or a fatalistic outlook, the common end result of lifelong drudgery and abuse. The full extent of abuse of women is unknown; the most that can be said of this enormous societal and often legal disgrace is that there is a growing awareness of it, and some societies, not necessarily the most affluent, have taken steps to reduce the incidence of woman abuse such as rape (Heise 1989). In one village in India, men who have raped women are disgraced publicly (Coyaji 1980). Nevertheless, rape remains a serious social problem worldwide. In a mass attack on school girls in Meru, Kenya, in 1990, over seventy girls were raped and twenty killed in a single episode (WIPHN News 1990). The head teacher was quoted as saying, "They did not want to kill them, they only wanted to rape them." Typically rape is not seen as a gender crime with women as the victims.

Rape and violence against women are used as instruments of political repression. The barbaric rape and forceful impregnation of over a half million women in Bosnia by Serbian soldiers and civilians was used for so-called ethnic cleansing and was a systematic part of the strategy. This activity is not new in countries such as Cambodia, Somalia, Peru, Liberia, and Uganda where abuse of women's rights have become part of the tactics of waging war. Until now the shame and blame was shouldered by the women victims. The barbarous violence against women is no longer to be tolerated. Military rapists in Bosnia are to be tried and punished by national criminal judiciary bodies (from a handout by the Women's Coalition against War Crimes, Council of Presidents meeting, 1993). Women's groups, as in Brazil, are forming shelters for battered women, and developing counseling for women and special rape crisis centres with special female police to assist victims (Baumslag 1989).

In some parts of India when a husband dies, the wife is expected to throw herself on his funeral pyre as an expression of extreme and blind devotion—a practice that persists although it has been outlawed. The dowry curse, or suicidal burning, still occurs in some areas, a consequence of social pressures forced on a wife whose husband or in-laws find her dowry insufficient. Of 4,000 burns cases admitted annually to one hospital, 75 percent were women, and of these, nine out of ten were dowry burnings. In Gujurat state, in India, 1,000 women alone were burned alive. The incidence is grossly underestimated (Heise 1989).

Wife beating throughout the world is widespread. It is often associated with alcohol abuse, but it is a gender crime. Unfortunately, in many countries, wife beating is accepted as a domestic problem. A proverb in Mahashtra State goes: "If the rain makes you shiver, and if the husband beats you, where can you complain" (Kanhere 1980). The trauma may be treated, but until the social issues are addressed, beatings will continue to be tolerated (UN 1989).

Occupational Health

In some societies, women are responsible for cloth dying and weaving in factories and are susceptible to bladder cancer from the aniline dyes used. They are also at risk from dust diseases. Women in agriculture exposed to insecticides or herbicide sprays are at risk of such disorders as sterility, stillbirths, and congenital defects in their offspring. Services geared to the care of working women should not only improve their health status but alert them to workplace risks and provide ways to protect themselves and their fetuses from harm. Such services should include measures to permit working women to breastfeed their infants.

In Africa, Asia, and Latin America, women are responsible for at least 70 percent of the food production, 50 percent of the animal husbandry. and 100 percent of the food processing and child rearing. Overwork combined with pervasive malnutrition and frequent childbearing opens the door to multiple afflictions. In most parts of Africa and Asia women work a double-day, sixteen hours per day with no leisure time or relief (Fig. 6.6). The load varies but poorer women, married and with more children, have the biggest work load. A Pakistani woman spends sixty-three hours a week on domestic work alone, while a Western housewife, despite her modern appliances, works just six hours less.

Women work harder than men whether they are Eastern or Western housewives or jobholders. When women do paid work they continue to also do the unpaid work they used to do. In the United States, partners of employed women give them less help (thirty-six minutes) than do partners of housewives (one hour and fifteen minutes). American women work twenty-one hours a week more than men (Wolf 1992).

New technology in agriculture generally does not benefit women. Before developmental interventions are intro-

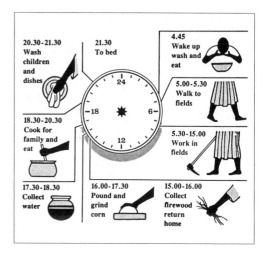

Figure 6.6. Women and work: a day in the life of a typical rural African woman. Source: UNICEF (1980).

duced, an analysis of women's work load should be undertaken. For example, technological developments like the plough, which increased leisure time for men, sometimes increased the fieldwork required of women, since the women had to plant and weed more land. As the number of planting seasons varies from region to region, so does the woman's work load (Boeserup 1970). If there are two planting seasons, women have even less leisure time. Looking at the mother's work load is helpful in assessing whether her diet is meeting her energy expenditures (Table 6.4).

Although females are heavily involved in agriculture from an early age, young girls in extension programs are taught domestic science while their male counterparts learn agricultural techniques. Furthermore, girls have little time for serious study. For example, in Upper Volta, seven-year-old girls work five and a half hours a day on household chores while their male siblings spend forty minutes on their work around the house (Mitchnik 1977).

It is not generally realized how little

Table 6.4. Energy Expenditure of Zambian Women During the Planting Season

Activity	Time spent (hours)	Energy expenditure (calories)
Walking and carrying baby (=3 mi./hr. with 10 kg. load)	0.50	102
Ploughing and hoeing (including periods of rest, standing)	9.50	1758–2328
Collecting firewood and carrying it home (=walking 3 mi./hr. with 10 kg. load)	1.00	204
Pounding grain or chopping firewood	1.50	315
Fetching water (= walking 3 mi./hr. to site and walking home 3 mi./hr. with 10 kg. load)	0.37 0.37	66 75
Cooking	1.00	102
Eating and sitting	1.00	69
Washing, clothes and children, or light cleaning	0.75	112
Sleeping	8.00	432
Total	24 hours	3235–3805

Source: FAO/WHO (1973). Artwork from *Development Forum,* July–August 1991.

Note: This table is not generalizable to all women. In different areas women's work load varies and the family size may also affect it.

leisure time women have, what onerous tasks are assigned to them, and how much energy is consumed. Women are the first to wake up, to prepare food for the family and prepare children for school; fetch up to 20 kilograms of water, which can take five hours a day (Masai Rift Valley women); gather as much as 20 kilograms of wood for cooking, at least a two-hour task (and much more in areas of extensive deforestation); make flour by grinding maize, millet, sorghum, or drying and pounding cassava, which entails an hour a day of extremely hard labor; and breastfeed, which can take up to five or more hours a day (Kitzinger 1980). Most calculations do not take this last activity into account. Washing, sewing, and sexual activity also take time. Women are usually the last to get to bed in the evening, the first to get up in the morning, and the least likely to find leisure time.

An analysis of the work load of women at the survival level or below shows little time available for child care, yet the health sector continues to make unrealistic demands on women's time. The mother is expected to act as a nurse/midwife, agent of change, incubator, caretaker and rearer, nutrient and immunity supplier, controller of the environs, educator, and income generator. Advocates of primary care should consider mechanisms for reducing women's physical labor so that they are able to provide more time for child care. Alternatives for working women may have to be considered. Where women are household heads, they often are forced to leave untrained youngsters to look after their infant siblings (Fig. 6.7). At the turn of the century, Dr. Josephine Baker in New York recognized that young girls were a "fertile source of mortality" (Rosen 1958) and started young girls' clubs,

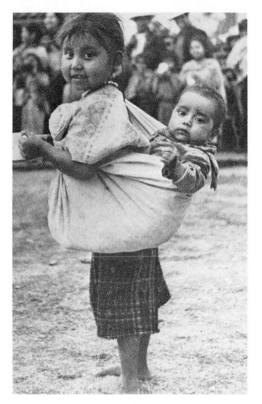

Figure 6.7. Children care for infants. Where mothers work, little children become little mothers and can be a "fertile source of mortality" unless trained. Little mothers' leagues among young children would give them practical instruction in child care and nutrition. Photograph from INCAP, Guatemala.

where she taught mothercraft. Day care centers at the work site can improve production and reduce childhood mortality. The approach and approval of management can make all the difference. Contented women are more continuous and productive workers.

In a cotton factory in Mozambique with a well-housed, well-staffed creche, there was a high rate of diarrhea and malnutrition among the children of employees, while in a nearby cashew nut processing plant, all of the children were healthy, despite the plant's being located in an old warehouse with grim and unsanitary conditions. It turned out that burglars had stolen the baby bottles from

the cashew processing plant some years before, and rather than ordering more, the management, in accordance with Mozambique law, allowed the working mothers to breastfeed their babies for two periods of a half-hour per shift; they also moved mothers to the part of the factory closest to the creche and encouraged breastfeeding ad libitum, and they allowed mothers to work in pairs for mutual support. These special arrangements benefited mothers, babies, workers, and management. At the cotton factory, in contrast, in the name of increased productivity, mothers were not allowed to leave their posts, and the infants were bottle-fed with disastrous results (Zambia Daily Mail 1981).

More often than not, the "maternity conventions" for pregnant and lactating working women in most countries listed in the International Labour Organization (ILO) in Geneva are "paper" regulations and not implemented. Creative programs should be developed that take into consideration the working population.

Health services have to be cognizant of the working conditions of women, both part time and full time, because health needs vary under different working conditions and in different seasons. Special support services for sick or handicapped women, such as respite care, appropriate time for alternate clinic schedules, home visiting, and home care, should be considered in providing continuity of care. Antenatal clinics for working mothers are useless if they do not reach those in need. Services for pregnant women may have to be offered in creative ways.

Personal Habits

Smoking can have adverse effects on maternal and child health. Because it results in high concentrations of carbon monoxide in fetal blood, it is one of the major causes of low-birthweight babies and prematurity in the United States (Jiminez and Newton 1979). In countries in Africa and Asia where high-tar cigarettes are vigorously promoted and smoking is a release from the drudgery and frustration of everyday life, cigarette smoking becomes another factor in the cycle of maternal and infant malnutrition (Last 1980). Heavy smokers have more than their statistical share of miscarriages, stillbirths, and premature babies. Twenty cigarettes per day smoked by a lactating mother can supply the equivalent of one cigarette's worth of nicotine to the nursing baby. Smoking is associated with a higher incidence of cancer of the cervix in women.

Even more deleterious than smoking is alcoholism, which is a problem even in developing countries. Alcohol is readily absorbed by fetal tissues. It is the second most commonly known environmental cause of problems in fetal development. The more alcohol a pregnant woman drinks, the more likely she is to harm herself and her unborn baby. Women who drink an average of two drinks a day have been reported to give birth to babies slightly smaller than average, and some babies may be born with fetal alcohol syndrome, characterized by growth retardation, weight loss, altered facial characteristics, and brain damage (Knuppel 1981). Low zinc levels have also been associated with the fetal alcohol syndrome (Rosso 1981).

NUTRITION

Impact of Maternal Nutrition

The nutritional relationship of women and infants is closely interacting (Jelliffe and Jelliffe 1989). In traditional societies, the child from the fetal stage up to age 2 or 3 years maintains a nutritional dependency on the mother. The discovery of the presence in breast milk of a wide range of species-specific growth modulators has revealed new and previously unappreciated aspects of the special value of human lactation. Moreover, the act of breastfeeding establishes an important emotional and psychological relationship between mother and child that includes emotional bonding and protection of the infant.

The mother too derives important benefits from breastfeeding, including speeding up uterine postpartum contractions and reducing iron-containing blood loss. Infant suckling increases birth spacing by preventing ovulation, thereby reducing the cycle of maternal nutrient drainage, which can worsen with each pregnancy. Equally important are the reported decreases in the incidence of breast cancer (Siskind et al. 1989), ovarian cancer (Gwinn et al. 1990), and urinary tract infections (Coppa et al. 1990) in breastfeeding mothers.

Maternal Malnutrition

For a number of reasons, women in developing countries are often at the edge of malnutrition. Poverty is the overriding factor, but there are others as well:

1. *Marginal or insufficient dietary intake:* Cultural taboos often restrict food availability for women during pregnancy and lactation. Even in Western cultures, the belief is common that men need a higher protein intake than women. The difference in dietary intake is accentuated in periods of seasonal food shortage. A study in Malawi showed that during times of food shortage, intake for men decreased by 10 percent, whereas for women it decreased by 25 percent (Baumslag et al. 1979). In areas where food is scarce, menarche is often delayed and lactation amenorrhea prolonged. Studies in Gambia and on the Kalahari !Kung indicate that birth seasonality is related to food intake, which is highest following the harvest (Prentice et al. 1983). Among the Kalahari !Kung, it was found that when they settled, food intake was higher and births more evenly distributed over time, confirming the relationship between nutritional status and fertility (Thomson et al. 1966; Wilmsen 1978).

2. *Unhealthy sanitary conditions:* A high prevalence of fever, diarrhea, and infectious parasitic and debilitating diseases is commonly associated with poor sanitation. In addition, women nurse the sick and dispose of all excreta; consequently, they are more exposed to infectious diseases. These acute and chronic diseases result in increased utilization of calories and loss of protein and other nutrients, exacerbating maternal malnutrition.

3. *Excessive energy expenditure:* The daily calorie intake is frequently not sufficient to cover women's heavy physical work load.

4. *Demands of growth, pregnancy, and lactation:* Generally one-third of all women are pregnant or lactating, making extra metabolic demands on tissues, despite recent evidence of considerable physiological adaptations. This burden is increased by frequent childbearing.

5. *Changing life-style:* The transition from rural to urban life and from nomadic to sedentary life has led to changes in dietary intake and patterns of work. Urbanization, migration, and industrialization have also had a major impact on the health and nutrition of human populations. When the !Kung Bushmen, for example, moved from a nomadic to a sedentary agrarian society, children were weaned earlier, the infant mortality rose, the birthrate increased, and the birth interval decreased; iron- and folate-deficiency anemia, previously unknown, began to appear. Women's status was altered because they no longer contributed in the same way to the community economy; men went out to work, and women stayed at home. Being dependent, they became more subjugated to men's decisions. The dietary intake changed from meat, nuts, and berries to a sugar, flour, and milk diet, affecting both the nutritional status and the customs of the mothers and, in turn, the infants (Baumslag and Watson 1978).

Repeated cycles of reproduction, infection, hard physical work, and nutrient drainage lead women to a state of maternal nutritional depletion (Fig. 6.8). The results can be specific (for example, increased prevalence of goiter or osteomalacia) or general (malnutrition, anemia, susceptibility to infection, fatigue, and decreased productivity). The maternal depletion syndrome is so common in Bangladesh that there is a vernacular name for it—*sutika* (Favin and Bradford 1984). Table 6.5 illustrates the population subgroups most at risk of malnutrition, and Table 6.6 illustrates the effects of malnutrition on mother and child. This nutritional vulnerability includes protein energy malnutrition, with acute forms resulting in kwashiorkor with edema.

Malnutrition and infection during childhood can have an adverse effect on childbearing and even on the weight of the infant. Mothers in many developing countries have chronic malnutrition, often dating back to childhood and exacerbated by pregnancy. In areas in Malawi, Guatemala, and Sierra Leone, as many as 25 percent of women have been found to have stunted growth (AID 1975; Baumslag and Watson 1979; Mata 1980). In Sierra Leone, more rural than urban women and twice as many pregnant as nonpregnant women were malnourished (AID 1975).

Low birthweight. A useful, although partial, indicator of maternal nutrition is low birthweight defined by WHO as less than 2.5 kilograms (WHO 1980b); it is a large problem in developing countries (Tafari 1981; Sterky and Mellander 1978). A WHO study in seven regions estimated that 22 million low-birthweight babies are born each year, 21 million of them in developing countries (Fig. 6.9). Within each country, there are large interregional differences, and undoubtedly genetic differences play a role. In Asia, the percentage of low-birthweight infants can range from 18 percent of all live births (Indonesia) to 50 percent (Bangladesh).

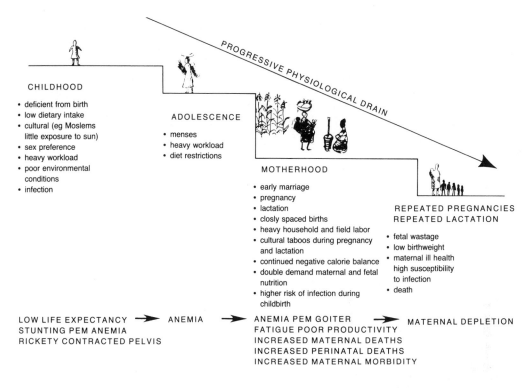

Figure 6.8. Maternal depletion syndrome.

South Asia has the lowest mean birthweight of all major areas (WHO 1991*b*). An early indicator of impending famine is the increased incidence of low-birthweight infants.

Low weight gain in pregnancy may precede the fall in birth weight. In the United States, the majority of low-birthweight babies are preterm. By contrast, in developing countries, 80 percent or more of low-birthweight babies are classified as small for gestational age (SGA) because of maternal infections in pregnancy, malnutrition, or specific deficiencies of iron, zinc, and/or folic acid and/or protein and calories (Jelliffe and Jelliffe 1989), as well as genetic factors.

Selective supplementation during pregnancy may be appropriate in some cases. Before the fetus's weight is affected, the mother must gain 6 kilograms. If weights are known before or early in pregnancy, a low weight for height of 10 percent or more below reference level or high weight for height of 20 percent above has been suggested as a rough indicator of under- or overnutrition, respectively (Rosso 1981). When caloric supplementation was given to women with low prepregnancy weight and low caloric intake (under 1700 calories), the percentage of low-

Table 6.5. Groups at Risk for Malnutrition

Nutritionally deficient group	Cause of problem
Smallholders—food crop producers and subsistence farmers	Insufficient food production
Smallholders—cash crop producers	Low earnings with poor distribution throughout year; income not necessarily spent on food
Landless poor	Low real income
Pastoralists	Vulnerability to weather, lack of food security
Urban unemployed or underemployed	Low real income

Source: Modified from Ghai et al. (1979).

Table 6.6. Some Effects of Inadequate Maternal Nutrition in Pregnancy

Maternal	Protein energy malnutrition[a]	Maternal depletion syndrome
	Specific nutrients	
	Iron, folate, B$_{12}$ (anemia)	
	Iodine (goiter)	
	Thiamine (beriberi)	
	Vitamin A (xerophthalmia)	
	or blindness)	
	Anemia, hemorrhage, sepsis	Maternal death
	Insufficient fat stores	Suboptimal lactation (insufficient volume)
Materno-fetal	Abortions	
	Stillbirths	
	Intrauterine growth retardation	
Infant	Prematurity	Possible growth retardation
	Low birthweight	Possible mental retardation
	Suboptimal neonatal stores	Defective immunity (susceptibility to infections)

Source: Modified from Jelliffe and Jelliffe (1985).

Note: The effects of inadequate maternal nutrition in pregnancy can become more marked with repeated reproductive cycles.

[a] Low caloric intake is the most common and important deficiency.

birthweight infants decreased significantly, and the viability of the infants increased (Lechtig et al. 1979). A Danish study on healthy women found that if fish oil was given in the thirtieth week of pregnancy, infants were heavier (by 107 grams) and the pregnancy longer (four days). This study suggested that doses of

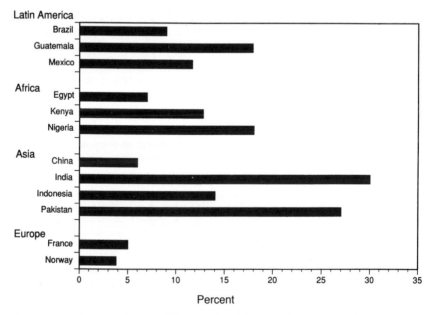

Figure 6.9. The prevalence of low birthweight in selected countries. In thirty countries, 15 percent or more infants have a low birthweight (less than 2,500 grams). Laos has a prevalence of 39 percent and India 30 percent. Source: WHO (1991a).

Table 6.7. Maternal-Fetal Risk Factors

Dietary	Caloric intake of less than 1600 to 2000 per day
Socioeconomic	Income less than $400 per capita per year Landless Unmarried Alcoholic Smoker Less than five years of education Heavy physical work load
Reproductive	Under 18 or over 35 years Over four pregnancies Unwanted pregnancies Twins or multiple births Birth spacing under one year Previous abortion or infant death
Medical	Illness (TB, STD, PID, amebiasis, schistosomiasis, infection)
Anthropometric	Under 5 ft. (150 cm) Arm circumference under 23 cm Weight gain of less than 20 lb. at the thirty-fourth week of pregnancy Prepregnancy weight of under 100 lb.

fish oil may prevent prematurity (Guardian 1992).

Two studies (Lechtig et al. 1979; Viegas et al. 1982), however, indicate that dietary supplements for all pregnant women do not always enhance uterine growth, and large amounts of protein may have a negative effect. Where specific nutrient deficiencies exist, supplementation of these nutrients will increase birthweight (Baumslag et al. 1970; Bergmann et al. 1980; Hibbard 1975; Iyengar and Rajalakshim 1975; Jameson 1976; Rosa 1970; Tafari 1981). The diagnosis must be made before therapy is initiated. Intervention must be appropriate and targeted to those in need through simple means of identifying risk factors (Table 6.7). Ideally women should have a caloric intake that covers their energy expenditure and physiological needs, as well as specific nutrients, such as folic acid and iron (Baumslag et al. 1979; Stein 1975) when pregnant or lactating (Naismith

1981). In some areas, women may have a caloric gap of up to 42 percent (Coyaji 1980) and during pregnancy may not gain any weight at all. As a result, lactation calories are not deposited. Nevertheless, lactation is surprisingly well sustained, even in overworked, poorly fed mothers in developing countries, usually enabling exclusive breastfeeding for four to six months. Attention needs to be given to diets in adolescence, pregnancy, and lactation and in careful follow-up. The mother's nutritional status must be maintained not only for the infant's nutrition but for the mother's health (Baumslag et al. 1970). Malnourished mothers can lose as much as 7 kilograms after a year of lactation, yet supplementary feeding programs often are directed to infants. Less than 15 percent of feeding programs provide supplements for mothers (Baumslag 1983). Additionally, supplementary feeding of infants may decrease suckling, which normally prevents ovulation, leading to the cycle of repeated depleting pregnancies (J. Trop. Pediat. 1982). Of note is the fact that it costs a tenth as much to provide the mother with lactation calories during pregnancy than to feed an infant with formula for six months.

Anemia. Women need three times more iron than men. Anemia has serious health consequences and can result in heart failure and maternal death, often due to a blood loss during delivery in an already anemic mother. Maternal death rates are five times higher in anemic than in nonanemic women. WHO reported that half of pregnant and more than a third of nonpregnant women are anemic. In Asia, for example, almost 60 percent of pregnant women are anemic (WHO 1992) (Table 6.8).

Most anemia is due to iron deficiency. However, anemia due to folic acid deficiency is not uncommon (Baumslag et al. 1970). For example, in a nutritional survey in Sierra Leone, folic acid deficiency was diagnosed in 10 percent of pregnant

Table 6.8. Estimated Prevalence of Nutritional Anemia in Women, around 1990 (percentages)

Region	Pregnant women	Nonpregnant women	All women
World	51	35	36
Developing countries	55	42	44
Developed countries	17	12	12
Africa	51	40	42
Asia	59	44	45
Latin America	41	30	34
North America	24	10	13
Europe	17	10	10

Source: WHO (1992).

Note: An estimated 42 percent of women in developing countries suffer from nutritional anemia (based on hemoglobin below 12 g/L for nonpregnant women and 11 g/L for pregnant women), compared with 12 percent of women in developed countries. This is both a direct and indirect cause of maternal mortality. In addition, it reduces work capacity, increases fatigue, and increases susceptibility to health problems.

women (AID 1975). Vitamin B_{12} deficiency may also be a cause of anemia in mothers and infants, as has been described in India among vegetarians whose normally adequate diets are limited by poverty. Therefore, treating anemia by blanket distribution of iron tablets, as if it were a uniform condition, can be expensive and harmful (Chalmers et al. 1990). Furthermore, in endemic areas, treatment of malaria is a more effective measure for anemia eradication than iron tablets. Ideally, there should be an investigative study to demonstrate the most prevalent forms of anemia. Where iron deficiency is found to be common, supplementation, especially during the last trimester of pregnancy, is beneficial and cost-effective for both mother and infant. Two studies in areas where there was evidence of folate deficiency showed that folate supplementation in the last trimester markedly reduced the number of low-birthweight infants (Baumslag et al. 1970; Hibbard 1975).

Some MCH clinics provide iron and folic acid supplements, but many do not. In Latin America, a physician put nails in water with lemon juice and used the rusty water as iron medicine, an original form of improvisation, particularly since

vitamin C helps increase absorption of iron from food sources (Cornell University 1983). Where the clinic is not well stocked, local sources of iron should be sought and may prove to be adequate and cheap. The use of an iron cooking pot can add substantially to iron intake.

There is a significant relationship between parasites, such as hookworm, and anemia. In Venezuela one-third of anemia cases are caused by hookworm. An infestation of hookworm can result in the loss of 6 milliliters of blood daily—about one-half liter per year. Wearing shoes is a preventive measure that may be more effective than iron tablets for adults and older children. For younger children, other skin surfaces should be kept away from potentially infected soil.

Goiter. Goiter is prevalent in many parts of the world, especially among pregnant women and young girls. It tends to occur in pockets—for example, in Malawi, Lesotho, Zaire, Nepal, Ecuador, and Peru. Goiter affects the metabolic rate and can result in infantile cretinism and mental retardation. It may be due to iodine deficiency—for instance, where rock salt is used or excessive quantities of goitrogen in some types of cassava or cabbage are consumed. When iodized salt is made available, the incidence drops. Programs are more difficult to carry out than often thought, partly because goiter is not usually lethal and partly because the effects on the newborn are extremely underestimated. Where iodized salt is unavailable, other methods for prevention can be tried, such as intramuscular iodized oil injections. In a village in Zaire where cretinism was common (1 to 7 percent), a single intramuscular injection of slowly absorbable iodized oil was shown to reduce goiter prevalence for a period of three to seven years at a nominal cost per person of U.S. $0.70 (Thilly and Delange 1977).

HEALTH SERVICES FOR WOMEN

Women, because of their social status, appear to have the least access to health call services. Most MCH health services make no provision for anything that is not predominantly infant related, and many services for women are not even available. In many developing countries, women in the 30 to 40 age-group want to stop having more children; the range is from 49 percent of this age group in Jamaica to 79 percent in Bangladesh. If services existed for these women, many unwanted births and unnecessary infant and maternal deaths could be prevented (Maine 1982). Services should also include screening and early treatment for cancer of the cervix, which has a high prevalence in these countries. These services should be included in MCH services and not form part of a separate program. Some MCH programs provide antitetanus toxoid for pregnant women as a preventive measure for the fetus. In some cultures, women fear injections in pregnancy and do not use this service.

Health services are underutilized for other reasons. The indiscriminate promotion of family planning has aroused suspicion of the health services. In some countries, such as India, women are not allowed to go to the clinics for fear that they may be sterilized. Other grounds for underutilization of services include the following:

1. Inappropriateness of services.
2. Male health professionals who are not acceptable to certain groups, particularly Muslim women. Patients may not go to clinics or hospitals without their husbands' permission.
3. Young girls used as primary care providers may not have as much credibility as older women. This is even more of a problem if the providers come from the cities or outside the locality. Health care professionals from outside the community are often mistrusted.
4. Services provided by the government may be worse than indigenous services. For example, an overcrowded maternity ward may be associated with a high mortality rate due to sepsis and lack of staff and supplies. TBAs may offer better services, including help with housework.
5. Some government services charge a fee and may require patients to purchase prescribed medicines, which they cannot afford. A visit to the district hospital on a referral basis may involve costly transport, or the treatment offered may be culturally unacceptable or substandard. The clinic or hospital may lack screening tests, health information, basic drugs, or mechanisms for referral.
6. Services farther away than two miles or three kilometers are inaccessible for mothers carrying infants or sick children. Rainy or excessively hot, humid weather and difficult terrain may present additional transport problems.
7. In most developing countries, women live in rural areas and the specialists

are in urban areas. In one large Asian country, for example, only 32 percent of the rural population live within a two-mile radius of any kind of health facility, compared with 98 percent of the urban population, who have easy access in terms of distance.

8. Services are not individualized.
9. Services that do exist tend to concentrate on childbirth. Antenatal clinics, modeled on the Western prototype, are usually run by midwives and have a limited supply of drugs and diagnostic procedures. Laboratory tests, if available, may not cover the needs of the local community.
10. The health providers may be rude and impersonal.
11. Male administrators and decision makers may not be aware of the special needs of women.
12. There may be a lack of continuity of services, unsuitable outpatient times, and an irregular supply of drugs.

Childbirth

In developing countries, women customarily assist other women in childbirth. The assistant may be a relative, an older woman, or a TBA. No generalization can be made about the practices and activities; these vary considerably. Rarely, as in some parts of Ghana, TBAs may be male. Most TBAs are self-trained and provide a variety of services: antenatal care, abdominal massage, fetal positioning, herbal remedy prescribing, and delivery services. They may also perform household chores and prepare meals, as well as advise on breastfeeding. In some cases, they may stay with the mother for forty days and provide services to the child throughout the first year.

In some developing countries, 80 percent or more women deliver at home; few are assisted by a trained midwife. In order to reduce the number of maternal deaths and complications during childbirth, TBAs expertise should be reinforced in short training periods with selected safe, culturally appropriate Western medical practices. TBAs are usually strong on emotional and social support for mothers and families but weak on hygiene; appropriate training can lead to a beneficial blend (Baumslag and Watson 1981; Bayoumi 1976). In seven countries studied, as many as 80 percent of deliveries were attended by these women, and by providing them with minimal training, infection rates were reduced and referral improved (Magnay-Maglacas 1981).

The percentage of deliveries attended by a trained attendant, however, is still far from satisfactory and newer data indicates that it ranges from 85 percent in countries such as Sri Lanka, Dominican Republic, and Trinidad, to less than 33 percent in Burundi, Guatemala, Mali, and India (DHS 1991; Zahr 1991), and less than 10 percent in Nepal.

Antenal Care

In one DHS report (1991), the percentage of births in which women received antenatal care ranged from 90 in Botswana, Zimbabwe, Sri Lanka, the Dominican Republic, Trinidad, and Tobago, to less than 50 in Mali, Morocco, Bolivia, and Guatemala. The urban–rural differences are marked in many countries. For example, in Bolivia the rural percentage is 50 and the urban 30. The definition of antenatal care is variable and ranges from one late visit to ten or more visits throughout pregnancy. There is still much debate on whether antenatal care can reduce maternal mortality or severe morbidity and the proof is hard to come by. In a challenge by Chalmers and Renfrew to identify aspects of routine care that actually improve maternal mortality and morbidity, responses from many parts of the world varied and a number of different solutions were suggested for the most local problems, including anemia, hypertensive disease of pregnancy, and unwanted pregnancy, but no firm evidence was presented (WIPH News 1990). There is, however, no question that quality childbirth makes a difference. In countries such as Costa Rica where the percentage of births accompanied by antenatal care is 91, Cuba, 100, and Botswana, 90, and where there is extensive health care coverage, infant and maternal mortality is low (Zahr 1991).

In developing countries, most attendance at antenatal clinics takes place in the seventh and eight month of pregnancy, and women usually average only one clinic visit per pregnancy. If the antenatal period is to be considered an important time for interventions and identifying at-risk mothers, other outreach techniques have to be developed for those at risk. These should include services such as home visits, "waiting stations," self-care education, and self-examination.

When mothers have no available health services, they devise their own ways of measuring their stage of gestation. Some women in South Africa express their breasts during pregnancy. The color of the secretion helps them decide how far they are in pregnancy. Where there is no midwife, the provision of delivery kits (metal cases with scissors, basins, cord tie, etc.) although expensive, has been useful. But the adapted Masai "matchbox maternity kit" (which contains a piece of soap, sterilized cord tie, and a sterilized blade in a matchbox) is cheaper, can reach more women, and is easier to carry than the delivery kit.

Antenatal clinics could reduce childbirth risk by selective screening. Weight charts for pregnant women are a useful screening tool for identifying women at risk. Difficulties exist if the date of the last menstrual period and the mother's prepregnancy weight are not known. The maternal home-based record lists more common conditions so women and health workers can recognize them and take appropriate action (Shah 1982; WHO 1991) (Fig. 6.10), including counseling and referral. This, however, requires regular

weighing for all married women during home visits. Some records use arm circumference as a screening measure. A combined record for pregnant women and for infants has also been developed for screening and counseling. Still, it is unclear which screening measures are the best predictors of risk (WHO 1991) and which antenatal and childbirth interventions are most effective (Enkin and Chalmers 1982; Chalmers et al. 1990).

Childbirth

Globally, births attended by trained personnel vary from 2 to 97 percent. In rural Nigeria, 2 percent of deliveries are attended by a physician or take place in a hospital, 52 percent are attended by an indigenous practitioner, 40 percent by a family member, and in 6 percent of cases the women deliver alone. There are vast urban–rural differences as well. In Korea, 49 percent of urban births are attended by physicians or midwives compared with only 6 percent of rural births. This does not imply that better services are provided by physicians. In the United States, women delivered at home by midwives had fewer lacerations and complications than women delivered in institutions (Mehl et al. 1976). But it does imply that hygiene supervision, as well as support, are essential. Primary health care workers can identify women at risk, and serious problems can be solved by referral staff and community resources. Even illiterate TBAs can record, refer to support services, and evaluate their program through the use of symbols and colored tokens. In Malawi, Bullough (1979) established a method of utilizing illiterate TBAs to refer women who had been in labor over a period of twelve to fourteen hours. The TBAs kept a simple record chart on which they could indicate if labor had extended a full day or a full night (Fig. 6.11a). In the Sudan, messages about childbirth emergencies between village midwives in remote areas and distant

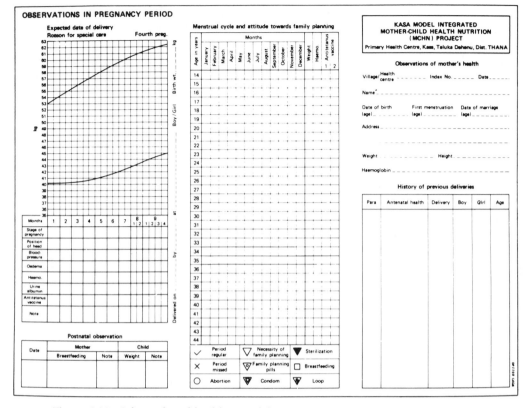

Figure 6.10. A home-based health record for pregnant women. Source: Shah (1982).

health facilities were transmitted by runners who carried tokens to the nearest facility to indicate the condition for which help was needed (Fig. 6.11b) (Magnay-Maglacas and Pizurki 1981). A good TBA would usually not let a labor exceed from one sunset to one sunrise, or vice-versa.

Supervised home deliveries and home visits in the first few days are effective alternatives to crowded and even unsanitary hospitals. If home conditions are poor, "birthing hut complexes" can be a highly satisfactory alternative. In Malawi, one TBA who received special MCH training combines traditional herbal remedies, ingenuity, and a minimum of government-provided sterile equipment to establish an effective system of maternal and child care in the bush. In her birthing complex, she had one hut for delivery and one for care of low-birthweight infants. She developed an ingenious system of using cardboard boxes as incubators. Temperature and humidity were regulated by bottles filled with warm water (Baumslag et al. 1979). This innovative technology helped reduce neonatal mortality.

WOMEN AND HEALTH POLICY

Universally women tend the sick and the old and provide love and care for infants and children. In traditional societies, they have been "allowed" to be TBAs and auxiliary health workers while the males are the "medicine men." In industrialized countries, women as well as men are medical doctors. At some medical schools

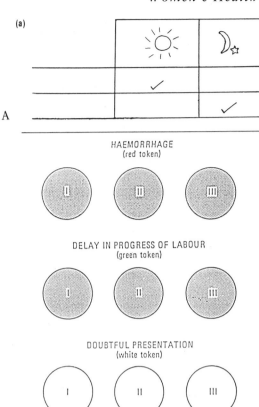

HAEMORRHAGE
(red token)

DELAY IN PROGRESS OF LABOUR
(green token)

DOUBTFUL PRESENTATION
(white token)

B I= 1st stage of labour; II= 2nd stage of labour; III= 3rd stage of labour

Figure 6.11. (A) Simple means of record keeping and communication. Source: Bullough (1979). (B) Red, green, or white tokens are carried to the nearest health facility to indicate the condition for which help is needed in childbirth. Source: Mangay-Maglacas and Pizurki (1981).

in the United States, a third to a half of the students are women. However, women occupy very few senior positions, and their influence in policymaking is negligible. One only has to look at the practice of breastfeeding, where the policy decisions continue to be made by men while women do the feeding.

Nevertheless, the influence of women in the resurgence of support for breastfeeding has been significant, exemplified by the La Leche League in the United States. Also, increasing numbers of lactation clinics are springing up in the United States and elsewhere, run by women health professionals, many of whom have nursed their own children.

If health care for all is to be achieved by the year 2000, women must share equally with men in key decision-making positions and service responsibilities. Allowing widespread, poor maternal health and nutrition to continue will have serious repercussions on future generations, on societal behavior, and on national policies. Clearly the solution requires a political approach at the highest government levels, with women participating in the establishment of priorities and implementing programs.

Maternal health can be improved by attention to education and services at home, community, and national levels (WHO 1980*d*). At an individual or group level, services and educational programs should be directed to hygiene during special periods (menses, delivery, the puerperium, and postpartum), adequate nutrient intake, and control of nutrient and electrolyte loss during infections. At a community level, provision of health services should include gynecological services for early detection of reproductive tract infections (RTIs) and STDs, PIV, cancer, treatment of prolapse, family spacing, infertility, and anemia. At a national level, women should be involved at all levels of administration, legislation, and decision making to provide constant vigilance over customs and practices that affect all mothers and infants. Programs need to be directed at improving women's knowledge and helping them exercise their rights. Adult literacy programs are essential to enable women to function at all levels of society and make correct decisions for their welfare and that of their children. Appropriate technology can be designed and implemented to improve women's status and health by reducing burdensome daily tasks. For example, protected wells can reduce the amount of time necessary to fetch water and decrease the incidence of waterborne disease; simple grain crushers and hand-operated mills can reduce the amount of time necessary for processing foods (Carr 1978; Darrow et al. 1981).

Women's and children's health is directly related to women's status in society, characterized in many parts of the world by their low social value, low income, illiteracy, and poor health care. Women are regarded as stages of pregnancy rather than as critical participants in their own and their families' health care. Because of their low status in many societies, women are denied basic services. Until women are allowed to participate more fully in society, they will remain victims of social oppression and exploitation. Society in general and the family in particular stand to benefit if women's mental and social well-being are improved.

REFERENCES

AID (1975). *Sierra Leone National Nutrition Survey, Office of Nutrition.* Development Support Bureau, Agency for International Development, Washington, D.C.

Baker, J. (1939). *Fighting for Life.* Macmillan Press, New York.

Baumslag, N. (1979). *Malawi Trip Report.* Report for the Agency for International Development, Washington, D.C.

Baumslag, N. (1983). *Africa Nutrition Position Paper.* Prepared for Africa Bureau, USAID, Washington, D.C.

Baumslag, N. (1992). Breastfeeding trends and influencing factors. *Child Health* 3(1), 39. *Ped Asso. J.*

Baumslag, N., and Sabin, E. (1978). *Perspectives in Maternal-Infant Nutrition.* Office of International Health, U.S. Department of Health, Education and Welfare, Rockville, Md.

Baumslag, N., and Vogl, L. (1989). *Violence against Women.* Women's International Public Heath Network, Bethesda, Md.

Baumslag, N., and Watson, D. (1981). Teenage pregnancy nutrition—fact or fiction. In *Nu-trition in Pregnancy,* pp. 20–35. Ed. J. Patrick Lavery. University of Louisville,

Baumslag, N.; Edelstein, T.; and Metz, J. (1970). Reduction of incidence of prematurity by folic acid supplementation in pregnancy. *Brit. Med. J.* 2, 16.

Baumslag, N.; Grace-Mason, L.; Roesel, C.; and Sabin, E. (1979). *Breast Is Best: A Bibliography on Breastfeeding and Infant Health.* Prepared for USAID, Office of International Health, Department of Health, Education and Welfare, Washington, D.C.

Bayoumi, A. (1976). The training and activity of village midwives in the Sudan. *Trop. Doctor.* 6, 118.

Bergmann, K. E.; Makosch, G.; and Tews, K. H. (1980). Abnormalities of hair zinc concentration in mothers of newborn infants with spina bifida. *Am. J. Clin. Nutr.* 33, 2145.

Berkeley, J. (1979). Epidemiological factors in maternal mortality. In *Maternal Services in the Developing World—What the Community Needs.* Ed. R. H. Philpott. Royal College of Obstetricians and Gynaecologists, London.

Blair, P. (1980). *Programming for Women and Health.* Prepared for the Office of Women in Development, Agency for International Development. Equity Policy Center, Washington, D.C.

Boeserup, E. (1970). *Women's Role in Economic Development.* George, Allen and Unwin, London.

Bronstein, A. (1982). *The Triple Struggle.* War on Want Campaign, London.

Brown, I. (1981). Perspectives in obstetric care for Zimbabwe. *Cent. Afr. J. Med.* 27(3),37.

Bullough, D. H. W. (1979). Discussion in maternity services. In *The Developing World—What the Community Needs.* Ed. R. H. Philpott. Proceedings of the Seventh Study Group of the Royal College of Obstetricians and Gynaecologists, London.

Campbell, O. M. R., and Graham, W. J. (1991). *Measuring the Determinants of Maternal Morbidity and Mortality.* London School of Hygiene and Tropical Medicine, London.

Carp, C. (1983). Seasonality, women's work and health. *Mothers and Children* 3, 10.

Carr, M. (1978). *Appropriate Technology for African Women.* African Training and Research Center for Women of the Economic

Commission for Africa, UNECA, Addis Ababa.

Ctr. Pop. Ops. (1992). *Adolescent Fertility in Sub-Saharan Africa.* Center for Population Options, Washington, D.C.

Chalmers, I.; Enkin, M.; and Keirse, M. (1990). *Effective Care in Pregnancy and Childbirth,* Vols. 1–2. Oxford University Press.

Coppa, G. V.; Gabrielli, O.; Giorgi, P.; Catassi, C.; Montanari, M. P.; Veraldo, P. E.; and Nichols, B. L. (1990). Preliminary study of breastfeeding and bacterial adhesion to uroepithelial cells. *Lancet* **335,** 569–71.

Cornell University (1983). Vitamin C improves iron nutrition in Philippine children. In *Research Reports.* Division of Nutritional Sciences, Cornell University, Ithaca, N.Y.

Coyaji, B. (1980). Indian women's deteriorating health. In *Health Needs of the World's Poor Women.* Ed. P. W. Blair. Equity Policy Center, Washington, D.C.

Darrow, K.; Keller, K.; and Pam, R. (1981). *Appropriate Technology Sourcebook,* vol. 11. Volunteers in Asia Publications, Stanford, Calif.

DHS (1991). Demographic and Health Surveys World Conference, *Proceedings,* vol. 2, p. 1645. Washington, D.C.

Ekelof, E. (1991). Working women. Health at risk. *Working Environment,* pp. 26–28.

Engle, P. L. (1983). The effect of maternal employment on children's welfare in rural Guatemala. In *Child Development and International Development: Research-Policy Interfaces,* pp. 57–75. Ed. D. A. Wagner. New Directions for Child Development, no. 20. Jossey-Bass, San Francisco.

Enkin, M., and Chalmers, I., eds. (1982). *Effectiveness and Satisfaction in Antenatal Care.* William Heinemann Medical Books Ltd., Philadelphia.

Favin, M., and Bradford, B. (1984). *Improving Maternal Health in Developing Countries.* APHA issues paper. Prepared for UNICEF by American Public Health Association, Washington, D.C.

FAO/WHO (1973). *Energy and Protein Requirements. Wld. Hlth. Org. Tech. Rep. Ser.,* no. 522. Geneva.

Freire, P. (1970). *Pedagogy of the Oppressed.* Continuum Press, New York.

Germaine, A.; Holmes, K. K.; Piot, P.; and Wasserheit, J. N. (1992). *Reproductive Tract Infections.* Plenum Press, New York.

Ghai, D.; Godfrey, M.; and Lisk, F. (1979). *Planning for Basic Needs in Kenya—Performance, Policies and Prospects.* International Labour Organization, Geneva.

Guardian (1992). Fish oil found to give longer pregnancies and heavier babies. *Guardian,* April 4.

Gwinn, M. L., et al. (1990). Pregnancy, breastfeeding and oral contraception and the risk of epithelial ovarian cancer. *J. Clin. Epidemiology* **43**(6), 559–68.

Harrison, P. (1982). *Inside the Third World: The Anatomy of Poverty.* 2d ed. Penguin Books, Harmondsworth.

Heise, L. (1989). Violence against women. *The Hamilton Spectator,* April 26, p. A7. Hamilton, Ontario, Canada.

Herz, B., and Measham, A. (1990). *The Safe Motherhood Initiative: Proposal for Action.* World Bank, Washington, D.C.

Hibbard, B. M. (1975). Folates and the foetus. *S. Afr. Med. J.* **49,** 1223.

Iyengar, L., and Rajalakshim, K. (1975). Effect of folic acid supplements on the birth weights of infants. *Am. J. Obstet. Gynec.* **122,**332.

Jameson, S. (1976). Variations in maternal serum zinc during pregnancy and correlation to congenital malformations, dysmaturity, and abnormal parturition. *Acta Med. Scanda.* (Suppl.) **593,** 21.

Jelliffe, D. B., and Jelliffe, E. F. P. (1985). *Child Nutrition in Developing Countries: A Handbook for Fieldworkers.* Office of Nutrition, Agency for International Development, Washington, D.C.

Jelliffe, D. B., and Jelliffe, E. F. P. (1989). *Community Nutritional Assessment.* Oxford University Press, Oxford.

Jiminiz, M. J., and Newton, W. (1979). Activity and work during pregnancy and the post partum period: A crosscultural study of 202 societies. *Am. J. Obstet. Gynec.* **135,** 171.

J. Trop. Pediat. (1982). Editorial: Contraceptive effect of breast feeding. *J. Trop. Pediat.* **28,** ii.

Kanhere, S. G. (1980). Violence against women is also a health problem. In *Health Needs of the World's Poor Women.* Ed. P. W. Blair. Equity Policy Center, Washington, D.C.

Kitzinger, S. (1980). *The Experience of Breast Feeding.* Pelican Books, New York.

Knuppel, R. (1981). Drugs, smoking, alcohol—influence in pregnancy. In *Nutrition in Preg-*

nancy, pp. 70–77. Ed. J. P. Lavery. University of Louisville, Ky.

Kwast, B. (1985). Epidemiology of maternal mortality in Addid Ababa; a community based study. *Ethiopian Med. J.* **23**(1).

Lancet (1983). Misuse of amniocentesis round the world, India. *Lancet* **i,** 812.

Last, J., ed. (1980). *Public Health and Preventive Medicine.* 11th ed, Appleton-Century-Crofts, New York.

Lechtig, A.; Klein, R.; Daza, C.; Read, M.; and Kahn, S. (1979). Effects of maternal nutrition on infant health: Implications for action. *J. Trop. Pediat.* **28,** 273.

Magnay-Maglacas, A., and Pizurki, J. (1981). *The Traditional Birth Attendant in Seven Countries: Case Studies in Utilization and Training.* Wld. Hlth. Org. Publ. Hlth. Pap., no. 75.

Maine, D. (1982). *Family Planning: Its Impact on the Health of Women and Children.* Center for Population and Family Health, Columbia University, New York.

Maine, D. (1990). *Safe Motherhood Programs: Options and Issues.* Center for Population and Family Health, Columbia University, New York.

Mata, L. (1980). *The Children of Santa Maria Cauque.* MIT Press, Cambridge, Mass.

Mehl, L. F.; Leavitt, L. A.; Peterson, G. H.; and Creevy, D. G. (1976). Home Versus Hospital Delivery: Comparisons of Matched Population. Paper presented at the annual meeting of the American Public Health Association, Miami Beach.

Mitchnik, D. (1977). *The Role of Women in Rural Zaire and Upper Volta.* International Labour Organization, Geneva.

MMWR (1993). *Morbidity and Mortality Weekly Reports* **41** (RR17).

Mosley, W. (1983). *Will Health Care Reduce Infant and Child Mortality? A Critique of Some Current Strategies with Special Reference to Africa and Asia.* Ford Foundation, Jakarta.

Naismith, D. (1981). Diet in pregnancy: Recommendations and realities. In *Applied Nutrition,* pp. 1–7. Ed. E. C. Bateman. Libbey, London.

PAHO (1982). *Health Conditions in the Americas, 1977–1980.* Pan American Sanitary Bureau, Pan American Health Organization, Regional Office of WHO, Washington, D.C.

PAHO (1990). *Health Conditions in the Americas.* Pan American Health Organization,Regional Office of WHO, Washington,D.C.

Peckham (1992). *Guardian,* April 25.

Pop. Ref. Bur. (1980). *World's Women Data Sheet.* Population Reference Bureau, Washington, D.C.

Pop. Ref. Bur. (1992). *1992 World Population Data Sheet.* Population Reference Bureau, Washington, D.C.

Prentice, A. M.; Whitehead, R. G.; Lamb, W.; and Cole, T. (1983). Prenatal dietary and supplementation of African women and birthweight. *Lancet* **i,** 489.

Puffer, R., and Griffiths, G. W. (1967). *Patterns of Urban Mortality in Latin America.* Report of the Inter-American Investigation of Mortality, Pan American Health Organization in Scientific Publication no. 151. Washington, D.C.

Rosa, F., and Turshen, M. (1970). Fetal nutrition. *Bull. Wld. Hlth. Org.* **43,** 785.

Rosen, G. (1958). *A History of Public Health.* MD Publications, New York.

Rosso, P. (1981). Prenatal nutrition and fetal growth and development. *Pediat. Ann.* **11,** 21.

Shah, K. P. (1982). Appropriate technology and perinatal care: The Kasa experience. In *Advances in International Maternal and Child Health,* 2: 1–15. Ed. D. B. Jelliffe and E. F. P. Jelliffe. Oxford University Press, Oxford.

Siskind, V., et al. (1989). Breast cancer and breastfeeding. Results from an Australian case-control study. *Am. J. Epidemiology* **130,** 229–36.

Stein, H. (1975). Maternal protein depletion and small for gestational age babies. *Arch. Dis. Childhood* **50,** 46.

Sterky, G., and Mellander, L., eds. (1978). *Birth Weight Distribution—An Indicator of Social Development,* SAREC Report no. R:2. Swedish Agency for Research Cooperation with Developing Countries.

Tafari, N. (1981). Low birthweight: An overview. In *Advances in International Maternal and Child Health,* 1: 105–27. Ed. D. B. Jelliffe and E. F. P. Jelliffe. Oxford University Press, Oxford.

Thilly, C. H. T., and Delange, F. (1977). Strategy of goitre and cretinism control in Central Africa. *Int. J. Epid.* **6,** 1.

Thomson, A., et al. (1966). Body weight changes during pregnancy and lactation in rural African (Gambian) women. *Brit. J. Obstet. Gynec.* **73**, 724.

Tietz, C. (1979). *Induced Abortion.* Population Council Fact Book, Population Council, New York.

UN (1976). *UN Demographic Yearbook, 1975.* United Nations, New York.

UN (1989). *Violence Against Women in the Family.* United Nations, New York.

UN (1990). *Women and Nutrition.* CC/SCN Symposium Report, Nutrition Policy Discussion Paper, no. 6. United Nations, New York.

UN (1991). *World's Women: Trends and Statistics.* Series K 1970–1990, no. 8. United Nations, New York.

UNICEF News (1980). Women of the world: The facts, development begins with women. *UNICEF News* **104**, 200.

UNICEF (1980). *Assignment Children.* Ed. P. E. Mandl. No. 49/50. UNICEF, Geneva.

UNICEF (1990). *World Summit for Children.* United Nations, New York.

UNICEF (1990a). *The Girl Child.* United Nations Children's Fund, New York.

UNICEF (1990b). *World Summit for Children, 77 Estimated HIV-infected Females.* UNICEF, New York.

UNICEF (1992). *Annual Report.* UNICEF, New York.

Viegas, O.; Scott, P.; Cole, T.; Mansfield, H.; Wharton, P.; and Wharton, B. (1982). Dietary protein energy supplementation of pregnant Asian mothers at Sorrento, Birmingham 1, unselective during second and third trimesters. *Brit. Med. J.* **285**, 589.

Wilmsen, E. N. (1978). Seasonal effects of Dietary intake on the Kalahari. *San Fed. Proc.* **37**, 65.

WIPHN News (1990). Does antenatal care make a difference? Vol. 8, Oct./Nov. (Women's International Public Health Network, Bethesda, Md.)

Wolf, N. (1992). How images of beauty are used against women. In *The Beauty Myth.* Anchor Books, New York.

Women in China (1982). Editorial: Why female infanticide still exists in socialist China. *Women in China* **5**, 1.

WHO (1980a). *Health and the Status of Women.* FHE/80.1. World Health Organization, Geneva.

WHO (1980b). The incidence of low birth weight: A critical review of available information. *Wld. Hlth. Stat. Q.* **33**(1), 97.

WHO (1980c). *6th Report on the World Health Situation (1973–1977).* Part 1: *Global Analysis.* World Health Organization, Geneva.

WHO (1980d). *Towards a Better Future, Maternal and Child Health.* World Health Organization, Geneva.

WHO (1982). *World Health Statistics Annual.* World Health Organization, Geneva.

WHO (1985). *Women and Breast Feeding.* Division of Family Health, World Health Organization, Geneva.

WHO (1986). Acquired immunodeficiency syndrome. *Weekly Epidemiology Record.* World Health Organization, Geneva.

WHO (1990). *AIDS Prevention: Guidelines for MCH/FP Programme Managers II.* AIDS of Maternal and Child Health, World Health Organization, Geneva.

WHO (1991a). *Child Health and Development: Health of the Newborn.* World Health Organization, Geneva.

WHO (1991b). *Weekly Epidemiological Record* **66**(47), 345–52.

WHO (1992). *Women's Health: Across Age and Frontier.* World Health Organization, Geneva.

WHO/UNICEF (1992). *Consensus Statement from the WHO/UNICEF Consultation on HIV Transmission and Breastfeeding,* April 30–May 1. World Health Organization, Geneva.

Zahr, A., and Royston, E. (1991). *Maternal Mortality—A Global Fact Book.* Division of Family Health, WHO, Geneva.

Zambia Daily Mail (1981). November 5.

7

Common Problems
in Children

*Whatsoever was the father of a disease, an ill diet was
the mother.*
GEORGE HERBERT, 1660

George Herbert's dictum is still too often true. It would also be true to say, "Whatever may be the cause of a disease, the result will be the malnourished state."

Patterns of disease depend first on the genetic endowment of the individual and second on the total environment—not so much the geographical situation as the protection and sanitation of the habitat, the economic situation, the establishment of law and order, various cultural and social attitudes, and the availability of food, worthwhile employment, and medical care. Their genetic factors aside, children are completely at the mercy of their environment. This includes particularly the attitudes, education, and economic circumstances of the mother and other members of the family.

Assessment of the problems of newborns, young children, and school-aged children, including adolescents, must include not only the clinical diagnosis but also traditional and existing attitudes, child care practices, educational level of household members, and the resources available to the family. It is important to have some statistical analysis of mortality and morbidity, of incidence, prevalence, and causation of disease, and of the availability and distribution of health services (Bennett 1979; du Florey et al. 1983). An epidemiological approach is called for, with information on families and measures of effectiveness.

THE NEWBORN

Mortality in the neonatal and perinatal periods is difficult to measure unless strict standards of agreed definitions and registration are maintained.

In many developing countries the perinatal mortality is 80 to 100 per 1,000 live births—four or more times greater than the national average of developed countries (Fig. 7.1) (WHO 1991a). There is increasing recognition that the perinatal and neonatal periods are a high source of mortality, especially in developing countries, and that much can be achieved through simple interventions. Of the estimated 13 million deaths of those under 5 years old, two-thirds occur in the first year of life, and half of these deaths occur in the first month of life. Furthermore,

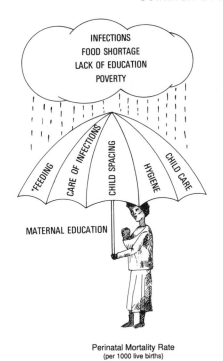

INFECTIONS
FOOD SHORTAGE
LACK OF EDUCATION
POVERTY

FEEDING · CARE OF INFECTIONS · CHILD SPACING · HYGIENE · CHILD CARE

MATERNAL EDUCATION

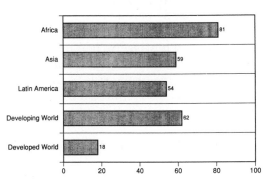

Perinatal Mortality Rate
(per 1000 live births)

Africa	81
Asia	59
Latin America	54
Developing World	62
Developed World	18

0   20   40   60   80   100

Figure 7.1. Estimates of perinatal mortality. Much can be done to reduce infant mortality that does not require sophisticated technology. Source: WHO (1991*a*).

perinatal mortality is estimated at half of the infant mortality.

Most of the infants born to the 500,000 women who die each year are among those who die in the perinatal period or infancy. This was realized in Sweden in the nineteenth century and later in Finland where, by placing trained midwives in the rural areas, maternal mortality dropped and perinatal mortality dropped rapidly shortly after.

Most inventions aimed at lowering perinatal or neonatal mortality must address maternal health and the social position of women because they are interrelated. Simple interventions antenatally, during childbirth and for the newborn, can make a dramatic difference through atraumatic and clean delivery, maintenance of body temperature, initiation of spontaneous respiration, and initiation of exclusive breast feeding shortly after birth (WHO 1991*a*). It will certainly be more fruitful for poorer nations to concentrate on facilities for prenatal and childbirth supervision and care and the neonatal period than on high-technology and intensive care for neonates (WHO 1991*b*).

In many less developed countries, particularly in rural areas, a baby who dies in the early hours or days of life may be buried without being registered as either a birth or a death. The pattern of infant mortality and the age-specific rates (neonatal, perinatal, postnatal) are important in order to develop appropriate practical programs but often difficult to obtain. Regional differences in the cause of neonatal mortality do occur. On some Pacific islands, 10 percent of newborns have hyperbilirubinemia; 5 percent die, and an equal number develop post-icteric brain damage. In parts of India, nearly 30 percent of neonatal deaths are due to birth asphyxia and another 20 percent to pulmonary causes (WHO 1991*a*). Controversial data suggest that the IMR is rising among disadvantaged groups in both the United States (among blacks) and in the former Soviet Union (in the southern eastern regions), and this has socioeconomic implications. However, the rising IMR may also be attributed to improved birth registration and medical care of nonviable infants.

In the United States, the infant mortality dropped from 21.8 in 1968 to 10.1 per 1,000 live births in 1987; the decline since has been only minimal. Among nations with lower rates in 1990 were Hong Kong and Singapore, with 7.4 and 7.0

deaths per 1,000 live births, respectively, and Sweden with 5.58 and Japan with 4.8 deaths per 1,000. The inability to eliminate infant mortality is paradoxical for a nation like the United States, which spends millions of dollars each year on scientific research and medical care and whose hospitals and neonatal intensive care units rank among the best in the world. The maldistribution of services for the poor, the misuse or abuse of technology, and adverse life-styles contribute to the large number of low-birthweight infants. WHO defines low birthweight as less than 2,500 grams and very low birthweight as less than 1,500 grams. Low birthweight is defined as less than 5 pounds, 8 ounces in the United States, where 7 percent of births are low birthweight and low birthweight contributes to 60 percent of deaths in the first year of life (NIH 1989). In the United States, some blacks have much higher infant mortality rates and a higher incidence of low-birthweight infants. The latter may be also due to an intergenerational effect.

In most developed countries, deaths in infancy from all causes has fallen, but in developing countries death rates in infancy are still high (Table 7.1). In some Latin American countries, deaths in infancy as a proportion of all causes is as high as 30 percent and in some Asian countries nearly 50 percent, especially in the rural areas where health care has not reached. China has made considerable progress in improving the health of mothers and children. In a study in Shunyi County, five major risk factors were identified—low birthweight, birth defects, hypertensive disorders of pregnancy, breech birth, and asphyxia—as contributing to the high perinatal mortality. Changes in training, introduction of clinical norms, reorganization of care, transport and exchange with community workers led to a marked reduction in perinatal mortality (WHO 1991a).

Late neonatal and postnatal deaths, uncommon in developed countries, are still leading causes of morbidity and mortality in developing countries. Studies in developing countries show that more than half of the deaths are infectious in origin and preventable. Furthermore, 60 to 75 percent are in low-birthweight infants (Kumari 1983). Puffer and Serrano (1973) found malnutrition to be an underlying cause in up to 57 percent of infant deaths in Latin America. Neonatal deaths are due mainly to low birthweight (including prematurity), infections, and congenital anomalies. Some of the risk factors and preventive measures for neonates are listed in Table 7.2.

Low Birthweight and Prematurity

Low-birthweight infants may be preterm (short gestational age) or term babies small for gestational age (WHO 1950, 1961; Sterky and Mellander 1978). There are

Table 7.1. Mortality Rates for Infants and Children Under Age 5, by Region

Country grouping	1991 population (millions)	Infant mortality rate	Under-5 mortality rate	Maternal mortality rate
Developing countries	4142	75	117	421
Least developed countries	460	119	198	737
East Europe	391	22	25	41
Developed market economies	837	14	18	34
Total	5370	68	104	370

Source: Adapted from WHO (1992).

Table 7.2. Practical Prevention of Neonatal Disease

	Prevention
Infections General septicemia, skin, respiratory	Breastfeeding
	Cleanliness by birth attendant and family at and after birth
	Minimum interference during birth (e.g., intravaginal maneuvers)
	Avoidance of indigenous dressing to cord
	Hospital admission for all neonates born by prolonged (48 hours) or difficult labor
Diarrhea	Breastfeeding (colostrum)
	Avoidance of neonatal feeds, herbal remedies, etc.
	Newborn by mother's bed, not in nurseries
	If artificial feeding absolutely necessary, great care with cleanliness or preparation
Ophthalmia neonatorum	Antenatal detection and treatment of maternal infection
	Routine prophylactic eye applications at birth
Tetanus	Cleanliness in cord care (e.g., cutting instruments, hands, dressing) ⎫
	Avoidance of dangerous indigenous cord dressing (especially if this contains animal dung) ⎬ Training of indigenous birth attendants
	Immunization of pregnant women or all women ⎭
Congenital syphilis	Antenatal blood test, and treatment of pregnant women if necessary
Birth trauma	Antenatal supervision and early referral of potential obstetrical problems (e.g., contracted pelvis, small stature, twins)
	Avoidance of local traumatic practices during delivery
	Avoidance of indigenous herbal oxytocins
Low birthweight (including prematurity)	Early detection and treatment of acute or chronic general or obstetrical disease or abnormality
	Improved diet in pregnancy with special reference to locally available foods (especially vegetable protein mixtures) zinc iron folate, protein
	Avoidance of excessive physical work
	Antimalarials during pregnancy
	Supplement of folic acid/iron/vitamin A if necessary in pregnancy
	Child spacing
	Avoidance of smoking

21 million low-birthweight infants born each year worldwide (one in six births), and of those, over 90 percent are born in developing countries (WHO 1991*a*). The incidence of low birthweight varies widely. In India and Pakistan, 30 percent of infants are so affected (WHO 1991*a*). Clinical impression in several parts of the

world is that many babies under 2,500 grams at birth are vigorous and more mature physiologically than expected. The developmental precocity of newborns in Africa (Geber and Dean 1958), rural Guatemala, and Mexico poses interesting, unresolved questions. As well as possible genetic and other prenatal influences, some of the precociousness even in the earliest days may be due to constant companionship with the mother, in contrast to the enforced isolation of the young baby that is practiced in many developed countries. Nevertheless, there is evidence that the lower the infant's weight the higher is the mortality (WHO 1992; Sterky 1978).

In Guatemala, more than half the infants born with a low birthweight (defined as less than 2,000 grams) died within the first year of life (Mata 1978). Approximately 45 percent of low-birthweight infants have congenital anomalies (WHO 1992).

In developed countries, two-thirds of all low-birthweight infants are preterm (less than thirty-seven weeks gestation) whereas in developing countries the reverse holds: three-fourths of all infants are full term but undernourished and small for gestational age.

Low birthweight may be due to several causes simultaneously: maternal malnutrition, close child spacing, and low socioeconomic status. Investigation is required into the differential diagnosis of various forms of low-birthweight babies—not only the cause of death but, especially, the initiating factors (Naeye et al. 1979).

In highly endemic malarial areas, the malarial parasite tends to congregate in the placenta even in immune mothers who themselves show no clinical ill effects, and at most a minor degree of parasitemia. Symptomless placental malaria leads to a lowering of birthweight by about half a pound (Jelliffe 1968).

In some areas, the percentage of low-birthweight infants is high, and from a general public health point of view, it is of practical value to define a level of special care based on birthweight, that can act as a guide to management (Jelliffe 1967). For example, in Kampala, Uganda, analysis of neonatal mortality for the previous two years among all births at Mulago Hospital and a one-year examination of all newborn babies for physiological maturity, particularly the suckling and swallowing reflexes needed for breast feeding, indicated that a birthweight of 4 pounds, 6 ounces could be taken as the special care level. This was the weight level below which special management was required, involving a warm environment, protection from infection, and, possibly, intragastric feeding. This weight level indicates possible time for discharge from hospital, but this must depend also on home conditions. Yet even with this lower level for babies needing special care, a much higher percentage is found in developing countries than in the Western world, and preventive measures are needed as a logical and economical approach.

With the many other large-scale problems facing health professionals in these countries, the priority level of a unit for premature babies (with low birthweight or requiring special care) is often debated, particularly in view of its potential expense in terms of equipment and staff. In the United States, cost estimates for the prevention of low-birthweight infants is between $14,000 and $30,000 (NIH 1989). The cost of caring for an infant under 2 pounds has been estimated at $40,287 (Pomerance et al. 1978). A more realistic approach is to concentrate attention on neonates between the special care level and about 2 pounds in weight. Babies above this range do not usually need special management; those of lower weight have an extremely high mortality even in ideal units and may be left with brain damage if they recover. The most important measure is to identify those at risk from whatever cause and to ensure that they receive continuing health care and supervision in the hospital, health center, and home.

The management of small neonates requiring special care in developing countries has to be based on the realization that the mothers are vital for the breast-feeding and survival of their offspring. Western practices that interfere with lactation (Jelliffe 1967; Kahn 1954) must be modified, with close mother-neonate contact from as early as possible for the initiation of breastfeeding and for warmth.

Birth Trauma

With the improvement in birth practices in Sweden has come a decrease in the incidence of spastic and ataxic cerebral palsy from 2.2 to 1.3 per 1,000 live births over a fifteen-year period (Hagberg et al. 1975). In developing countries, TBAs sometimes employ methods of delivery that are vigorous, toxic, and extremely damaging (Jelliffe 1978a). The umbilical cord may be dragged dangerously, cut with a dirty instrument, and dressed with a variety of unsuitable substances. Many deaths in West Africa have been the result of extensive incisions on newborns; deaths occur from hemorrhage, exposure, and sepsis.

Neonatal Disorders

Tetanus neonatorum. This preventable infection still kills many babies in developing countries. Even with early diagnosis (easily made on clinical appearance), the treatment is prolonged and expensive and must be highly skilled. The full incidence of the condition is not known in more remote regions, but in some areas it is thought that as many as 20 to 40 percent of neonatal deaths are due to tetanus neonatorum (Schofield et al. 1961).

The disease is easily preventable by hygienic practices at the time of delivery. A clinic may issue an envelope containing

a razor blade, a length of ligature, and a dressing; or the birth attendant can be taught to use scissors flamed in the fire for cutting the cord and a sterile dressing. Modern maternity hospitals use a clip on the cord and leave it undressed. It dries up and falls off quickly and cleanly with this treatment. But in some home conditions, it is probably safer to use a dressing until the skin has healed. A valuable additional method of prevention is to immunize the mother against tetanus during her antenatal period (Kretchmer 1969; Schofield et al. 1961). In areas where tetanus incidence is high and antenatal services limited, mass vaccination campaigns of childbearing-age women are highly recommended (Lancet 1983b); it is estimated that they have reduced the number of deaths due to tetanus neonatorum from 800,000 to 550,000 (WHO 1992).

Septicemia. This can occur in the home and in hospitals. The condition is common and needs to be treated with antibiotics even if only suspected.

Conjunctivitis. This may be due to the gonococcus or other organisms (especially chlamydia). Classical prevention has been with the use of 1 percent silver nitrate eyedrops shortly after birth. Unfortunately, silver nitrate is not effective against nongonococcal infections, and a 1 percent solution rapidly becomes concentrated in hot, dry climates when antibiotics run out. In Samoa during an epidemic of hemorrhagic conjunctivitis, breast milk squirted in infants' eyes was effective (MMWR 1982).

Diarrhea. Diarrhea is not common where the infant is kept close to the mother and is breastfed by her without delay and on demand. Where babies are kept in a separate nursery away from the maternity ward, are bottle-fed, are handed around to various relatives to be put to the breast, given chewed-up rice or banana early in life, or given a purgative, diarrhea may be frequent, troublesome, and dangerous.

Congenital syphilis. This often appears to be a curiously rare condition. Even in areas where serologists report that 80 percent of parents have a positive serology, remarkably few babies are born with, or develop, the obvious signs or symptoms of congenital syphilis. It is possible that even the more specific tests for syphilis are still returning false-positives because of the number of infective and parasitic diseases that are, or have been, present. In some areas, yaws still affects the serological reactions, both as a result (or as a recrudescence of an old infection) or as new cases appear after "eradication." Nevertheless, especially among migrants and in urban slums, congenital syphilis should be looked for. It may easily be overlooked by those unfamiliar with its range of clinical manifestations.

Congenital abnormalities. The incidence seems to vary in different countries. In the United States, the percentage of deaths from congenital abnormalities increased from 6.4 percent in 1900 to 20.5 percent in 1989 (NCHS 1992). Abnormalities range from minor deviations—such as rudimentary extra digits, which are common in equatorial Africa (Applebaum 1970; Williams 1946), an erupted tooth, or a fold above the inner canthus, often found among Chinese—to a major abnormality incompatible with life. In parts of Africa, any deviation from the normal was once regarded with dread, and it was customary for such babies to be destroyed. Now, many parents come eagerly to special centers, where available, to have abnormalities corrected. Whether these abnormalities are reported depends on the attitude of the parents and the effectiveness of treatment.

Jaundice. Severe jaundice of the newborn is usually due to septicemia. If there is any possibility of such a diagnosis, treatment should be instituted prior to receipt of blood culture results.

Respiratory distress syndrome. RDS in all its forms and degrees of severity is more common in premature and low-birthweight infants than in those who are up to standard weight and development. It is responsible for a high proportion of neonatal deaths all over the world but may be less common in developing countries. A new study shows that inositol (present in colostrum) prevents not only RDS but also retinal damage in preterm infants (Hallman et al. 1992).

Other disorders. Other disorders of the newborn occur as elsewhere. Severe neonatal anemia, sometimes requiring transfusion, can occur in communities where the umbilical stump is not tied, particularly if the cord has been cut with a sharp razor blade or if the cord is tied too early.

Prevention of Neonatal Disorders

Many of the conditions afflicting newborns in developing countries can be prevented or at least made much less frequent. The key lies in improved antenatal care, education, and supervision (particularly of the maternal diet), which must include recognition and treatment of diseases, together with cleaner, more skillful midwifery, particularly through the training of TBAs; with child spacing through family planning; and with ensuing breastfeeding. It is essential to undertake adequate follow-up through widely distributed health centers and supervision in the homes of visiting nurses and auxiliaries. Even the simplest medical and health supervision can effect improvements and reduce mortality in newborns. All health personnel involved must appreciate the importance of breastfeeding including the special significance of colostrum.

THE YOUNG (UNDER 5) CHILD AND SCHOOL-AGED CHILD

Young children have a very high proportion of problems in health and medical care. In developing countries three major disorders make up the bulk of illness among young children: diarrhea, respiratory disorders, and malnutrition. All are interdependent. Many of the cases of malnutrition result from diarrhea, with malabsorption and maldigestion; respiratory disease is often a terminal condition in malnourished children. Each year diarrhea-related dehydration claims the lives of 3 million children, and yet it is often underestimated as a major contributor to malnutrition and mortality (Grant 1984). The death of ten people from starvation or a flood will excite rapid action, but the death of a thousand children from diarrheal disease has often remained unnoticed. However, with the widespread use of ORT (oral rehydration therapy), both recognition and effective, low-cost rehydration treatment have become possible.

Diarrhea

Diarrhea is a symptom or sign and not a disease; it is caused by many factors (Gordon et al. 1964; Jelliffe and Stanfield 1970; Baumslag et al. 1979). It is serious and fatal in young children, especially if they are malnourished. Severe diarrhea in infancy is seen largely among bottle-fed infants; infants who are exclusively breastfed on demand do not succumb (McClelland et al. 1978; Pittard 1979). During a cholera epidemic in Bahrain, cholera occurred seven times more frequently in bottle-fed than in breastfed children (Gunn 1979). The peak incidence of diarrhea occurs between the ages of 6 months and 2 years, depending on when weaning occurs. Diarrheal diseases are perpetuated by poverty, malnutrition, and poor sanitation.

The immediate danger of diarrhea is dehydration, which is a problem in about 10 percent of acute cases and life-threatening in about 1 percent of cases. Shock or coma and death result when the fluid losses equal about 10 percent of body weight. The degree of dehydration is best assessed by clinical signs. Inelasticity of the skin, dry mouth, sunken eyes, and hypotonia are late clinical signs. Early diagnosis is based on a history of three or more loose stools and/or vomiting.

Malnutrition that occurs after repeated episodes of diarrhea is the long-term problem. Puffer and Serrano (1973), in their study of Latin American mortality, found that diarrhea and malnutrition were inextricably bound together. Children in developing countries have an average of six to twelve episodes of diarrhea per year (Grant 1984), and a poorly nourished child is twice as likely to suffer from diarrhea as a well-nourished child (Baumslag et al. 1979). Conversely, diarrhea causes or adds to malnutrition. The combined process of poor diet and recurrent infection can lead the child in a downward spiral toward further malnutrition, chronic infection, and death.

When infants develop diarrhea, their chances of survival depend on the availability of prompt medical care, the correction of dehydration, and the continuation of breastfeeding or appropriate feeding for older children. Bottle feeding, early mixed feeding, insanitary practices, and delay in rehydration or even wrong treatment (such as purgation or the withholding of fluids, thought, erroneously, to rest the bowel) are responsible for the high death rate in infants and children in many developing countries.

Cultural beliefs sometimes add to the problem. In parts of West Africa and Latin America, a sunken anterior fontanelle in infants is treated by holding the baby upside down. (It should be noted that a depressed anterior fontanelle is a late sign of diarrheal dehydration.) In Guatemala, some mothers believe that if a baby sucks at the breast too hard or if the nipple is withdrawn too abruptly, the suction will create a vacuum in the baby's head, causing the fontanelle to sink. In parts of Africa, diarrhea is blamed on the mother's infidelity or on the "evil eye." In Somalia it is believed that a certain bird causes diarrhea by flying over the child at night. Health workers should incorporate local beliefs into health education activities to encourage early rehydration.

Investigation does not always reveal classical pathogens or newly recognized bacteria or viruses. Some cases may be due to alterations in bowel flora (Mata 1965). Others may be caused not so much by infection as by malabsorption, maldigestion, or irritation and rejection of unaccustomed or unsuitable foods introduced accidentally or unwisely. Diarrhea may result from excessive feeding, wrong timing, or emotional upset. Several causes may be operating at once, especially in the weanling (Gordon, 1964). Consumption of green mangoes or other fruits or of cereals such as millet, sorghum, or maize insufficiently pounded, winnowed, or cooked may give rise to diarrhea. The incidence is often seasonal; in Egypt, 75 percent of diarrheal deaths occur (McCord 1979) during the summer months, when fly breeding increases.

Where pathogens can be identified, contaminated water, food, and milk are likely sources. Acute episodes of food poisoning may be encountered in individuals, families, and communities. These may be due to anything from toxic herbs to rat poison mixed with flour or even the consumption of a cow infected with anthrax.

There is still insufficient evidence to show how much diarrhea is due to infections and infestations (including measles and malaria), the physical characteristics of food, or congenital or acquired deficiency of lactase or other enzymes (McCracken 1970). Health workers must differentiate between watery stools and dysentery (containing blood and mucus)

and between acute and chronic diarrhea. Chronic cases are more difficult to treat, and attention to the diet is a most important factor in recovery. A great deal of information can be gained from stool gazing (Dammin 1964; Jelliffe and Stanfield 1970).

Treatment. The discovery that glucose dramatically enhances the absorption of water and salt, even in a damaged bowel, has revolutionized the technology needed for rehydration. ORT has proved so safe and effective that it can be given in the home by nearly anyone with minimal training. Once the routine use of ORT is established, mortality from diarrheal dehydration can be virtually eliminated. Severe cases still require intravenous or intragastric rehydration; however, even in these cases, ORT can be life-saving when it is used as an early stopgap measure, especially in unserved areas. In some countries, the problem has become so widespread that rehydration centers have been organized (Jelliffe 1968; Jelliffe 1970). Mothers and child caretakers should be taught to give oral rehydration solution (ORS) if a child has three or more watery stools in a day. As a rough measure, for each stool passed, two cups of ORS should be given. In young patients with severe diarrhea, cup and spoon feeding in small quantities is recommended to reduce the risk of vomiting (Fig. 7.2). Mothers should continue breast feeding, and children should be given as much food as can be tolerated in addition to ORS, especially after initial rehydration (often four to eight hours) (Jelliffe 1989a).

ORS can be prepared commercially or at home. WHO recommends a rehydration formula of sodium chloride (3.5 grams), sodium bicarbonate (2.5 grams), potassium chloride (1.5 grams), and glucose (20 grams) per liter of water. For home preparation of 1 liter of ORS, 5 cups of water, 8 teaspoons of sugar, and 1 teaspoon of salt should be used. It is

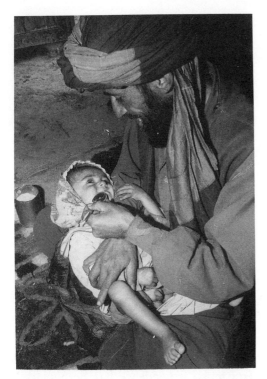

Figure 7.2. Oral rehydration therapy. A Pakistani father gives oral rehydration salts (ORS) to his child. Mothers often have heavy work loads, and other family members may have more time to give ORS. They should be trained and supervised by a health worker. UNICEF photograph by Bruce Thomas.

most important to provide sugar, salt, and water in the correct proportions. A prepackaged standardized WHO mix is produced by UNICEF for use at home and in health centers. Some countries are producing their own mix. Problems have arisen in areas where standard containers measure less than a liter, and local measures have had to be adapted. Critics argue that a standardized solution should not be used because the salt content is too high for infants under 3 months.

In some areas, packets of ORS are unavailable, and other methods have been developed for home preparation of a solution. These include a "pinch and scoop" measure (using a standardized three-finger pinch of salt and a small scoop of sugar to barely cover the palm of the hand, for one drinking glass of water), using a special two-ended plastic spoon (one end for sugar, the other for salt), or a homemade measuring spoon (Fig. 7.3) (Baumslag et al. 1979; Werner and Bower 1982). Home methods for preparation are not always satisfactory, since a mother may give a more concentrated solution in the belief that more is better. Also, measurements made at home are not always precise and sometimes contain too much salt (Ebrahim 1982), which can cause brain damage due to hypernatremia.

Where sugar is unavailable, substitutes have to be found. Oral rehydration has long been practiced in traditional forms by mothers who give rice water, coconut water, carrot juice, or bean and chicken soup for diarrhea. Research in Asia shows that rice-based ORS is not only effective in the treatment of dehydration but may be better nutritionally than the simple sugar, salt, and water mix (Patra et al. 1982). Much recent investigation has endorsed the value of cereal-based oral rehydration, especially rice (Molla et al. 1989). These local remedies are readily available and more cost-effective than prepackaged mixes. The world demand for packaged ORS is estimated at 2.4 billion yearly, at a cost of eight to twelve cents or more per packet (Baumslag et al. 1979; Ebrahim 1982). There is no way that enough packets can be produced and distributed to rehydrate all the children with diarrhea.

ORT treats the hazards of dehydration, not diarrhea itself. Drugs are usually contraindicated, except for specific infections, such as cholera, shigella, amebiasis, and giardiasis (WHO 1990*a*). The prevention of malnutrition and the elimination of the causes of diarrhea are the ultimate goals. There has been a loss of perspective by prescribing a mass solution. With the focus on rehydration, the root causes are forgotten, and prevention can become subordinate rather than primary.

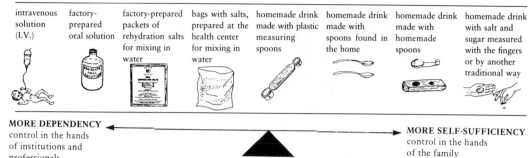

| intravenous solution (I.V.) | factory-prepared oral solution | factory-prepared packets of rehydration salts for mixing in water | bags with salts, prepared at the health center for mixing in water | homemade drink made with plastic measuring spoons | homemade drink made with spoons found in the home | homemade drink made with homemade spoons | homemade drink with salt and sugar measured with the fingers or by another traditional way |

MORE DEPENDENCY
control in the hands
of institutions and
professionals

MORE SELF-SUFFICIENCY
control in the hands
of the family

Figure 7.3. A range of rehydration methods for children with diarrhea. Food-based oral rehydration is the cheapest and most cost-effective method. It is also nutritionally more adequate and reduces the number of stools, an important consideration for mothers and other caretakers. With all methods, the earliest return to feeding is indicated. Source: Werner and Bower 1982, 1992.

Providing oral rehydration packets is only a stopgap measure. What is needed is continuity of care. Currently, the method of separately funding ORT as a vertical program makes it difficult to integrate nutrition and other health activities into primary health care.

While it has been advocated by health-care providers that the mother provide this primary care intervention, it may not be possible as the mother may be ill, or away from her family for long periods during the planting season. The problems that lead to diarrhea are primarily social and environmental, not only chemical (Zurbrigg 1984). Properly educated mothers, supervised day care centers, and responsible child caretakers could make a difference. The idea that the mother has only the sick child to care for is misplaced. Task analysis may be helpful to improve the awareness of health care providers. For treatment to be effective, causes must be determined.

Prevention. According to Gordon et al. (1964),

The present-day approach to the control of diarrheal diseases has given too much emphasis to the obligations and duties of public health agencies and little recognition to the fact that control depends to a great extent on individuals. The stress has been too much on what society should do for the individual and not on what the individual must, of necessity, do for himself, as good epidemiological evidence shows.

Too much dependence has been placed on the package approach to oral rehydration rather than on the prevention of the root causes of diarrhea. First, the cause should be identified; then a course of action should be planned. If pollution of commercially produced infant foods, fecally contaminated water source, reliance on bottle feeding, malabsorption, or malaria is identified, then appropriate preventive measures should be taken.

Breastfeeding, especially when it is exclusive, plays a critical role in the prevention of diarrhea and of malnutrition (Jelliffe 1978b). A number of factors tend to reduce the incidence of breastfeeding in a community:

1. "Modern" fashion and fear of undesirable changes in the shape of the breast ("loss of the figure") among urbanized families. For example, in Ethiopia, the dress that buttons down the back requires major gymnastics for the baby to reach the breast.
2. Advertising pressures in favor of bottle feeding.

3. Episiotomies and cesarean section, which some mothers find excessively painful. They dread trying to sit up for breastfeeding.
4. Separation of mother and baby after delivery.
5. Delay in offering the breast milk to the baby. The delay of twenty-four to forty-eight hours is less often practiced now.
6. Feeding at four-hour intervals. If the baby is with the mother, the demand for suckling is very irregular at first. But most couples settle into a reasonable pattern if this is not frustrated by "four-hourly dictatorship." Frequent sucking is the key to establishment of lactation.
7. Ignorance, possessiveness, or impatience on the part of the doctors and nurses responsible for obstetric and maternal services. Conversely, overemphatic propaganda, without accompanying advice and support, may lead, paradoxically, to interference with the let-down reflex and the establishment and the continuation of lactation.
8. Supplementary feeding with sweetened milk or water or even formula, which may give the infant a distaste for less sugary feeds and far more difficult flow of breast milk. When a bottle is used, the problem is compounded because bottle feeding requires a different sucking mechanism, and moving from breast to bottle confuses the infant as well as providing a fertile source of pathogens, including rota virus (Jelliffe 1978*b*). Mixed feeding of bottle and breast (the "triple nipple syndrome") (Latham et al. 1986) leads to lactation failure (Fig. 7.4).
9. A physical problem. The infant may have a blocked nose, be oversedated from maternal anesthetic, have thrush or slight stomatitis (making sucking painful), have a structural defect such as cleft palate, or is unable to suck due to severe retardation. These conditions are uncommon yet must be considered when there is a problem.

Most of the barriers to breastfeeding are not physiological; thus, effective breastfeeding can be promoted or at least protected.

ORT involves more than just giving ORS packets for replacing fluid. It must also include nutrition education and preventive measures to reduce diarrheal disease. The discovery that mothers' recipes for diarrheal control, such as rice water or chicken and carrot soup, are effective, not only for replacing fluid loss but for reducing the number of stools passed (a real problem for mothers) and providing nutrients, has led to the promotion of food- or cereal-based ORT (Elliot 1990).

The following points should be emphasized in the prevention of diarrhea:

1. Infant feeding
   a. Encourage exclusive breastfeeding for six months. Provide complemented breastfeeding for up to two years, together with attention to maternal nutrition and a high-protein weaning diet, with gradual transition to an adequate adult diet.
   b. Introduce mixed feeding gradually at age 6 months, and avoid peppery, spicy, coarse, undercooked, bulky, or watery and indigestible food for young children. Ensure nutrient requirements are met, especially the need for foods that are calorie dense.
   c. Avoid long intervals between meals, and bulky and irregular, monotonous, contaminated, or stale food (Williams 1938; Wiseman 1964).
2. Environmental health
   a. Promote hygiene and health measures. Spread of fecally contaminated food and water can be markedly reduced by hygienic measures, particularly contamina-

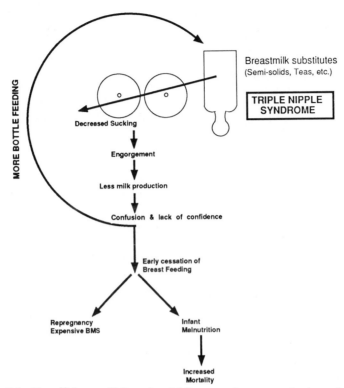

Figure 7.4. "Insufficient milk" cycle. Adding supplementary feeds to breastfed infants can cause a decrease in sucking and in milk production. When breastfed infants are given supplementary feeds, there is nipple confusion, a decrease in sucking at the breast, and a resultant decrease in milk production.

tion of supplemented foods, through boiling water, washing hands, adequate cooking of meals shortly before eating, and proper waste disposal. Rapid provision of medical attention and avoidance of dietary restrictions when the child is ill reduce the risk of diarrheal dehydration and malnutrition (Mata et al. 1965).

b. Encourage safe disposal of waste. An index of the sanitation in any community is the frequency with which shigella occurs in children. In parts of Guatemala where waste disposal is a problem, Mata found the incidence to be three to four times more frequent than for other enteropathogens (Mata 1978). In Costa Rica the gastroenteritis mortality rate dropped rapidly when the water supply was improved (Fig. 7.5).

c. Encourage control of pests: flies, rats, mice, cockroaches, and mosquitoes.

d. Involve the community in improving the environs through social engineering, especially with regard to malaria and measles immunizations.

3. Health and nutrition

a. Keep children under regular and frequent supervision at a health center or home. Persuade the mother to bring young children

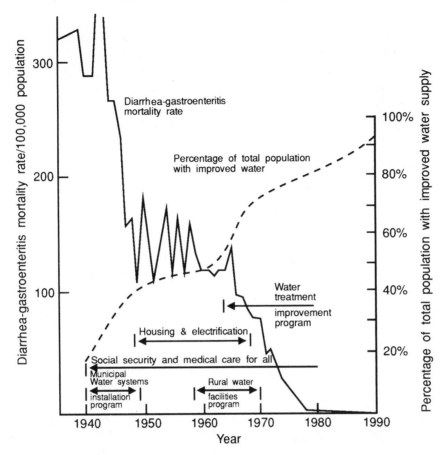

Figure 7.5. Relationship of availability of potable water to diarrhea/gastroenteritis mortality rate. Between 1980 and 1989, Costa Rica increased the availability of potable water from 84 percent to 93 percent, and the diarrheal mortality rate fell to 5.4. Sources: Isley (1982); PAHO (1990).

with her to the antenatal clinic, and make sure the children are examined as well.

b. Take the child for treatment as soon as any disturbances appear. Start with replacement of fluid straightaway—two cups of fluid for every stool passed (ORS if available or scoop-pinch home method). Continue feeding breastmilk if breastfeeding or other foods to maintain nutritional status.

c. Ensure the child's admission to hospital (with the mother in serious cases) and follow up on discharge.

Respiratory Tract Disorders

These are very common as a cause of death in countries with a high child mortality rate, but the incidence of respiratory disorders in well-to-do, well-born, well-fed, well-cared-for young children is also high worldwide. In fact, "chubby, cheerful, and catarrhal" babies are possibly more commonly found in the United Kingdom in unskilled workers than in professional and managerial workers, less easy to account for, and often very difficult to treat. It is true that they generally recover from, or more likely grow out of, their problems. Asthma is more common in the "overdeveloped" countries than in developing areas, and in the latter it will very often become less frequent when intestinal helminths have been treated. The possibility of tuberculosis always must be considered. Children who are breastfed have less tendency to allergic conditions than those who are bottle-fed and those fed on a soya-bean milk less than those fed on cow's milk.

In the developing areas, babies may be exposed to soaking rain and chilling breeze and have inadequate clothing and housing, with smoky conditions and overcrowding. These conditions all contribute to respiratory disorders that are common all over the world. Malnourished children and those with any severe disease are prone to pneumonia, which may be terminal, or to severe or fatal forms of whooping cough or measles.

Diagnosis is essentially clinical; often pneumonia can be diagnosed by inspection alone, especially indicated by rapid breathing and "insuction" during respiration. Sedatives and soothing cough syrups must be used with the greatest discretion.

Treatment. In bacterial pneumonia, medical treatment is indicated, usually penicillin or sulfonamides, together with appropriate sedatives or antispasmodics. Even for viral infections, antibiotics are sometimes useful because secondary bacterial infection is not uncommon.

Nursing is of the utmost importance in both the hospital and the home, and the mother must be taught what to do:

The nasal passages must be kept clear so that the child can suck.

Spoon-feeding with expressed breast milk may be necessary.

Only small and frequent portions of fluid or semisolid foods should be given. The child must be encouraged to eat as much as possible.

Maintaining fluid intake is important. In dry areas, humidity can be increased by hanging wet clothes around the room or using a steaming kettle (Morley et al. 1961).

The child should be slightly propped up in a well-ventilated room. A restless child should be held, talked to, and soothed but not carried about on the back.

Prevention. Prevention of whooping cough and measles through immunization has reduced the incidence of active respiratory infections (ARI). Exclusive breastfeeding is protective against ARI. Nonbreastfed infants are from 3.6 (in Brazil) to 5 times more at risk of ARI than breastfed infants (Black 1991). Young infants should be kept away from crowds as much as possible. In many areas, the incidence of upper respiratory infection is higher during months of celebrations, when large crowds gather (Morley 1961). Better housing will result in less overcrowding, and the protection of babies from cold and exposure during the rainy season will help. Finally, early treatment, especially of pneumonia, as a result of prompt recognition by parents and health workers is an important measure of secondary prevention. Parents and community health workers should be taught to recognize that fast or strained breathing is a danger sign, indicating that treatment is urgently needed. Recent publications by WHO stress the need for correct diagnosis for appropriate treatment (WHO 1990c).

Other Main Diseases

A few of the more common and damaging conditions have been selected here for special mention. Multiple diagnosis is the rule rather than the exception. The major disorders—diarrhea, respiratory disorders, and malnutrition—may be complicated by other pathological conditions. Among the most common are intestinal parasites, tuberculosis, malaria, certain infectious diseases, skin infections, accidents, dental problems, eye diseases, and oral sepsis.

Intestinal parasites. Diarrhea and dysentery; acute, chronic, subacute, and recurrent abdominal discomfort; intussusception, rectal prolapse; and considerable malabsorption can be caused or complicated by various, often multiple, infestations (Grant et al. 1963; Jelliffe 1967). Of these, roundworms, hookworms, whipworms, tapeworms, threadworms, *Entamoeba histolytica, Giardia lamblia,* and *Strongyloides* are perhaps the most prevalent (De Silva 1948; Scragg 1960).

The identification and treatment of these parasites are not as easy as books on tropical medicine often suggest, and reinfection is difficult to avoid. Most people ultimately develop some sort of immunity to these parasites, but young children are at great risk. "Tropical" medicine has paid much attention to the study of the life histories and the anatomy of intestinal parasites. Less attention was originally given to their effect on children, their distribution, and the economic treatment and practical prevention of them. A microscope is indispensable for examination; health centers should have one at hand. It is important to realize that the "worm burden" is critical—that is, the number of parasites relative to the child's size.

Amoebic dysentery can be a very damaging condition in young children; amoebic liver abscesses have been described as early as 15 months. The stool must be examined fresh. If this condition is diagnosed, children respond well to standard medical treatment (Grant 1963; WHO 1990*b*).

The presence of liver abscesses (due mainly to ascaris and to amoebiasis) is generally not diagnosed except where health professionals are alerted by post-mortem findings (Fig. 7.6) (Jelliffe and Stanfield 1970; Scragg 1960).

Older vermifuges were toxic and needed

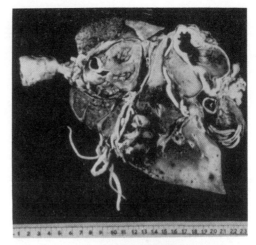

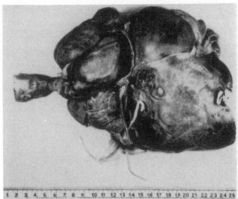

Figure 7.6. Ascaris, a cause of malnutrition. A child of about 6 years, admitted with emaciation and in extremis, died in two hours. At post-mortem, the internal organs were found to contain many ascaris. They were present in the thorax, pericardium, and peritoneum and were forming liver abscesses. This condition could not even be imagined without an autopsy. The child had been diagnosed as malnourished. Photographs by the late Dr. L. S. de Silva, Singapore (1937).

to be used with care. The real need has always been the availability of a cheap single dose of a tasteless wide spectrum antihelminthic drug. This has not been achieved completely, but mebendazole and similar compounds are effective against most major intestinal helminths (WHO 1990*b*).

Preventive measures (Jelliffe 1970) must

be modified according to the environment and the life history of the various types of parasite. The following preventive measures are helpful:

1. Improved personal and domestic hygiene in the homes, especially hand washing.
2. Improved environmental hygiene and housing, water supply, and excreta disposal.
3. Improved nutritional knowledge of markets, food handling, meat inspection, and food preparation and presentation, especially for fruit and vegetables. Thorough cooking of meat and fish for prevention of hydatid and other tapeworms.
4. Protection of skin from infected soil (use of shoes or sandals). Introduction of playpens, a railed-off corner of the veranda, or other safety area for toddlers.
5. Supervision, advice, and treatment readily available in health centers and homes.
6. Precautions with respect to domestic (dogs and cats) and farm (cattle, pigs, and sheep) animals that may be vectors or hosts for some infestations.
7. Countries where schistosomiasis is a threat or a problem must give a great deal of attention to protection of their water supplies. As in other matters, the excretory practices of the public determine the efficacy of protection.

Tuberculosis. In young children, tuberculosis is clinically different from the infection in older children and adults. There are also management problems peculiar to the young child, and signs and symptoms are indefinite and nonspecific. Many patients, particularly those with malnutrition, may give false negative tuberculin reactions. Sometimes tuberculosis presents as a loss of weight, even in the absence of obvious malnutrition or poor food intake. At other times, it is the cause of a prolonged fever or a bronchopneu-

monia that fails to clear. Often the onset of tuberculosis in children is masked by malnutrition or an acute infection, particularly measles.

Because tuberculosis is not easy to diagnose in children, it is easily missed. Therefore, all admissions to the children's ward should be routinely screened for tuberculosis. BCG (bacille Calmetle-Guérin) vaccination can be used as a diagnostic test. Positive cases should be followed up in the homes, and contacts diagnosed and, if possible, treated. Spitting habits must be controlled, though this may involve great effort.

On both economic and humanitarian grounds, prevention is the logical approach to tuberculosis. Case finding, diagnosis, and treatment must be pursued. In high-risk populations, BCG vaccination may be advised for newborn infants as a routine measure. If a baby is born to a sputum-positive mother, lactation can be maintained, with the baby vaccinated, and given prophylactic izoniazid.

Tuberculosis is still widespread in many poverty areas, especially urban slums, where rates are much higher than in the rest of the city (Ebrahim 1983). Findings of a tuberculosis prevention trial in India raised doubts about the effectiveness of BCG as a preventive measure (Tuberculosis prevention trial 1979). A WHO committee has recommended that BCG vaccination be undertaken only after an epidemiological review. If 5 or more percent of children between 10 and 14 years have been affected, BCG should be given at birth (WHO 1950). Thus the prevalence of tuberculosis in the community is an important indicator. Bhandari and Mandowara (1982) found that continued contact with a tuberculosis patient was the most important cause of tuberculosis in vaccinated children. Treatment of index cases is thus very important, and studies underscore the need for case finding through positive smears and short-term treatment with an intensive two-month, four-drug regime (izoniazid, rifampicin, purazimanide, and strepto-mycin), followed by six months of izoniazid and thiacetazone (Styblo 1983). Difficulties with ensuring treatment include cost and obtaining the individual's cooperation for this prolonged period. BCG alone does not seem to be the answer. Moreover, drug resistance has emerged as a new problem in many areas.

Malaria. Despite the emphasis of the 1950s and 1960s on worldwide malaria eradication, it is now clear that this is not practical. The expense of protection against malaria in remote, sprawling areas and the development of resistant mosquitoes and insensitive plasmodia have produced unexpected and serious complications.

In highly endemic areas, malaria is caused mainly by the parasite *Plasmodium falciparum.* The clinical picture and age affected depends on the degree of immunity in the community. In nonimmune communities, disease can occur in 4-week-old infants and presents with fever, irritability, refusal to feed, hepatosplenomegaly, anemia, unexplained jaundice, and convulsions (Choudhary et al. 1964). Usually, in hyperendemic areas, malaria is a problem between the ages of 6 months and 3 years, when children have lost the immunity acquired from the mother across the placenta and have not yet built up their own protective antibodies. During this same period, many other stresses occur, so that there is great need for supervision and medical care (Pringle 1966). Anemia is common in infants affected with malaria. Children who are transfused run the new added risk of contracting AIDS.

In nonimmune children, chemoprophylaxis is required, using the locally most effective drug whenever possible. In indigenous children in a highly endemic area, malarial suppression in early childhood may lead to interference with the development of active immunity. Probably the most logical, if dangerous, ap-proach is to treat suspected or proved cases as urgently as possible. The choice of the drug used will depend on the local situation regarding sensitivity or resistance of the plasmodia responsible.

The availability of prompt treatment, the use of mosquito nets impregnated with low-cost insect repellent, screening, and control of domestic mosquito breeding by minimizing local stagnant water sources will also help to reduce transmission. The search goes on for antimalarials to which the parasites have not yet become resistant (Lancet 1983*a*). The ancient Chinese remedy artemesinin and its derivatives offer new possibilities.

Measles. Measles and pertussis are killing diseases and conditioning infections in the etiology of malnutrition (Morley 1973). In developing countries 900,000 children die from measles each year. Malnourished and severely ill hospitalized children are most susceptible (Benenson 1980). The virus apparently does not vary in different parts of the world; any differences lie in the nutritional state of the children, in the delay in receiving medical attention, and in the presence or absence of nursing care. The main causes of severe illness in measles in children in these countries are secondary infections of the respiratory tract (including pneumonia), diarrhea, severe malnutrition (including cancrum oris), and blindness.

Measles presents a peculiarly difficult practical problem because it is extremely infectious, especially in crowded children's outpatient departments where cases are likely to convert the area into an infection center. Children with measles who require admission to hospital in the highly infectious forty-eight hours after the onset of the rash should be isolated to prevent the spread of infection to others, especially malnourished children, and also to avoid secondary infection with other organisms. In severe cases, extensive desquamation of the skin occurs, often signaling a poor prognosis.

Measles causes severe photophobia; a variety of eye damage is estimated to occur in 0.8 to 2.8 percent of cases (Koblinsky 1982). Lesions vary from photophobia to corneal ulceration and blindness. The cause is not well established in all cases, but coincidental vitamin A deficiency is the commonest. Some believe zinc may be the primary deficiency; others believe the origin is *Herpes simplex,* and still others argue it is caused by noxious agents used by traditional practitioners—for example, sourwood concoctions, which produce severe chemical conjunctivitis (Imperato 1969).

Measles is preventable through immunization with live attenuated vaccine, best given to infants between 9 and 12 months of age. In Gambia, where a heat-stable vaccine (one dose) was used, effective immunization was achieved, as ascertained through the health and growth charts carried by mothers (Hull et al. 1983). There are still problems with costs and logistics, especially maintaining the "cold chain." Recently, some African countries with high vaccine coverage levels (70 percent or more) have reported measles outbreaks. In order to prevent this disease from recurring, it has been recommended for densely populated urban communities that high doses of measles vaccine should be given at age 6 months and if necessary again at 2 years. The matter is still contentious (Cutts et al. 1991).

Whooping cough. Although it is now one of the less important diseases of temperate countries, whooping cough, or pertussis, still causes as much death and disability among children in developing countries as it once did in Europe.

Little, if any, maternal immunity is transmitted to the fetus through the placenta; in areas where children are carried on their mothers' backs, they often catch whooping cough when they are still only a few weeks old because of increased exposure. The disease is frequently unrecognized, for under the age of 1 year, children do not "whoop"; it is only the persistent nature of the cough, often with cyanotic attacks, that suggests the diagnosis. Some sticky sputum is produced, and mothers often say they have to pick it from the children's mouth. In older children, some help in diagnosis may be had from the general course of symptoms and the association of vomiting with the cough. To start with, there is a catarrhal stage, followed by a rapid spasmodic cough that is often accompanied by choking or vomiting. After this follows the true whoop.

Diagnosis is not easy, and for this reason the full mortality rate from whooping cough is unknown. Nor is it easy to tell which child will die, for a child may be sleeping peacefully on his mother's back between attacks, only to die in the next paroxysm of coughing. Convulsions in an infant with whooping cough are a serious prognostic sign and justify immediate hospital admission. Early diagnosis is essential, for in the first five days of the cough, a short course of chloramphenicol or tetracycline will often eradicate the disease. After the first week, medicine is of no avail in stopping the whoop, though penicillin may be useful in reducing secondary infection.

Like measles, the fever, anexoria, and vomiting of pertussis rapidly precipitate a child into a state of malnutrition, particularly in the first year of life. This usually can be prevented by encouraging mothers to feed their children well during the illness. They should be persuaded to give another feeding half an hour after a vomit, to give extra milk by cup and spoon, and to modify the spasms with a sedative, such as phenobarbital. Mothers should be warned about these tablets lest they are all given at once, and codeine preparations should never be used.

Nursing care is just as important in pertussis as in measles. All health workers should be able to give careful and patient advice and, if possible, practical demonstration and help in the homes to mothers and others who are looking after these ill children. Whooping cough may give rise to spasms that are terrifying for the patients and for their attendants.

The young child with whooping cough (or any other severe respiratory condition, for that matter) should not be kept shut up in a dark, overcrowded, smoke-laden hut or be carried about on an adult's back or hip. The child must be protected from rain, cold breezes, and sudden changes of temperature. Sponging down with tepid water once or twice a day will help. Clothing must be lightweight, clean, and not constricting, and the child should be kept warm. During the attack, the child may be held and comforted but never slapped on the back. Food—semisolid, and smooth, nutritious, warm or cold, and acceptable—should be given in small quantities. The child who vomits should be fed soon after so as to be able to absorb something before the next attack.

Whenever an older child is seen with pertussis, inquiries should be made about any others in the family with coughs. The others can be treated with chloramphenicol or tetracycline on the assumption that they probably have pertussis too. Immunization offers an economical, safe, and effective approach to prevention and can best be given in the first six months of life. Research is underway for a safe vaccine, such as the acellular vaccine pioneered in Japan (Kimura and Kunosaki 1991).

Other Infectious Diseases

Diphtheria. Diphtheria is unknown in some rural areas, but with increasing urbanization, cases are now occurring more frequently in many parts of developing countries. As long as routine immunizations are practiced and this is included in the DPT (diphtheria pertussis-tetanus) vaccine used, there is unlikely to be widespread infection.

Poliomyelitis. With efficient immunization with oral vaccine, the incidence of this disease should be minimal. It is usually much more common than appreciated but has some promise of being eradicated, as was the case with smallpox.

Typhoid. This is by no means rare and is once again spreading, particularly in South America. Fortunately, typhoid tends to be a milder disease in children than in adults. Children often do well if diets are maintained. Treatment with chloramphenicol is usually prescribed and generally is effective.

Cholera. In countries where cholera exists, it is extremely important to ensure adequate protection and treatment for children, for example, by breastfeeding. Failure to observe the susceptibility of children to this and similar diseases is due to the fact that so many of them die before reaching hospital that their numbers are underestimated. Early oral rehydration in cases of cholera is proving to be effective.

Rheumatic fever. This is not strictly infectious but is more common than is generally appreciated in some of the diverse ecologies covered by the word *tropics.*

Eye diseases. Severe eye diseases are often common: corneal ulcers from trauma or wind-blown sand (exacerbated by sun glare), untreated conjunctivitis (including in newborns), trachoma and xerophthalmia (severe), and vitamin A deficiency. These conditions may lead to blindness, but fortunately most are preventable (Table 7.3).

HIV infection. HIV infection, eventually manifesting as the fatal disease, AIDS, is occurring increasingly in many developing areas of the world, notably in central and east Africa and Thailand. In young children, the condition usually presents as unexplained marasmus or pneumonia,

Table 7.3. Preventive Measures for Some Common Blinding Disorders and Management at the Primary Health Care Level

Disorder	Primary prevention	Secondary prevention			Tertiary prevention
		Recognition	Initial treatment	Referral	
Trachoma	Education Hygiene Conjuctivitis treatment	Conjunctival signs of trachoma	Topical treatment (tetracycline eye ointment)	Systemic treatment of severe cases Trichiasis	Possible measures include corneal transplantation (often bad results in these circumstances) or optical iridectomy, or low vision care for optimal use of residual vision
Xerophthalmia	Breast-feeding Nutrition education Measles vaccination Vitamin A prophylaxis	Night blindness Ocular signs	High dose of vitamin A	Cases of corneal involvement	
Conjunctivitis in the newborn	Education of mother Antenatal care Prophylaxis in newborn (Credé or similar)	Acute purulent conjunctivitis	Cleansing plus topical antibiotics	Urgent referral for definitive treatment	
Corneal ulcers	Hygiene Treatment of minor trauma Awareness	Creamy spot on cornea in painful red eye	Initiate topical treatment	Urgent referral for definitive treatment	
Superficial trauma	Education and awareness Protective measures and devices	Foreign body on cornea or conjunctiva Superficial scratch on cornea	Remove foreign body Topical antibiotic treatment	Referral if severe corneal involvement (painful red eye)	

Source: Thylefors, B. (1991). *WHO Forum* 12, 78.

with inevitably fatal outcome. Children usually contract the virus transplacentally or from maternal blood or secretions during birth. In some older children, sexual spread (including rape and incest) may be the cause. In Bangkok and some other cities, HIV infection has been found in young prostitutes.

Another tragedy with AIDS is that affected children may be left as orphans if their parents die.

Controversy has arisen regarding the possible spread of HIV virus in breast milk. It is possible as a very rare occurrence, but the balance in risks clearly favors the continuation of breastfeeding rather than the dangers of bottle feeding (WHO 1992).

Skin Diseases

Infrequent or inadequate bathing because of restricted water gives a dry, inelastic quality to the skin, often with encrusted dirt, and renders it liable to infection. Inadequate fat in the diet may also affect the texture of the skin and its resistance to infection and to nutritional dermatoses. In some areas, children are overclothed in garments that are dirty and infested with lice, fleas, bedbugs, and ticks.

Skin infections occur in overcrowded and unsanitary conditions, particularly where water shortages limit washing or bathing facilities. Skin sepsis, boils, and septicemia can be a serious problem. Parents must be taught and given help to eradicate the infection in the home.

Children are particularly susceptible to leprosy. It is most important that the condition be identified and treated without delay (PATH 1989; Kinnear-Brown 1960).

Dental Care

Much human unhappiness is associated with dentition—from the time of eruption of the teeth until final extraction, and beyond. Nutrition and diet affect the teeth, but there are many other factors, including genetics.

Until recently, the intake of sweets and refined carbohydrates in traditional diets was minimal, so caries were uncommon. There were, however, a number of cases of gingivitis and pyorrhea, and quite young people (aged about 30 to 40) might become edentulous. Recently, diets in towns and especially among schoolchildren have become higher in sugar and refined foods. School dental surveys show that dental caries have increased. Infants who are bottle fed (especially those that are bottle propped) on sweetened orange juice or sweetened beverages develop rampant "feeding bottle" or "milk bottle" caries. Their teeth rot away, leaving soft, black roots (Drinnan 1973). Services directed to oral hygiene require attention and expansion and health education on bottle propping and overuse of sticky, sugary foods. Infants exclusively breast-fed do not have malocclusion (Labbok 1987).

Fluorine deficiency or excess may be a problem. When fluoride is added to the water supply in small, harmless amounts, it has a considerable proactive effect against dental caries. In large amounts it discolors teeth and causes ossification of tendons and bones.

More attention should be paid to dental hygiene education in the training of doctors, nurses, and midwives, in health education in schools, and in teacher-training colleges. The training of dental auxiliaries or hygienists, pioneered in New Zealand, was a major advance. This work should be expanded. Training should include due attention to indigenous practices, such as the use of the chewing stick (for cleaning teeth) or the Hindu ritual postmeal mouth rinse with water.

Accidents

Burns and scalds, injuries, home accidents, and poisoning are common accidents. Preventive measures promoted through health education have reduced accident rates. Burns, in particular, can cause deformity, death, and a drain on health services. They are largely preventable. Simple precautions such as fireguards, keeping toddlers and children away from cooking areas, raising fires on stones or bricks, and careful use of paraffin lamps or candles can be promoted through health education. Each area has its own hazards—the sari in India and grass skirts in Papua New Guinea that catch in open cooking fires (Sinha 1974; Buchanan 1972), for example. Through an epidemiological approach, the appropriate preventive measures for health education and identification of groups at risk can be determined (Wilson et al. 1991).

In some studies, a quarter of the burn cases occurred in children with epilepsy (Barss 1983). Epileptics are an underserved group who suffer enough without having severe burns added to their problems. In some traditional cultures, epilepsy is blamed on sorcery or witchcraft, and treatable causes of convulsions such as cysticercosis and tuberculosis are missed. If the cause of epilepsy is treatable, then fireguards alone are not enough.

Child Abuse

There is increasing awareness of child abuse and neglect (including the battered child syndrome) in developing countries, especially in urban areas. Abuse and neglect are probably partly a result of rapid urbanization and a breakdown of the traditional extended family, which in the past provided a stable, supportive community. Also, what is perceived as acceptable in one culture may be considered abuse in another. For example, Vietnamese refugees in the United States are sometimes falsely accused of child abuse because health professionals are unfamiliar with the folk medicine practice of *cao gio*, or "scratch the wind," in which a hot coin is rubbed over the skin to free the body of "bad winds," producing abrasions in linear patterns. Many traditional practices may indeed have adverse physical or psychological consequences, but they are performed in the belief that they are beneficial or necessary and are not intended to harm (Primosch and Young 1980).

The effects of child abuse are far-reaching. In urban communities in Nigeria, child neglect (a form of child abuse) can play a major role in the etiology of malnutrition (Jinadu 1980). Abusive practices of crippling, blinding, or starving in order to put a child to work as a beggar are seen in countries as diverse as Niger, Egypt, and Sri Lanka (De Silva 1981). A 2-year-old child with marasmus in Colombo, Sri Lanka, was deliberately starved by his mother for begging purposes (Fig. 7.7). His older brother (7 years old) appeared to be in robust health. Child selling is another practice that often results in abuse.

There are certain signs indicating abuse: a delay in seeking medical care, bruises and fractures in unusual places, and accident histories that do not adequately explain the injury, among others (Table 7.4). All fractures in children under 2 years of age must be viewed with suspicion, especially if in unusual areas or if multiple. Sexual assault is another form of child abuse; sexually transmitted disease or trauma to the external genitalia is strong evidence.

Individual signs are not always signif-

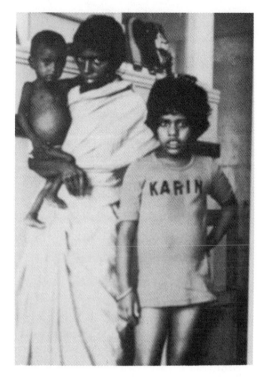

Figure 7.7. Malnutrition and child abuse. This mother and her 7 year old are in good health. The 2 year old is not; he was deliberately starved for begging purposes. Photograph courtesy of Dr. T. Branch, Sri Lanka.

icant, but clusters of signs warrant investigation of family, home, and environment (Child Protection Assessment Board 1977). The health care professional, on home visiting and speaking to neighbors, has a unique opportunity to recognize and assist abused children. Special attention must be given to the training of health professionals in the management of child abuse. It is a delicate situation, and the child will not be helped by episodic deprecatory or judgmental attitude towards the parents. The health worker must find relatives or other suitable guardians for the child while finding ways to help the abuser. Counseling and support groups are sometimes effective. Many countries have passed legislation making

Table 7.4. Selected Child Abuse Risk Factors and Indicators

Psychosocial	Family history of abuse
	Unwanted or "abnormal" pregnancy or infant
	Change in family life circumstances (alienation, single parent, stepparent)
	Alcohol or drug addiction
	Emotional stress, unemployment or economic stress
	Neonatal separation, or within first six months of life
History and observations	Unexplained injury, especially a fracture in a child under 2 years
	Inadequate or inconsistent accident history
	Parental reluctance to discuss injuries
	Suspicious history of previous accidents, repeated burns or scalds, "easy" bruising
	Evidence of neglect (repeated skin infections, dirty clothing, poor hygiene)
	Failure to thrive
	Abnormal emotional behavior ("cringe or crave")
Physical examination	Multiple abrasions, lacerations, in unusual places
	Burns, especially on buttocks or soles of feet, cigarette burns
	Bite marks, belt lashes
	Old healed lesions—burns, lacerations, old fractures
	Sexually transmitted diseases
	Head injuries

it possible to remove children from life-threatening situations.

A high percentage of prison inmates claim to have been abused as children. Usually abused children become abusive adults (Magnason et al. 1983). Failure to acknowledge child abuse as a problem is the major barrier to its prevention and treatment.

CONCLUSION

The changing pattern of diseases in children must be studied in order to organize effective services that focus on priority problems as judged by prevalence, mortality, and cost of treatment versus the prevention and feasibility of management with limited resources. Much that affects the physical, mental, and social well-being of children depends on the parents and on conditions in the home. Adolescents need to be provided with health care, and, where necessary, special programs should be designed for their problems, which may include drug addiction, unwanted pregnancies, malnutrition, and risky sexual behavior.

REFERENCES

Applebaum, R. M. (1970). The modern management of successful breast feeding. *Pediat. Clin. N. Am.* **17**, 203.

Bang, A. T., et al. (1990). Reduction in pneumonia mortality and total childhood mortality by means of a community-based intervention trial in Gadchiroli, India. *Lancet* **336**(8079), 201.

Barss, K., and Wallace, K. (1983). Grass-skirt burns in Papua New Guinea. *Lancet* **1**, 733.

Baumslag, N.; Mason, L. G.; Davis, R.; and Sabin, E. (1979). *Diarrheal Disease and Oral Rehydration: Education, and Welfare.* Office of International Health, Washington, D.C.

Baumslag, N.; Edelstein, T.; and Metz, J. (1970). Reduction of the incidence of prematurity by folic acid supplementation in pregnancy. *Brit. Med. J.* **1**, 16.

Benenson, A. S., ed. (1980). *Control of Communicable Disease in Man.* 13th ed. American Public Health Association, Washington, D.C.

Bennett, F. J., ed. (1979). *Community and Health Action—A Manual for Tropical and Rural Areas.* Macmillan, London.

Bhandari, B., and Mandowara, S. L. (1982). A study of tuberculosis in BCG vaccinated children. *Indian Pediat.* **19**, 865.

Black, R. E. (1991). *Prevention of Pneumonia Morbidity or Mortality by Interventions*

Against Host Risk Factors. Prepared for the International Consultation on Control of Acute Respiratory Infections, Washington, D.C.

Blair, P. (1992). *Integrated Child Development Services*. USAID, Washington, D.C.

Brown, R. E. and Sandhu, T. S. (1966). Autopsy survey of perinatal deaths in Uganda. *Trop. Geogr. Med.* **18**, 292.

Buchanan, R. C. (1972). The causes and prevention of burns in Malawi. *Cent. Afr. J. Med.* **18**, 55.

Chalmers, I. (1980). Better perinatal health Shanghai. *Lancet* **i**, 1–37.

Child Protection Assessment Board (1977). Suspected non-accidental injury, child abuse or neglect. *Aus. Fam. Physician* **6**, 1179.

Child Survival (1992). *A Seventh Report to Congress on the USAID Program*. USAID, Washington, D.C.

Choudhary, S. P.; Dabi, D. R.; Sing, R. N.; Theraja, S. L.; and Dammin, G. J. (1964). The pathogenesis of diarrhea. Disease in early life. *Bull. Wld. Hlth. Org.* **31**, 29.

Cutts, F. T.; Henderson, R. H.; Clements, C. I.; Chen, R. T.; and Patriarca, P. A. (1991). Update. Principles of measles control. *Bull. Wld. Hlth. Org.* **69**(1), 1–7.

Dammin, G. J. (1964). The pathogenesis of diarrhoea. Disease in early life. *Bull. Wld. Hlth. Org.* **31**, 29.

De Silva, C. C.; Fernando, P. V. D.; and Gunaratne, C. D. H. (1962). The search for a prematurity level in Colombo. *Ceylon, J. Trop. Pediat.* **8**, 29.

De Silva, L. S. (1948). Ascariasis and its dangers. *Med. J. Malaya* **3**, 41.

De Silva, W. (1981). Some cultural and economic factors leading to neglect, abuse and violence in respect of children within the family in Sri Lanka. *Child Abuse and Neglect* **5**, 391.

Drinnan, A. (1973). Family dentistry. In *Family Care*. Ed. N. Baumslag. Williams and Wilkins, Baltimore.

du Florey, V. C.; Burney, P.; D'Souza, J.; Scrivens, E.; and West, P. (1983). *An Introduction to Community Medicine*. Churchill Livingstone, Edinburgh.

Ebrahim, G. J. (1979). *Care of the Newborn in Developing Countries*. Macmillan, London.

Ebrahim, G. J. (1982). *Child Health in a Changing Environment*. Macmillan, London.

Ebrahim, G. J. (1983). Editorial: Primary care and the urban poor. *J. Trop. Pediat.* **29**, i.

Egsmose, T. (1969). *Epidemiological Studies of Some Tuberculosis Control Measures in a Developing Country*. Munksgaard, Copenhagen.

Elliott, K. and Attawell, K. (1990). *Cereal Based Oral Rehydration Therapy for Diarrhea*. International Child Health Foundation, Columbia, Md.

Geber, M. and Dean, R. F. A. (1958). Psychomotor development in African children: The effects of social class and the need for improved tests. *Bull. Wld. Hlth. Org.* **18**, 421.

Gordon, J. E.; Behar, M.; and Scrimshaw, N. S. (1964). Acute diarrhoeal disease in less developed countries, 3. Methods for prevention and control. *Bull. Wld. Hlth. Org.* **31**, 21.

Grant, J. (1984). *The State of the World's Children*. UNICEF, New York.

Grant, L. S., et al. (1963). A survey of parasitic infection in two communities in Jamaica and a drug trial on positive cases. *W. Ind. Med. J.* **12**, 185.

Gunn, R. (1979). *Cholera in Bahrain: Bottle Feeding as a Risk Factor in Infant Cholera*. 28th Annual Epidemic Intelligence Service Conference, Center for Disease Control, Atlanta.

Hagberg, B.; Hagberg, G.; and Oslow, I. (1975). The changing panorama of cerebral palsy in Sweden, 1954–70. *Acta Pediat. Scand.* **64**, 187.

Hallman, M.; Bry, K.; Hoppu, K.; Lappi, M.; and Pohjavuori, M. (1992). Inositol supplementation in premature infants with respiratory distress syndrome. *New England J. Med.* **326**(19), 1233.

Hull, H. F.; Williams, P. J.; and Oldfield, F. (1983). Measles mortality and vaccine efficacy in rural West Africa. *Lancet* **i**, 972.

Imperato, P. J. (1969). Traditional attitudes towards measles in the Republic of Mali. *Trans. R. Soc. Trop. Med. Hyg.* **63**, 768.

Isely, R. B. (1982). Evaluating the role of health education strategies in the prevention of diarrhoea and dehydration. *J. Trop. Pediat.* **28**, 253.

Jelliffe, D. B. (1967). *Prematurity in Obstetrics and Gynaecology in the Tropics and Developing Countries*. Edward Arnold, London.

Jelliffe, D. B. (1992). *Child Health in the Tropics*. 6th ed. Edward Arnold, London.

Jelliffe, D. B., and Jelliffe, E. F. P. (1978*a*). Worldwide care of the mother and the new-born child. *Clin. Obstet. Gynec.* **5**, 64.

Jelliffe, D. B., and Jelliffe, E. F. P. (1978*b*). *Human Milk in the Modern World*. Oxford University Press, Oxford.

Jelliffe, D. B., and Jelliffe, E. F. P. (1989*a*). *Dietary Management of Young Children with Acute Diarrhea*. World Health Organization, Geneva.

Jelliffe, D. B., and Jelliffe, E. F. P. (1989*b*). *Community Nutrition Assessment*. Oxford University Press, Oxford.

Jelliffe, D. B., and Stanfield, P., eds. (1970). *Diseases of Children in the Subtropics and Tropics*. 3d ed. Edward Arnold, London.

Jelliffe, E. F. P. (1968). Low birth-weight and malarial infection of the placenta. *Bull. Wld. Hlth. Org.* **38**, 69.

Jinadu, M. K. (1980). The role of neglect in the aetiology of protein-energy malnutrition in urban communities of Nigeria. *Child Abuse and Neglect* **4**, 227.

Kahn, E.; Wayburne, S.; and Fouche, M. (1954). The Baragwanath Premature Baby Unit—An analysis of the case records of 1000 consecutive admissions. *S. Afr. Med. J.* **28**(45), 3.

Kimura, M., and Kunosaki, H. (1991). Pertussis vaccines in Japan—A clue toward understanding of Japanese attitudes to vaccines. *J. Trop. Pediat.* **37**(1), 45.

King, M.; King, F.; and Martodipoero, S. (1978). *Primary Child Care: A Manual for Health Workers*. Oxford University Press, Oxford.

Kinnear-Brown, J. A. (1960). The role of leprosaria and treatment villages in mass campaigns in tropical Africa. *Int. J. Leprosy* **28**, 1.

Koblinsky, M. A. (1982). *Severe Measles and Measles Blindness*. Prepared for USAID Office of Nutrition, by International Center for Epidemiologic and Preventive Opthamology, Johns Hopkins University, Baltimore.

Kretchmer, N. (1969). Child health in the developing world. *Pediatrics* **43**, 4.

Kumari, S.; Pruthi, P. K.; Mehra, M. D.; and Gujral, V. V. (1983). Infection scoring in early neonatal infection. *Ind. J. Pediat.* **50**, 177.

Labbok, M. H., and Hendershot, G. E. (1987). Does breastfeeding protect against malocclusion? An Analysis of the 1981 child health supplement to the National Health Interview Survey. *Am. J. Prev. Med.* **3**, 227.

Latham, M., et al. (1986). Infant feeding in urban Kenya: A pattern of early triple nipple feeding. *J. Trop. Pediat.* **32**(6), 276.

Lancet (1983*a*). Editorial: Malaria control and primary care. *Lancet* **i**, 963.

Lancet (1983*b*). Editorial: Prevention of neonatal tetanus. *Lancet* **i**, 1253.

Lechtig, A.; Habicht, J. P.; Delgado, H.; Klein, R. E.; Yarborugh, C.; and Martorell, R. (1975). Effect of food supplementation during pregnancy on birth weight. *J. Pediat.* **56**, 508.

Longo, L. W. (1982). The health consequences of maternal smoking: Experimental studies and public policy recommendations. In *Alternative Dietary Practices and Nutritional Abuses in Pregnancy*, pp. 135–9. Food and Nutrition Board, Committee on Nutrition of the Mother and Pre-School Child, National Academy Press, Washington, D.C.

McClelland, D. B. I.; McGrath, J.; and Samson, R. R. (1978). Antimicrobial factors in human milk. *Acta Paediat. Scand.*, Special Suppl. **271**, 1–20.

McCord, C. (1979). *Oral Fluid Treatment for Diarrhea in Menoufia Governorate, Egypt*. Report from the American Public Health Association, Washington, D.C.

McCracken, R. (1970). Origins and implications of the distribution of adult lactase deficiency in human populations. *J. Trop. Pediat.* **17**, 7.

McKigney, J. I. (1968). Economic aspects of infant feeding practices in the West Indies. *J. Trop. Pediat.* **14**, 55.

Magnason, E.; Grant, M.; and Wilde, J. (1983). Child abuse: The ultimate betrayal. *Time*, September 5.

Mata, Leonardo, J. (1978). *The Children of Santa Maria Cauque: A Prospective Field Study of Health and Growth*. MIT Press, Cambridge.

Mata, L. J.; Urrutia, J. J.; and Gordon, J. E. (1965). Diarrhoeal disease in a cohort of Guatemalan village children. *Trop. Geogr. Med.* **19**, 247.

MMWR (1982). *Morbidity and Mortality Report* **3**, 31.

Molla, A. M.; Molla, A.; Nath, S.; and Khatun, M. (1989). Food based oral rehydration salt solutions for acute childhood diarrhoea. *Lancet* **ii**, 429.

Morley, D. C. (1973). *Pediatric Priorities in Developing Countries*. Butterworth, London.

Morley, D.; Woodland, M.; and Martin, W. J. (1961). Measles in Nigerian children. *J. Hyg. (Lond.)* **61**, 115.

Naeye, R. L.; Tafari, N.; Marnoe, C. C.; and Judge, D. M. (1979). Causes of perinatal mortality in an African city. *Bull. Wld. Hlth. Org.* **5**(7), 63.

NCHS (1992). Death rates and the percentage of total death rates for the 15 leading causes of death: United States 1989. *Monthly Vital Statistics Report, Maryland* **40**(8), Suppl. 2, 5.

NIH (1989). *Infant Mortality 1989 Research Accomplishments.* National Institutes of Health, Bethesda, Md.

PAHO (1982). *Health Conditions in the Americas 1977–1980.* Scientific Publication no. 427, Pan American Health Organization, Washington, D.C.

PAHO (1990). *Health Conditions in the Americas.* 2 vols. Pan American Sanitary Bureau, Pan American Health Organization, Washington, D.C.

PATH (1989) Leprosy. *Health Technology Directions* **9**(3), 1 (on disc).

Patra, F. C.; Mahalanabis, D.; Jalan, K. N.; Sen, A.; and Banerjee, P. (1982). Is oral rice electrolyte solution superior to glucose electrolyte solution in infantile diarrhoea? *Arch. Dis. Childhd.* **57**, 910.

Payne, D.; Grab, B.; Fontraine, R. E.; and Hempal, J. H. G. (1976). Impact of control measures on malaria transmission and general mortality. *Bull. Wld. Hlth. Org.* **54**, 368.

Pittard, W. B. (1979). Breast milk immunology—A frontier of infant nutrition. *Amer. J. Dis. Child.* **133**, 83.

Pomerance, J. J.; Ukrainski, C. T.; Ukra, T.; Henderson, T. H.; Nash, A. H.; and Meredith, J. L. (1978). Cost of living for infants weighing 1000g or less at birth. *Pediatrics* **61**, 908.

Primosch, R. E., and Young, S. K. (1980). Pseudobattering of Vietnamese children (Cao Gio). *J. Amer. Dent. Asso.* **101**, 47.

Pringle, G. (1966). The effect of social factors in reducing the intensity of malaria transmission in coastal East Africa. *Trans. Roy. Soc. Trop. Med. Hyg.* **60**, 549.

Puffer, R. R., and Serrano, C. V. (1973). *Patterns of Mortality in Childhood.* PAHO Scientific Publication no. 262. PAHO/WHO, Washington, D.C.

Rosa, F. W., and Turshen, M. (1970). Fetal nutrition. *Bull. Wld. Hlth. Org.* **43**, 785.

Schofield, F. D.; Tucker, V. M.; and Westbrook, G. R. (1961). Neonatal tetanus in New Guinea. Effect of active immunization in pregnancy. *Brit. Med. J.* **2**, 785.

Scragg, J. (1960). Amoebic liver abscess in children. *Arch. Dis. Childhd.* **3**(5), 171.

Simmonds, S.; Vaughan, P.; and Gunn, S. W. (1983). *Refugee Community Health Care.* Oxford University Press, Oxford.

Sinha, R. N. (1974). Burns in tropical countries. *Clin. Plastic Surg.* **1**, 121.

Sterky, G., and Mellander, L., eds. (1978). *Birthweight Distribution—An Indicator of Social Development.* SAREC Report no. R:2. Stockholm.

Styblo, K. (1983). Tuberculosis and its control: Lessons to be learned from past experience, and implications for leprosy control programmes. *Ethiop. Med. J.* **21**, 101.

Tafari, N. (1978). Prime causes of perinatal mortality in a developing society. In *Birth Weight Distribution—An Indicator of Social Development*, pp. 20–28. Ed. G. Sterky and L. Mellander. SAREC Report no. R:2. Stockholm.

Thylefors, B. (1991). Preventing Blindness. *WHO Forum* **12**, 78.

Tuberculosis prevention trial (1979). Madras trial of BCG vaccines in South India for tuberculosis prevention. *Ind. J. Med. Res.* **70**, 349.

USDHEW (1979). *Smoking and Health.* Report of the Surgeon-General, U.S. Department of Health, Education and Welfare, U.S. Public Health Service Publication no. (PHS) 79-50066. Washington, D.C.

Werner, D., and Bower, B. (1982). *Helping Health Workers Learn: A Book of Methods, Aids, and Ideas for Instructors at the Village Level.* Hesperian Foundation, Palo Alto, Calif.

Werner, D., and Bower, B. (1992). *Helping Health Workers Learn.* 2d ed. Hesperian Foundation, Palo Alto, Calif.

Williams, C. D. (1938). Child health in the Gold Coast. *Lancet* **i**, 97.

Williams, C. D. (1946). Rickets in Singapore. *Arch. Dis. Childhd.* **21**, 37.

Wilson, M. H.; Baker, S.; Teret S. P.; Shock, S.; and Garbarino, J. (1991). *Saving Children.* Oxford University Press, New York.

Wiseman, G. (1964). *Absorption from the Intestine*. New York.

WHO (1950). *Report of the Expert Group on Prematurity*. Wld. Hlth. Org. Tech. Rep. Ser., no. 217.

WHO (1961). *Public Health Aspects of Low Birth Weight*. Wld. Hlth. Org. Tech. Rep. Ser., no. 217.

WHO (1970). *Genetic Factors in Congenital Malformations*. Wld. Hlth. Org. Tech. Rep. Ser., no. 438.

WHO (1980*a*). *WHO—BCG Vaccination Policies, Report of a WHO Study Group*. Wld. Hlth. Org. Tech. Rep. Ser., no. 652.

WHO (1980*b*). *Sixth Report on the World Health Situation, 1973–1977. Pt. 1: Global Analysis*. World Health Organization, Geneva.

WHO (1990*a*). *The Rational Use of Drugs in the Management of Acute Diarrhoea in Children*. World Health Organization, Geneva.

WHO (1990*b*). *Drugs Used in Parasitic Diseases*. World Health Organization, Geneva.

WHO (1990*c*). *Acute Respiratory Infections*. World Health Organization, Geneva.

WHO (1991*a*). *Child Health and Development*. Health of the Newborn EB 89/26. World Health Organization, Geneva.

WHO (1991*b*). *Technical Bases for the WHO Recommendations on the Management of Pneumonia in Children at First Level Health Facilities*. World Health Organization, Geneva.

WHO (1992). *Implementation of the Global Strategy for Health for All by the Year 2000*. 2d ed. World Health Organization, Geneva.

Worthington-Roberts, B. S.; Vermeersch, J.; and Williams, S. R. (1981). *Nutrition in Pregnancy and Lactation*. 2d ed. C. V. Mosby, St. Louis.

Zurbrigg, S. (1984). *Rakku's Story: Structures of Ill-Health and the Source of Chance*. George Joseph Publishers, Madras, India.

8

Nutrition and Malnutrition

*If you learn your "nutrition" from a biochemist, you are not
likely to learn how essential it is to blow a baby's nose before
expecting him to suck. Or to realize that a child needs cuddling
just as much as calories.*
CICELY D. WILLIAMS, 1973

The subject of nutrition is of universal importance in sickness and in health, physically, mentally, and socially. It is economically urgent. Most of humankind's struggles over the centuries have been to secure food for individuals and their families.

Hunger is the most innate of urges, yet the differences among hunger, fasting, starvation, food shortages, imbalance, and greed are poorly described and ill understood. Nothing promotes a sense of security more than a meal of accustomed food. Apart from biochemistry, nutrition plays very little part in the training of doctors and nurses. Medical training is shaped in the well-fed countries, where nutrition studies concentrate on rare metabolic disturbances, adequate nutrition is (wrongly) taken for granted, and abnormalities are more commonly related to excessive intakes of calories, sugar, and fat ("malnutrition plus"). Biochemistry is a respectable intellectual subject, while clinical malnutrition, especially community aspects of nutrition, is often complicated and

imprecise and holds little academic prestige.

Problems of malnutrition mostly occur in developing or politically unstable countries. Malnutrition is often the result of a number of adverse factors, all of which need to be identified. If prevention is to be the goal, the causes of malnutrition in communities served and in individuals need investigation.

In the United States, national board examinations for medical students contain few questions on infant feeding and nutrition. Government health documents worldwide often pay very little attention to nutrition. For example, a 135-page manual on nutrition published some time ago by the Ministry of Agriculture, Fisheries and Food in the United Kingdom devoted only three-quarters of a page to malnutrition. In medical schools globally, little attention is paid to clinical nutrition except high-tech parenteral nutrition.

Great advances have been made in the biochemistry of nutrition and in the potential of food production since 1970s, but in spite of extensive undertakings in nutrition research in underprivileged areas, there is little evidence of improvement in nutrition status among children or in the nutrition training of medical and auxiliary staff. In fact, child health improves in areas where there are good services—for example Singapore, Kerala State, Costa Rica, and Cuba—and not just where nutrition is researched. Child health has improved due to more equitable allocation of resources.

The main problem is that many experts are willing to study the food but not the consumer. They are inclined to spend a great deal of time in laboratories and not nearly enough time in wards observing the features or the attitudes of sick babies, and less time still in the homes listening to those who grow, provide, and prepare the food. Until this pattern of behavior is changed, health professionals will continue to be ignorant of the community's nutrition and deliver expensive and often damaging feeding programs (Fig. 8.1).

The business of the young is to grow and mature; the growth cannot take place without food. For the young, therefore, the digestive system is especially important and determines a much larger proportion of the total physiological economy than it does in an adult. During intrauterine life, nutrients for life, growth, and development are supplied by the umbilical vessels. A dramatic change takes place at birth when the circulation is rerouted; the lungs instead of the umbilical vessels become responsible for ventilation, and the digestive system takes over the whole vast problem of nutrition. Nature has provided mammals with specialized nutriment for infants, and science has been unable to improve on this fluid or even come close, though vast efforts have been made to reproduce or to synthesize breast milk.

The progress from a milk to an adult diet is apparently just as hazardous as from the uterus to milk, probably because it is more prolonged and subject to human vagaries and control. Few human beings go through life without occasional attacks of colic, "indigestion," or worse. In young children, gastrointestinal problems, especially diarrhea and vomiting, if not prevented or treated early, can easily cause mortality from dehydration. In addition, serious gastrointestinal conditions—for example, intussusception, rectal prolapse, intestinal obstruction—are more common in young children (Williams 1962).

BIOLOGICAL NEEDS

The young have comparatively higher requirements than adults for all nutrients—including calories, minerals, vitamins, and protein (Jelliffe 1968). Because they have to develop their body tissues rapidly, they have a relatively higher need for protein and for the various building blocks necessary for growth and development. If growth is rapid, there is a high demand for all nutrients, including vitamins. The baby who is fat and growing fast may develop the most severe form of rickets or beriberi if the proportion of vitamins and other nutrients is unbalanced. In the young, dehydration or hypoglycemia occurs all too readily. The young have high demands and slender reserves, but if changes are introduced gradually, they adapt. Absorption may become more efficient, metabolism more economical, and bowel activity more orderly (Booyens and McCance 1957).

In subacute and chronic cases of malnutrition, the body may respond by adapting to a diet astonishingly low in protein, without obvious damage and even without growth retardation. In kwashiorkor, the muscle mass is consumed to supply the metabolic need for protein. Immunologically the young child is outgrowing the passive immunity endowed by the mother and is acquiring his or her own. This period is fraught with a multitude of signs and symptoms that are

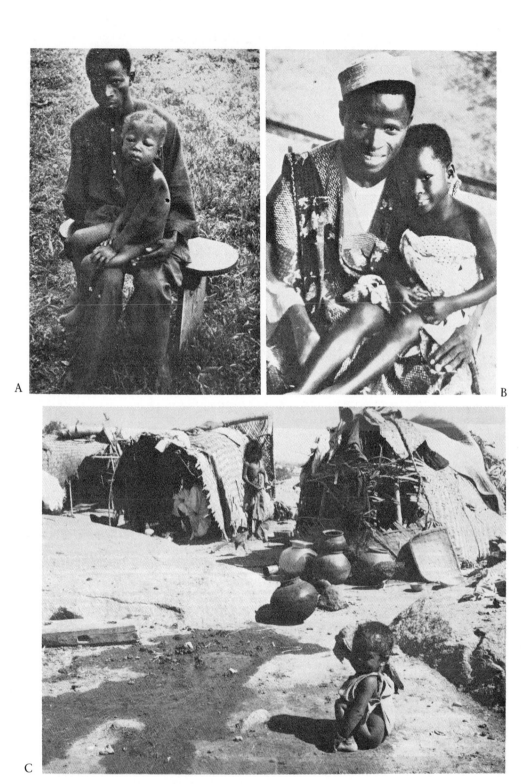

Figure 8.1. Good and bad nutrition. Chronic severe case of kwashiorkor in Western Nigeria: before (A) and after (B) five months of treatment. Note the father's expression. Photographs by David Morley. (C) This child remains in good health while being breastfed, but the environment will be a source of concern as soon as weaning begins. UNICEF photograph, India.

difficult to explain and treat but unwise to ignore. The need to produce immunoglobulins further increases the demand for special nutrients. It is certain that many children who go through periods of failure to thrive, to the distraction of all interested parties, may grow up normal and even exceptionally tough. Children who are deprived of proper nourishment, particularly early in the first year or in fetal life, may suffer some restriction of mental development.

In most parts of the world, urbanization is on the increase. Currently more than one-third of all children in the developing world live in urban slums under appalling conditions—overcrowded shacks, no safe water, rudimentary sanitation, and poor health services—despite their proximity to relatively sophisticated health care. In these areas, the incidence of child malnutrition is high, particularly of marasmus, notably associated with the trend to expensive bottle feeding, heavily advertised by formula manufacturers, which many people cannot afford (Fig. 8.2). The problem is compounded by the change to easily stored refined flours and the transition from a largely food-growing livelihood to a mainly cash economy (Jelliffe 1985). A study in the southern highlands of Tanzania showed an increase in malnutrition when there was a change from subsistence farming to cash cropping. Nutritional levels were highest among families who still clung to a subsistence economy. Earnings had to exceed a certain level before the nutrition status improved (Fig. 8.3). Cash croppers used earnings to purchase alcohol, shoes, radios, and tin roofs; family food purchase was a secondary consideration (Jacobsen 1978).

Projections for the year 2000 indicate that more than half the urban population worldwide will be living in slums. The health situation will worsen unless a concerted effort is made to provide continuous basic services, especially to vulnerable groups. Urgent measures are needed, for when a population is demoralized, it is far more difficult to assist.

INDIVIDUAL VARIATIONS

Animals vary enormously in their conversion factors, or ability to metabolize grass or fodder into milk or their bodies. The same applies to human beings, even those in the same family, brought up on the same food and exposed to the same diseases, environmental hazards, and psychological stresses.

Nutrition demands vary from time to time in the same individual, according to age, activity, and endocrine and physiological or pathological changes (Fig. 8.4) (Beaton 1983; Booyens 1957; Keen 1979). The saying that one man's meat is another man's poison is true. Individual variations are just as important as, and perhaps more so than, biochemical analysis. A baby with a low blood sugar of 50 milligrams may show symptoms and signs of hypoglycemia, while another with a blood sugar of 60 milligrams may show neither. On the other hand, a malnourished child who has been inoculated for tuberculosis may not convert from negative to positive until his or her nutritional state improves.

HABITUATION

Survival to adulthood indicates that the individual has become accustomed to certain prevailing diets and environmental hazards. Habituation depends on food availability, domestic or tribal and cultural traditions, and individual variations. It is extremely rare to find a baby who has difficulty in getting used to mother's milk (though he or she always has to get used to the mother as a person). It is not so rare to find children who begin by rejecting cow's milk or other foods until they become habituated. The weaning period is always a

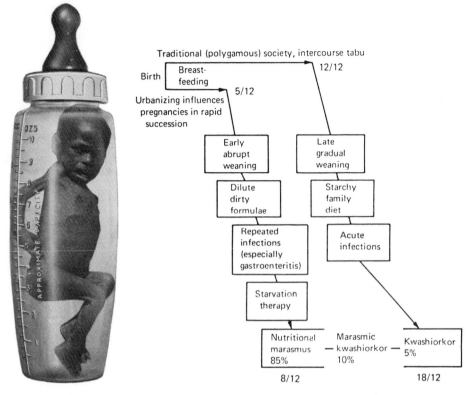

Figure 8.2. Relationship of malnutrition and early cessation of breastfeeding. Sources: Chetley (1979); McLaren (1966).

time of some anxiety, and sometimes may be hazardous or even disastrous.

There has been much discussion about lactase deficiency in African and other children, but lactase deficiency is not prevalent among the Hausa, Masai, Wag-

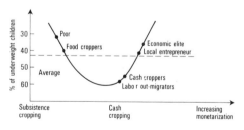

Figure 8.3. Malnutrition and economics. The proportion of underweight children, and thus those with malnutrition, increases as farmers move from subsistence to cash cropping and monetarization. Source: Jacobsen (1978).

ogo, Ankole, and other African tribes who keep cattle. In some areas in Africa, probably because of the tsetse fly or other pests, there are no cattle. If animal milk, a customary traditional food, is unavailable, lactase deficiency will be found in a proportion of older children and adults. Some children are conservative in their food habits, and their unwillingness to try new foods may produce physiological limitations.

Another example of habituation has been reported as a form of child abuse in malnourished infants in England receiving fad diets (Roberts 1979). In these cases, the adults appeared normal, but their infants or children fed on macrobiotic diets were not only in a wretched condition but also B_{12} deficient, with neurological signs and symptoms. Even

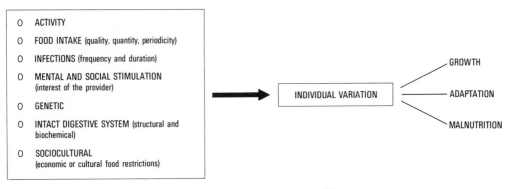

Figure 8.4. Nutrition status modifiers.

in a technologically sophisticated country like England, improved nutrition knowledge and monitoring are essential.

Lacto-vegetarians and even vegans know that this form of diet can be satisfactory if it is balanced and carefully prepared, if adequate in amount, and if the vulnerable groups are well supervised. It has been found that the local Indian bread (chapati) can be used as part of a suitable weaning diet if it is soaked in water. Some of these unusual diets may show a highly satisfactory nutrient analysis, but the form in which they are presented may be unsuitable for the young.

DIGESTION AND ABSORPTION

All food introduced by mouth is subject to a large number of processes. Human beings vary greatly in the efficiency of these processes, which depend on, for example, healthy gums, teeth, mucosa, and digestive organs. Infective, degenerative, and genetic conditions, as well as the character of the food and even the emotional atmosphere in which food is eaten, affect the physiological processes.

It is possible to measure food intake with some accuracy, but variation in the combined processes of mastication, deglutition, fermentation, digestion, absorption, metabolism, and excretion is

not easy to measure. A considerable proportion of the nutrients may be lost with the feces. It is known that some pigs on farms in Asia and sleigh dogs in the Arctic may depend in part on human feces for their food. To a certain extent, food-deficient communities can adapt to food shortage by physiologically increased food absorption and utilization. Limitation of food intake may, in itself, lead to improved powers of absorption, as well as to economy of metabolism in ways not currently understood.

The most careful analysis of food composition and body composition will not improve nutrition. The most useful guide to the state of nutrition is to examine the patient and make certain the diet is adequate. It is also necessary to examine carefully all the causes leading to malnutrition (Fig. 8.5) and to provide continuity of care and supervision for children during the years of growth and development aimed at the most significant risks.

THE DIMENSION OF THE PROBLEM

The question of the magnitude and cost of the nutritional problems affecting young children is complicated by different classifications of malnutrition and by diver-

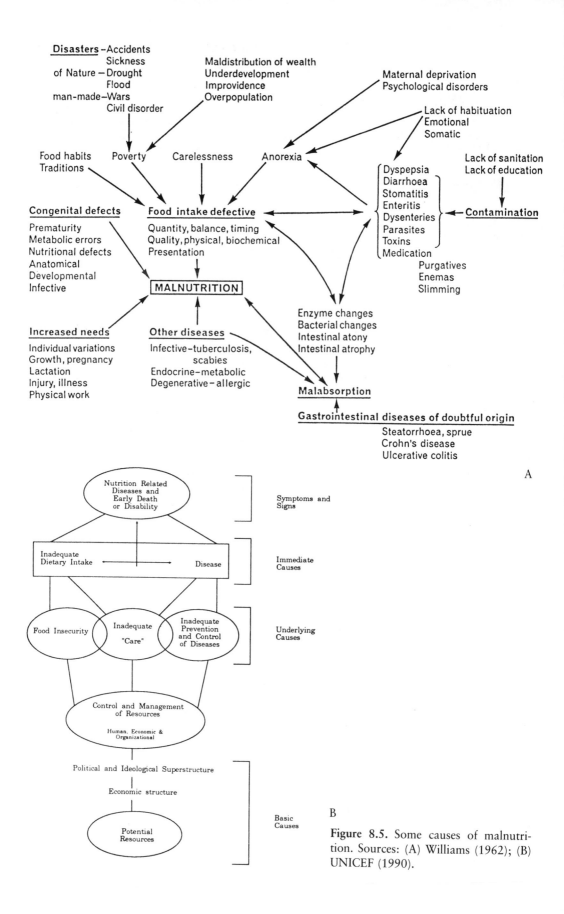

Figure 8.5. Some causes of malnutrition. Sources: (A) Williams (1962); (B) UNICEF (1990).

gences in the definition of age groups. Most workers use the term *preschool child* for the postinfancy period of 1 to 4 years. However, some include all children from birth to the fifth birthday; to others, the group may be defined as beginning at the second birthday; and to still others, the period may be extended up to the seventh birthday (Jelliffe 1968, 1992). And certainly the term *preschool child* is unsatisfactory in areas where a high percentage of children never go to school. Moreover, the risks and problems during the usually prescribed period of 1 to 4 years are by no means uniform within this age span or from region to region.

Basic to the problem is the fact that sometimes in early life young children are in a transitional state both biologically and culturally (Jelliffe and Jelliffe 1990). They have moved from the protection of fetal life, both uterine and exterogestate, but have not yet acquired biological and developmental protection against the hostile environment that enables older children and adults to live in balance with the local ecology. It may be a time of multiple stresses; even the most apparently fit may not survive. Some of the pathological processes are no more selective than an earthquake or a war.

The dominance of malnutrition in child health in less developed regions cannot be overestimated. The high incidence of cases of gross malnutrition admitted to hospital wards in some countries is paralleled only by a large number of severe cases who never reach modern medical care and by a very much greater occurrence of moderately affected children in the community itself, both receiving and not receiving health services. It is common for 20 percent of pediatric admissions to be suffering from severe malnutrition in the form of kwashiorkor or marasmus, and for one- to two-thirds or more of the young-child population at large to show marked failure to thrive and growth retardation—for example,

weight-for-height levels below the third percentile (approximately 80 percent of reference level) (Jelliffe and Jelliffe 1990a). In the developing world, one in three children remains malnourished, and this commutes to 60 percent of child deaths (USAID 1992).

Malnutrition is responsible for millions of deaths annually, not only directly but in combination with or as a result of multiple infections (Tomkins 1989). The diagnostic label given will often be arbitrary and reflect the interests or preconceived ideas of the particular group in which the death occurs. In fact, many children admitted with infections or diarrhea are also malnourished, and the cause of admission to hospital or of death should always list all the conditions present, preferably with an attempted assessment of the primary and the secondary causes (Table 8.1).

Cumulative stresses in fact operate in the etiology of most forms of malnutrition in this age group. Severe anemia, a common and important hospital problem, is frequently due to multiple causes, including malnutrition, infections, worms, and malaria. "Weaning" diarrhea is the end result of varying mixtures of alimentary infection, malnutrition, maldigestion, and poorly absorbed diet. It must always be borne in mind that there is individual, and possibly community, variation in nutrient need and metabolic efficiency and also that an excessive dietary intake may lead ultimately to obesity, diabetes, gout, cardiac disease, and, particularly in early years, allergic disorders. Allergy and obesity are now tending to be seen in children of the urban elite.

It is not surprising that supplementary feeding programs, even large-scale ones, have generally had disappointing results. Except in cases of disaster, malnutrition calls for individual and community investigation and for management of the causes responsible locally rather than for mass feeding programs.

Table 8.1. Analysis of Diseases, Childrens Wards, Singapore General Hospital, August 1937–July 1938

	Primary				Secondary			
	Ages 0–1 year		Ages 1–6 years		Ages 0–1 year		Ages 1–6 years	
	Admission	Died	Admission	Died	Admission	Died	Admission	Died
Respiratory diseases	312	179	114	54	338	328	83	66
Malnutrition	93	60	34	24	5	3	5	4
Keratomalacia	3	3	9	1	6	4	2	
Beriberi	604	289	53	35	59	39	4	2
Scurvy	2		1	1				
Rickets	30	14	2	1	10	7		
Anemia	65	35	14	8	60	29	22	16
Enteritis	344	201	46	25	154	107	22	12
Dysentery	7	2	17	8	2	2	7	3
Worms	16	11	117	40	4	2	33	9
Tuberculosis	45	39	88	70	3	3	3	3
Skin sepsis	148	71	31	9	34	19	18	5
Diseases of newborn	51	40						
Congenital defects	116	76	21	2	4	2	2	
Accidents	10	1	66	6				
Burns and scalds	6	1	19	2	1	1		
Eye conditions	23		26		6	2		
Ear, nose, and throat	27	4	38	5	10	3	2	
Meningitis (excluding TB)	28	23	14	13	17	17	4	3
Convulsions	8	3	2		9	3	2	1
Urinary infections	28	12	15	4	13	7	6	3
Tetanus	82	80	3	3				
Malaria	10	8	20	9				
Diphtheria	17	5	12	5	2		1	1
Typhoid			23	8				
Gonorrhea	11	3	13		1		4	
Congenital syphilis	32	27	2	1	2			
Endocarditis and pericarditis	1	1	4	3	1	1		
Other diseases	24	3	24	2	5	1	5	4

Source: Williams (1938*b*).

Note: Children admitted for observation, as lodgers, and those not yet discharged are not included in this table.

CAUSES OF MALNUTRITION

Food shortage is by no means the only or the most usual cause of malnutrition. In most cases, the diagnosis of severe malnutrition is obvious, but the cause is not so clear-cut, particularly in children where the malnourished state is the endpoint of the cumulative effect of a vast number of nondietary as well as dietary factors, including diarrhea, worms, tuberculosis, and maternal deprivation (Brown 1966). In each area, the type and extent of the problem and local causes must be identified (Fig. 8.5). Many causal factors have been recognized, and seven or eight may be present simultaneously.

Innumerable studies have pointed to social and environmental factors associated with poor nutritional status in children, such as poverty (especially with maldistribution of wealth and, with worldwide recession, national debt inflation), family size, mother's literacy level, single-parent households, maternal deprivation, and many other factors, including child neglect or abuse (Mata 1978; Jelliffe and Jelliffe 1984*a*; Alleyne et al. 1977*a*, 1977*b*; DeMaeyer 1976; Kielman 1978; Whitehead 1977). These may result in inadequate food intake. In the rainy season in particular, when planting is done, the problem is compounded by food shortage and a high incidence of infections, especially malaria.

In some cases there may be sufficient food available but the quality is inadequate. For example, where kwashiorkor is highly prevalent, low-protein, bulky foods such as cassava or plantains are the sole staples. Where there is importation of cheap overmilled white rice, local parboiled rice is less used, and beriberi may occur. An often underappreciated need is for compact calories to meet the metabolic needs of young children with small stomach capacity. In areas of chronic food shortages, food supplementation has led to uncontrolled distribution of skimmed milk, which has been responsible for increased xerophthalmia and blindness (unless fortified with vitamin A), discouraging breastfeeding as well as local food production and encouraging dependency. In poverty areas, as a result of inequitable distribution of resources, notably money and land, the poor suffer even though enough food is produced (Lappe and Collins 1979).

Cultural practices may restrict the use of locally available nutritious foods. For example, eggs in some areas are not eaten lest they make females infertile. Other cultural attitudes include withholding food from a baby with diarrhea in the belief that the bowel needs a rest or giving an infant small feedings because of an umbilical hernia, in the belief that too much food will push the bowel out (as among the Tswana of southern Africa). In other places "evil spirits" are blamed or the wife's infidelity. Some mothers may starve during pregnancy, "eating down" to avoid large babies and complicated deliveries. Many pregnant mothers fear that their breast milk will poison nursing infants. In an analysis of random milk samples of pregnant lactating women in Zaire (Vis and Hennart 1978), the breastmilk

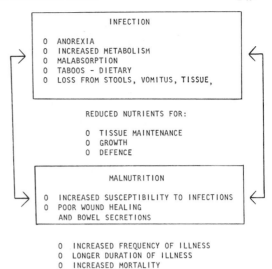

Figure 8.6. Interaction of malnutrition and infection.

showed a sudden change in composition with pregnancy. When the milk returned to a colostrum-like composition, some infants developed a mild "lactation diarrhea." This has also been noted by pregnant lactating mothers of the La Leche League. Little attention has been paid to the cultural attitudes of child care providers. Their attitudes, tastes, preferences, and knowledge have a great bearing on child feeding practices.

A lack of clean water and sewage disposal is associated with infections, and these in turn exert a major negative effect on infants' nutrition, particularly those not breastfed. Infections by a variety of mechanisms cause nutrient loss and increase the demand for nutrients (Fig. 8.6). In some studies, measles has been found to be a precursor of over half the cases of kwashiorkor. Measles causes not only weight loss but also a drop in albumin levels and a decrease in immunity (Alleyne et al. 1977*a*). In malnourished children, especially those under 3 years of age, the effects are devastating. To add to the problem, malnourished children are often immunologically deficient (Chandra 1983) and thus more susceptible to infections. In such diverse locations as Guatemala, Gambia, and Uganda, diarrhea in malnourished children is five or more times as frequent as in their well-nourished counterparts, and diseases such as pneumonia are nine times more frequent. Roundworms and hookworm also contribute to stunted growth and deterioration of nutritional status. It has been calculated that a roundworm population of 100 can result in a nutrient loss equivalent to four eggs per week. Programs that provide supplementary feeding may be feeding the worms, not the children.

The causes of malnutrition can vary with geography and culture and even within a single village (Williams 1957), as the following cases of malnourished children in Ghana demonstrate:

1. Aged 4 months. Mother died in childbirth. The grandmother, who had not had a baby for sixteen years, tried to breastfeed the child, but her milk was insufficient. She said that cow's milk gave the child diarrhea.
2. Aged 6 months. Being breastfed, but the mother had severe anemia. The dispensary was nineteen miles away. She had attended once and was given medicine for malaria but no iron and no instructions about food.
3. Aged 1 year. The mother and her three children were deserted by the father. She worked very hard trying to grow food; the family was living mainly on a little maize, sweet potatoes, and green leaves.
4. Aged 2 years. Parents kept cattle and chickens but believed that milk and eggs were bad for the child.
5. Aged 3 years. Child was getting quite a good diet but suffered from repeated attacks of gastroenteritis and from roundworms.
6. Aged 3 years. Child was getting a fair amount of food but getting thinner. Perhaps tuberculosis was a problem.
7. Aged 4 years. The total quantities of food probably were adequate, but the child got practically nothing to eat until the evening, when he ate an enormous meal. His abdomen was distended, and he frequently had severe stomachache. The mother worked very hard, but the maize was badly ground, and she had no time to carry enough wood or water for cooking it properly.
8. Aged 7 years. The well-to-do parents had land, cattle, and cash crops, but this child spent most of his day herding the goats and got food only at irregular intervals. Last year, his brother died in the hospital with malnutrition and pneumonia.

GENERAL MALNUTRITION

The most common form of malnutrition in the world today is that associated with diarrhea, as well as with an inadequate diet in the young child. Observations show that the peak incidence of gastroenteritis is followed by that of malnutrition, often in the clinical form of marasmus (wasting, emaciation) or growth failure (Meneghello et al. 1960). Abdominal distension is common and is both a cause and a sign of malabsorption. Muscular atony and atrophy affect both the intestinal and the abdominal muscles (Fig. 8.7).

The side effects of malnutrition include some variable hypoglycemia, some anemia, hypothermia, hypotonia, and mental apathy. As the stores of nutrients in the body are depleted, the metabolic processes become more labile. Some degree of edema is often present. The type, distribution, and severity must be noted and the urine tested for albumin. In areas where the most severe cases of malnutrition are seen, a proportion arrive at the hospital in extremis. The duration of the diarrhea, for example, is often more accurately judged by clinical examination than by the mother's observations.

Nutritional disorders present a wide variety of clinical pictures according to

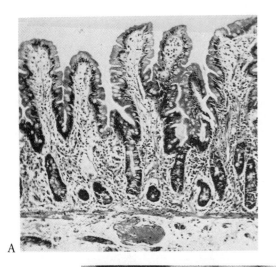

A

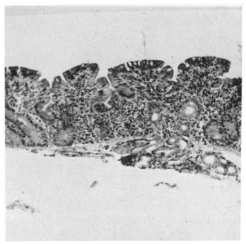

B

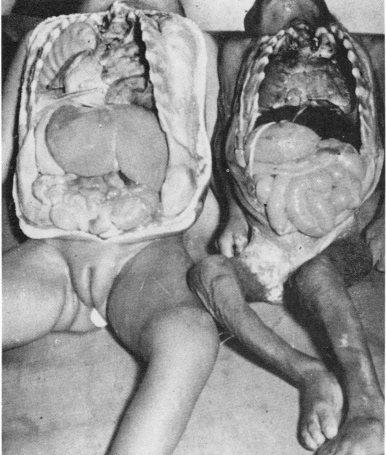

C

Figure 8.7. Effects of malnutrition on the digestive system. (A) Small intestine; normal villi. (B) Small intestine, kwashiorkor; gross atrophy of villi (muscles are also atrophied—not shown). (C) Postmortems: (left) kwashiorkor; edema, depigmentation, liver enlarged and fatty, subcutaneous fat present; (right) marasmus: emaciation, no subcutaneous fat, liver small and dark. Photograph courtesy Dr. B. E. R. Symonds.

the type and severity of the deficiency or multiple deficiencies, the age of the patient, the duration of the disease, and the environment of the patient (Williams 1938a; WHO 1981; Jelliffe and Jelliffe 1990).

SPECIFIC FORMS OF MALNUTRITION

There are variety of classifications used to describe malnutrition; however, no classification is satisfactory. For practical purposes, clinical malnutrition can be considered as:

1. Balanced overnutrition (for example, obesity).
2. Unbalanced overnutrition (for example, hypervitaminosis).
3. Balanced undernutrition (for example, marasmus).
4. Unbalanced undernutrition (for example, kwashiorkor and avitaminosis).

Most types of malnutrition are mixed, and pure textbook cases of one particular nutritional disease are uncommon. A number of children are subject to disease that interferes with ingestion and absorption or to infections and degenerative conditions that create excessive metabolic disease. Some cases, especially in the very young, are acute and need regular supervision.

Severe malnutrition is the predominant form of malnutrition that contributes to the high mortality and morbidity of children under age 5 in developing countries and to mental and physical impairment in those who survive (Fig. 8.8).

Kwashiorkor

The disease called kwashiorkor in the Ga language of Accra, Ghana (Williams 1933, 1938a), means "the disease of the deposed baby" and has attracted worldwide attention for sixty years. In 1933,

classical kwashiorkor was first described in the literature as a "well marked syndrome" of the "deposed" infant (i.e., taken off the breast), distinctly different from pellagra and "an amino acid or protein deficiency could not be excluded" (Williams 1933). The so-called experts, however, continued to call it 'infantile pellagra' even when it did not respond to nicotinic acid, and in some areas it was even confused with congenital syphilis. Child welfare clinics in Uganda, for example, treated 90 of 100 patients as having congenital syphilis. Incredible as it seems, this state of ignorance and disbelief continued until 1952, when irrefutable evidence in the form of low serum albumin established kwashiorkor as a distinct clinical syndrome. It is not surprising that Trowell and associates (1982), in their history of kwashiorkor, warn that highly specialized "experts" should never be consulted about the status of a new idea in medicine.

The most acute form of the disease is generally found in a child of 10 to 24 months who has had an excessively carbohydrate diet containing relatively little protein. A slight loss of weight may be later masked by edema and enlargement of the liver. Coldness of the extremities is well marked, and the child is miserable but apathetic. When anorexia and/or diarrhea set in, there is a loss of weight in spite of the edema. This marasmic stage may be due to malabsorption rather than to a deficiency in caloric intake. Chronic cases show depigmentation of skin and hair, with the hair losing its luster, becoming straight, dry, and sparse. In late stages of the disease, the skin shows depigmentation, as well as the typical "flaky paint" rash, particularly in areas of pressure or irritation (Fig. 8.9). The condition is often precipitated by measles or other forms of infection or stress and complicates other diseases. During the terminal stages, there may be purpura in addition to the typical rash. Degenerative changes occur in the intes-

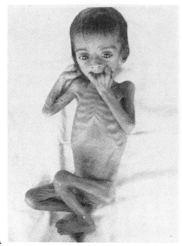
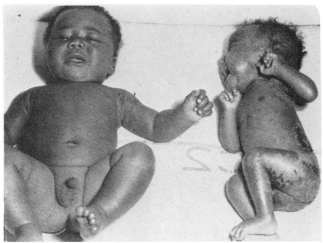

A

B

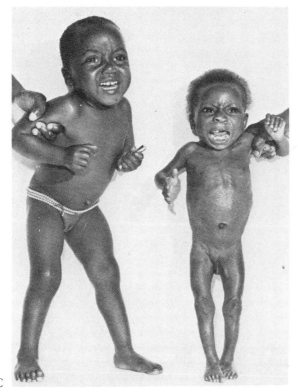

C

Figure 8.8. Types and causes of malnutrition. (A) Marasmus in 3-month-old Trinidadian infant, following bottle feeding with diluted contaminated cow's milk formula. Photograph courtesy of Dr. B. E. R. Symonds. (B) Twins: one normal (left) following breastfeeding and adequate supplementary foods, contrasted with the other (right) with kwashiorkor, following artificial feeding and largely carbohydrate gruels as weaning foods. (C) Uganda twins: one normal growth (left) and one with late marasmus (right) resulting from severe untreated cleft palate.

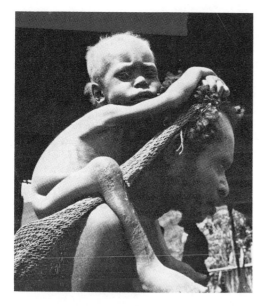

Figure 8.9. Child with kwashiorkor in New Guinea highlands. A severe and chronic case of kwashiorkor, showing depigmentation of skin, "flaky-paint" rash, depigmentation and thinning of hair, edema of feet, and emaciation, due probably to anorexia and to malabsorption. Photograph by Dr. H. A. P. C. Oomen.

tinal tract and in the muscles (Wiseman 1964).

Kwashiorkor appears to be due to a number of other causes and not protein malnutrition alone. Hendrickse (1988) has proposed that afloxin may be a causative agent. *Cancrum oris* or *noma* sometimes appears in malnourished populations. It is usually found in children between ages 2 and 4 years. It is a terrifying condition, unknown in a well-nourished community. Initially, there is gangrene of the cheek, later affecting the gums and bones of the mouth (Fig. 8.10).

Marasmus

This condition, seen in children whose weight is markedly below normal for their length, is described as a state of balanced starvation. A general deficit of protein and energy has occurred, leading to severe wasting of subcutaneous fat and

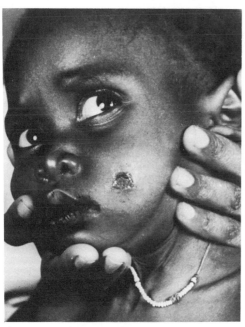

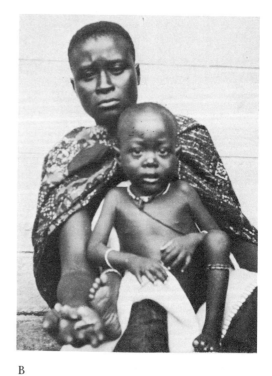

A   B

Figure 8.10. *Cancrum oris.* (A) Early *Cancrum oris,* Africa. (B) Healed *Cancrum oris.* Mother's right hand holds left mandible, which was sloughed out.

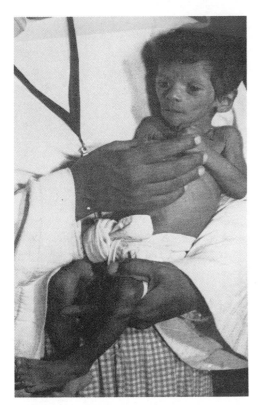

Figure 8.11. Marasmus. If MCH services are effective, no child should have to reach this condition before being admitted to hospital. This marasmic infant does not display the misery seen in kwashiorkor, and there is comfort in contact. WHO photograph, India.

muscle tissue. It often occurs between the ages of 6 months and 18 months (Fig. 8.11). The marasmic child appears as a wizened old man in appearance, with loss of most fatty tissue, shriveled buttocks, and emaciated limbs. Many of the signs of kwashiorkor, such as edema, skin rash, and hair discoloration, are absent. There is a general slowing of all body processes in response to the starvation, so the condition does not produce the biochemical imbalances of kwashiorkor and is not considered as serious or difficult to treat. The marasmic child is often hungry and willing to eat when offered foods.

Kwashiorkor is distinctly different from marasmus (Table 8.2), but mixed forms do occur (Cameron and Hofvander 1983; Jelliffe 1984*a*).

Anemia

Anemia is common in young children all over the world but especially in developing countries. It is often due to a number of simultaneously occurring factors, including dietary deficiencies (especially iron), bacterial and parasitic infections, genetic abnormalities, such as sickle cell anemia in African children, and cord blood loss (through premature tying of the cord, 46 milligrams of iron per 100 cubic centimeter of blood can be lost) (Baumslag 1992).

Iron needs are high in early childhood because of the rapid increase in the total number of red blood cells and in muscle mass that occur with normal development. Iron deficiency results when these needs are not met because of dietary inadequacy (for example, with prolonged unsupplemented human and cow's milk or iron-poor staples) or from blood loss (for example, infection with hookworm, or bilharziasis), often associated with low iron stores (for example in twins, prematures, babies of iron-deficient mothers), and possibly with malabsorption, especially in protein-deficient diets.

Where dietary deficiency is the cause, the form of iron available may be as important as the quantity (USAID 1979). Although breastmilk has less iron than cow's milk, the bioavailability of iron in breast milk is 49 percent compared with only 10 percent in cow's milk. Furthermore, the addition of ascorbic acid can enhance iron absorption two- to fivefold. Vitamin C–rich foods in later infancy can greatly increase iron absorption.

If the dietary iron intake is insufficient, local foods can serve as iron sources. Many villagers in Africa and Asia eat dark-green leafy vegetables (DGLV) high in iron content. In southern Africa, women seek out certain green plants called wild spinach *(morogo)*. The Wogogo of Cen-

Table 8.2. Principal Features of Marasmus and Kwashiorkor

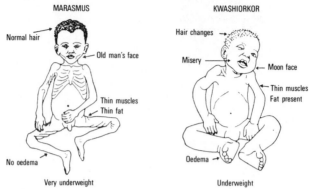

Features	Marasmus	Kwashiorkor
Essential features		
Edema	None[a]	Lower legs, sometimes face, or generalized[a]
Wasting	Gross loss of subcutaneous fat, "all skin and bone"[a]	Less obvious; sometimes fat, blubbery
Muscle wasting	Severe[a]	Sometimes
Growth retardation in terms of body weight	Severe[a]	Less than in marasmus
Mental changes	Usually none	Usually present
Variable features		
Appetite	Usually good	Usually poor
Diarrhea	Often (past or present)	Often (past or present)
Skin changes	Usually none	Often, diffuse depigmentation; occasional, "flaky-paint"[a] or "enamel" dermatosis
Hair changes	Texture may be modified but usually no dispigmentation	Often sparse—straight and silky, dispigmentation—greyish or reddish
Moon face	None	Often
Hepatic enlargement	None	Frequent, although it is not observed in some areas
Biochemistry/pathology		
Serum albumin	Normal or slightly decreased	Low[a]
Urinary urea per g of creatinine	Normal or decreased	Low[a]
Urinary hydroxyproline index	Low	Low
Serum-free amino acid ratio	Normal	Elevated[a]
Anemia	May be observed	Common; iron or folate deficiency may be associated
Liver biopsy	Normal or atrophic[a]	Fatty infiltration[a]

Source: Jelliffe (1968).

[a]The most characteristic or useful distinguishing features.

tral Province, Tanzania, make flat cakes of pounded dried green leaves, which they string around the cooking place for easy access when cooking. In urban areas, these greens are not so readily available, and selective supplementation may be necessary. Iron cooking pots and drinking water may be other sources of iron.

In areas where malaria is endemic, chloroquine or other effective antimalarials may be required rather than iron supplements. Routine iron supplementation may be contraindicated in areas where malaria is endemic. Not infrequently, folate deficiency may also be present. If the diet has enough iron but anemia is prevalent, phytates may be interfering with iron absorption, or there may be blood loss. Iron tablets may produce black stools and sometimes even "indigestion," anorexia, and loose stools or constipation.

Avitaminosis A

Xerophthalmia, now widely recognized as one of the chief causes of blindness in the world (McLaren 1963; Pirie 1983), is often associated with protein energy malnutrition. Clinical deficiency can be precipitated by infections, particularly measles. Moreover, some of the reduction in circulating retinol levels is due to zinc deficiency. A study in Hyderbadad showed that zinc therapy exclusive of other supplements raised circulating vitamin A levels in children with kwashiorkor (Shingwekar et al. 1979).

Xerophthalmia may appear as early as nine days after birth. Low Vitamin A stores in the mother, infections, twins, or prematurity may account for some early cases, but most are due to the young babies' being bottle-fed on unsuitable foods. The most common of these are sweetened condensed milk and skimmed milk powders that have not been fortified with vitamin A, or the milk may be too diluted to provide a proper diet. Breastfed babies are protected in early infancy because colostrum is high in vitamin A.

Xerophthalmia is too often ignored in small babies. It begins with small ulcers and a matte surface called dryness of the cornea, which produces no pain, lacrimation, or discharge unless secondarily infected. The small baby lies with eyes shut; unless the eyes are carefully inspected, the condition will be missed until the sight is seriously damaged by scarring or destroyed by rupture of the softened, gelatinous eyeball (keratomalacia). Response to treatment with vitamin A is rapid if the condition is caught in time.

In later childhood, children may be seen with xerophthalmia—thickened and wrinkled conjunctivae that progress to corneal opacities. Some children may develop Bitot's spots. The response to treatment with vitamin A is not very rapid. In older children and adults, avitaminosis A may first present as night blindness. Sommer and associates in a study in Indonesia (1986) found that not only did vitamin A distribution in high–vitamin A deficiency areas lead to reduction in the incidence of blindness but also resulted in a lower childhood mortality rate in high risk populations (Daulaire et al. 1992).

Iodine Deficiency

Iodine deficiency is so easy to prevent that no child should be born mentally handicapped for that reason. Recent evidence indicates a much wider spectrum of disorders from iodine deficiency than previously realized (Table 8.3). It is estimated that more than 400 million people in Asia alone, as well as millions in Africa and South America, are at risk.

Iodine-deficiency disorders include goiter at all ages, especially in females (in the Philippines it was found to be eight times higher in girls aged 7 to 14 years than in boys of the same age [MARHIA 1991]); increased stillbirths; perinatal and infant mortality; fetal effects, presenting as endemic cretinism (Fig. 8.12) or as

Table 8.3. Iodine Deficiency Disorders

Fetus	Abortions[a]	
	Stillbirths[a]	
	Congenital anomalies[a]	
	Increased perinatal mortality[a]	
	Increased infant mortality[a]	
	Neurological cretinism ⟶	Mental deficiency[a]
		Deaf mutism[a]
		Spastic diplegia[a]
		Squint[a]
	Myxoedematous cretinism ⟶	Dwarfism
		Mental deficiency[a]
	Psychomotor defects[a]	
	Fetal hypothyroidism	
Neonates	Neonatal hypothyroidism	
	Neonatal goiter	
Child and adolescent	Juvenile hypothyroidism	
	Goiter	
	Impaired mental function[a]	
	Retarded development[a]	
	Cretinism	
	Myxoedematous	
	Neurological	
Adult	Goiter with its complications	
	Hypothyroidism	
	Impaired mental function[a]	

Source: Hetzel (1989).

[a] Items indicated are nonspecific and can be caused by many other pathological conditions.

mental deficiency, often with deaf mutism; and spastic diplegia.

Although this disorder is preventable, it is estimated that the prevalence of surviving cases of cretinism is 6 million cases. There are another 20 million with measurable mental retardation attributable to iodine deficiency (WHO 1991). Prevention is practicable through iodinization of a commonly used food, usually salt, or by intramuscular injections of iodized oil. Diagnosis is mainly by clinical examination, with decreased iodine as a biochemical test if laboratory facilities are available (they usually are not).

Beriberi

Infantile beriberi is usually found among rice-eating populations, particularly where overmilled white rice is eaten with insufficient supplements. It has become less common with health education and fortification of white rice. The mother may show no clinical signs of beriberi, although her breast milk shows levels of thiamine insufficient for the rapidly growing infant. In its earliest manifestations, acute infantile beriberi may be suspected from the presence of oliguria, or anuria, flabbiness, anorexia, bradycardia and cyanosis, and edema. In the acute stage, the infant may have convulsions and become pulseless and comatose or develop cardiac failure. Prompt treatment with thiamine is very effective and will be followed by copious diuresis (Williams 1938b). If not treated early, it can result in sudden death.

Although infantile beriberi appears to be less common than in the past, the chronic manifestations need to be known by health professionals to avoid misdiagnosis. These include a typical cry from

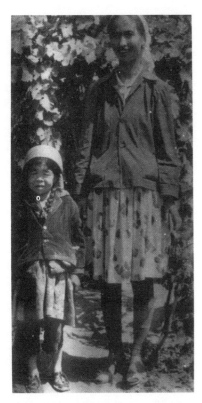

Figure 8.12. Iodine deficiency. A cretin woman together with a "barefoot doctor" of the same age from the Hetian district of Xingjian, China. Photograph courtesy of Dr. Ma Tai, Tianjin, China (1986).

The disease is easy to prevent and easy to cure if it has not become chronic. Mothers and families should be taught that pregnant and lactating women and young children should eat undermilled or enriched rice, with soya and other beans, eggs, pork, yeast, liver, and fresh green vegetables.

It is possible that failure to thrive, as well as some cardiac emergencies, may in fact be due to unrecognized thiamine deficiency. A simple test is to give a small dose of thiamine; if this produces a diuresis, there is probably some B_1 deficiency.

Scurvy

This is caused by the lack of vitamin C or ascorbic acid. This vitamin is present in human breastmilk, citrus fruit, tomatoes, papaya, and mango and highly concentrated in the guava and West Indian cherry. It is also present in green leafy vegetables but may be destroyed by overcooking. Scurvy is, in fact, rare in the tropics, but cases do occur, particularly in urban areas. It may be more common in the future among bottle-fed babies.

Rickets

Rickets has become more common recently in some tropical and subtropical countries (Jelliffe and Jelliffe 1990; Jelliffe 1984a; Williams 1946). Young children may not be given vitamin D in their food or as supplement and may not be exposed to sunlight because of living urban conditions, or may be purposely kept indoors for cultural reasons—for example, for purposes of purdah, to avoid the evil eye, or to keep the skin fair. Diagnosis is usually based on clinical observations (enlargement of costochondral junction, epiphyses of the wrists, and bossing of head) since radiological examination is often difficult to obtain. Metabolic changes that increase the likelihood of anemia and gastrointestinal and

edema of the larynx, dilation of the right heart followed by hypertrophy, anorexia or aphonia, meteorism, and failure to gain weight. There is marked flabbiness of the muscles and restlessness. Even where there is no obvious external edema, autopsy will show edema of the internal organs, particularly of the gallbladder. These cases respond well to treatment with thiamine. Chronic cases, in which there are nervous manifestations and severe right-sided cardiac hypertrophy, often fail to respond in spite of large doses of thiamine enterally and parenterally.

If the mother is thiamine deficient, the baby may develop an acute form of beriberi. The baby should not be taken off the breast, but the mother should be given massive doses of thiamine.

respiratory disorders are more immediately serious than the bone changes (Fig. 8.13), though these, if they persist to later life, may create pelvic narrowing and difficult childbirth in affected females.

Pellagra

This disease is rare in children and does not occur in those on a milk diet. In the past, cases have been described in children more than 4 years of age in Italy, the southern United States, Egypt, southern Africa, and India. In the past it has been confused with protein malnutrition; the two diseases may, of course, occur together.

Pellagra begins with the classical dermatosis (on the face and neck, hands and forearms, feet and legs to just above the knee) but only if the skin is exposed to the sun. The onset may be acute, with painful redness and blistering, although chronic cases show dry, branny desquamation. In the early stages, and even with marked dermatosis, the child is running about and not at all depressed. This is followed by diarrhea with emaciation; finally, dementia may set in. The disease is found mainly among people on a maize diet but has occurred in others—for example, European prisoners in Singapore during World War II living on a rice diet. It responds to treatment with nicotinic acid and improved diet, provided the degenerative changes have not become irreversible.

Zinc Deficiency

There is an increased awareness of the importance of zinc as an essential nutrient. Dwarfism, failure to thrive, delayed wound healing, and increased susceptibility to infections have been found in zinc-deficient children. Children with marginal zinc intakes and with high phytate diets are at risk. In Jamaica and Peru, children recovering from clinical malnutrition have gained weight at accelerated rates when given zinc supplements (Golden 1981). The importance of zinc may in-

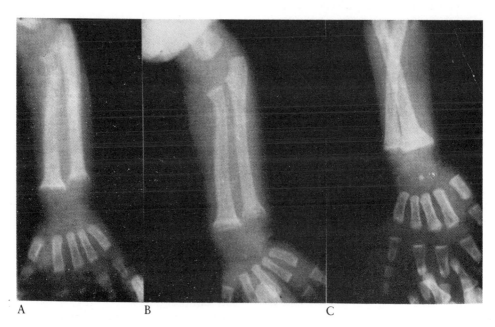

A   B   C

Figure 8.13. Bone changes in rickets. Rickets in an infant of 8 months who had been kept in a dark cubicle. (A) Initial finding: cupping of the epiphysis and decreased mineralization. Marked improvement at (B) 3 weeks and (C) 6 weeks after treatment.

crease as foods become more refined and processed. Maternal zinc deficiency in pregnancy may affect birthweight and result in congenital malformations. Furthermore, zinc deficiency causes anorexia and affects taste and smell. Zinc is abundant in meat but is also present in legumes and cereals (WHO 1973).

In this chapter, the discussion has focused on vitamin and micronutrient deficiencies, but excessive intake of micronutrients does occur and can be harmful (Jelliffe and Jelliffe 1984a; Cameron and Hofvander 1983). Most problems arise when there is no supervision. For example, in the United States a daily high-level pyridoxine (vitamin B_6) consumption (Shaumburg et al. 1983) has resulted in ataxia and severe nervous system dysfunction.

Obesity

In some of the industrialized countries, obesity is the most common form of malnutrition. Obesity can create physical, mental, and social problems especially in pregnancy, in children, and in old age. Obesity is often associated with or is the cause of diabetes, hypertension, and cardiac emergencies and needs serious and persistent treatment.

The overfed baby presents a definite syndrome and is usually chubby, cheerful, and bronchitic. It is often hard to convince the proud parents that danger lurks in this apparently delightful child. But it is advisable to control excessive weight gain. Antibiotics can usually be used to treat any serious chest complications, but it is better to control the weight by sensible minor adjustments in the diet than to rely on medication.

It was found among the Eskimos that changing life-styles and refined foods high in sugar and fats increase the prevalence of dental caries, obesity, and obesity-related complications. Obesity is nine times more prevalent in low-income females in the United States than it is with

low-income males (Akesode and Ajibode 1983). Obesity and the sequelae are also becoming more prevalent in developing countries and, in contrast to developed countries, it is more frequent among higher socioeconomic classes who have greater access to sugar and fats (Schaefer 1971; ICN 1992).

Anorexia Nervosa

This dangerous form of wasting disease was well known to the Victorians but rare in Western cultures in the early years of this century. It is now seen frequently, mainly in young females. It may occur in cases where there has been a history of childhood trauma, such as physical or sexual abuse (Torem 1990). It often starts with some emotional stress or with overenthusiasm for fashionable thinness. Vomiting and the excessive use of laxatives are usual. Cases that are identified early generally respond to treatment if the physical, mental, and social aspects are treated adequately. Many of the cases become irreversible and even fatal. There is no effective treatment. Psychiatric care is required.

MEASUREMENT OF NUTRITION

Weight for height and age, weight loss, and weight gain are the most common methods of assessing nutritional status, body build, and progress in growth and development. The sitting height compared with total height is another measure (Fig. 8.14). Mid-arm circumference and skinfold thickness have also been widely used (Jelliffe and Jelliffe 1990) and are particularly useful in community settings.

Weight depends not only on food intake but also on infections that cause fever, increasing metabolism and diminishing body reserves. Infections may be acute, such as measles, or chronic or re-

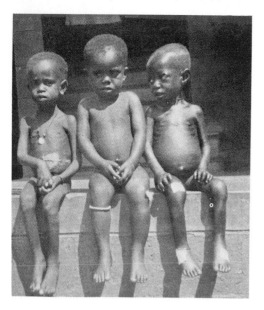

Figure 8.14. Sitting height, a potential screening measure. Child in center; aged 2½ years, had been brought regularly to a weighing center for supervision and advice; growth and development were excellent. The children on either side; each aged about 4 years, were brought in from the bush, both suffering from serious failure to thrive, malnutrition, and malabsorption. The child on the left was admitted to the hospital and improved after four months of treatment. Parents refused admission of the child on the right, who died shortly after. Photo taken in Ghana, 1934.

current, like tuberculosis. They may be generalized, like typhoid, or localized, like otitis media.

Gastroenteritis, anorexia, dysentery, and even maldigestion lead to malabsorption, as well as diarrhea and vomiting. Dehydration may cause sudden severe loss of weight. The body of the child is more labile than that of an adult, and a disease such as cholera can cause rapid death. In some epidemics, it is said that children seldom reach the hospital. Pain and discomfort caused by injury or fear may give rise to insomnia and weight loss. Parental deprivation or neglect is a frequent cause of "faltering" in weight. Fear may give rise to diarrhea, or to vomiting, or both.

Of all the conditions that produce the malnourished state, unsuitable foods, infections, and infestations are probably the most common and therefore require the most frequent measurement. Some diseases, on the other hand, may give rise to weight gain. Nephritis and cardiac failure may cause water retention. Edema may be obvious in advanced cases of protein malnutrition, but in early cases it is difficult to detect and may mask the loss of weight. Small quantities of fluid may collect in the peritoneum, thorax, and pericardium and be detected only at necropsy.

Chronic malnutrition can cause abdominal enlargement (although the potbellied toddler is overemphasized in descriptions of malnourished populations). Several factors lead to the potbelly. First is the excessive consumption of coarse, fermentable, indigestible food, which is easily identified by examining the stools. In many cases, the timing of the food is at fault. Because the mother is working all day, the toddler has very little food in the morning, and by the time the mother has collected the wood and the water, pounded and winnowed the grain, and boiled the meal, the child is ravenous and eats voraciously. After the evening meal, the child carries a distended abdomen. The food is poorly digested and poorly absorbed. Protein malnutrition will also cause degeneration of intestinal muscles and the digestive enzymes. Intestinal parasites may cause further enlargement of the abdomen and increase in weight. Ascaris is the worst offender. A child of 3 years who weighed 24 pounds had 255 ascaris, which weighed 3 pounds, or almost 10 percent of his combined weight.

Each child's growth needs to be followed regularly and carefully and the results discussed with the mother. Growth charts, such as the Road to Health chart, serve as valuable educational tools and promotion of the infant's health, provided they are explained and understood. In Soweto, South Africa, mothers called the growth chart "River of Life." Use should be made of cultural concepts.

There are three useful measures of nutritional status: diet history, anthropometric (arm circumference, skinfold thickness), and biochemical. However, it is important not to concentrate on anthropometric measures alone but also to note the general appearance, activity, and development of the child and the mother's history.

PREVENTION OF MALNUTRITION

The prevention of malnutrition calls for more understanding of the causes for adaptation to the local epidemiology (Williams 1938*b*; Alleyne et al. 1977*b*; Beaton and Bengoa 1976). The following are important approaches:

Ensure equity of food distribution and food reserves at the national and household levels ("food security").

Encourage and protect breastfeeding.

Improve weaning practices by using local foods.

Screen for infants and children at risk from malnutrition, and give them special attention.

Provide nutrition and rehabilitation, especially in households.

Integrate nutrition into primary health care.

Ensure regular supervision in clinics and visiting in homes by inspection and growth monitoring.

Ensuring equity of food distribution requires a national food and nutrition policy. Policymakers and planners must be aware of the problems and encouraged to develop appropriate food and nutrition policies guided by medical advice and combining the activities of all groups involved with respect to supplies and personnel (Beaton and Bengoa 1976; Jelliffe

1974). Food fortification and supplementation may also be necessary.

In drought-stricken areas or where there are long hunger periods, measures such as temporary price fixing, food ration stores, production of higher-yielding crops, and access to markets have made more food available to those most in need. In cases of acute food shortages, there may be a need for supplementary feeding. In Lesotho, special grain stores for emergency reserves have been set aside (as was done in ancient Egypt). Food conservation, storage, and improved small-scale village-level agricultural methods have also helped local independence and food continuity (McDowell 1978; Beaton 1983). At the household level, improved food preservation and storage, use of gardens (where possible), and other measures have extended the food supply. The measures used depend on the locale and require analysis before locally appropriate programs are formulated. An ongoing epidemiological approach at all levels is called for.

To encourage optimal feeding practices, pregnant mothers need to be monitored through serial weighing using locally appropriate relevant levels. Because infant feeding starts in utero, maternal nutrition is of particular concern, and selective supplementation for malnourished mothers should be available in a form and method of distribution that ensures that such foods are not lost to other less needy family members. A second way is to encourage and protect breastfeeding (Fig. 8.15). The importance of breastfeeding cannot be overemphasized. In Brazil, when bottle-fed infants were compared with exclusively breastfed infants, the relative risk of diarrhea in the former was found to be 14.2 greater than in the latter, and pneumonia 3.6 times greater (Victora 1987). In Scotland Howie et al. (1990) found that infants breastfed for thirteen weeks or more had a reduced risk of diarrhea and respiratory disease during the first year of life. Exclusive

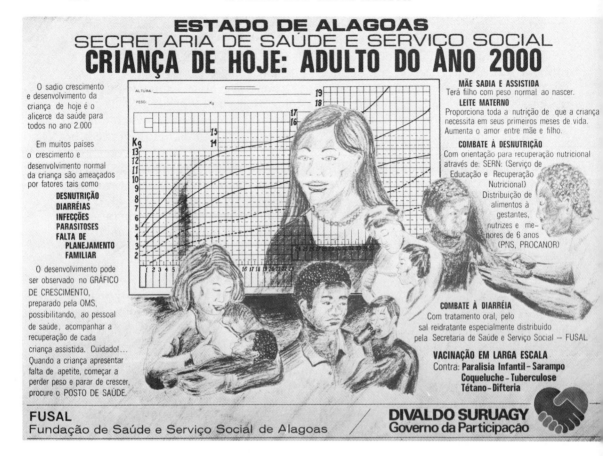

Figure 8.15. Encouraging breastfeeding. Brazil has recognized the importance of breastfeeding and good nutrition as part of its Health for All program. This poster was produced by the state of Algoas, Secretary of Health and Social Service, Brazil.

breastfeeding has been found to reduce the risk of noninfective conditions and may even enhance intelligence (Lucas et al. 1992).

Breastfeeding relates to several important aspects of health and growth (Fig. 8.16). In developing countries exclusive breastfeeding for six months is critical (Cameron and Holfvander 1983; Jelliffe 1974). From birth onward, the difference between formula-fed and breastfed infants is marked. A study in New Delhi among low-birthweight infants demonstrated the association between feeding expressed human breast milk and a reduction in the incidence of infections and deaths compared with a cohort fed care-fully prepared sterile formula (Narayanan et al. 1981). There is also evidence that exclusively breastfed infants of well-nourished mothers have normal growth patterns for up to nine months (Helsing and King 1992). Even when the mother is malnourished, the decline in growth velocity is usually not before age 4 months and in part reflects a physiological normal growth deceleration. Nevertheless, in view of the high rates of bacterial contamination of artificial feedings in developing countries, irrespective of whether they are formula or water-starchy beverages, extended lactation is still a better alternative. It is imperative to monitor the infant's growth and development and

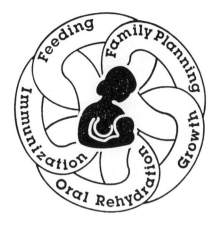

Figure 8.16. Breastfeeding, the focal point of infant health. It is important for adequate growth in infancy; it provides protection against some infections and a form of passive immunization for the baby through the mother; it prevents diarrhea and should form part of oral rehydration; it is the natural form of family planning but needs reinforcement with technological contraceptives; by adding human milk to weaning foods, it forms part of weaning multimixes.

to use the infant as his or her own standard.

At the time of weaning—ideally 6 months of age—semisolid food is introduced; breastmilk as a complement can still contribute an additional 25 percent to the caloric intake. There is no question that in developing countries malnutrition is more prevalent in bottle-fed infants than among breastfed infants; the relative risk is four to six times as high (Helsing and King 1982; Jelliffe 1968).

A number of developing countries have implemented country-wide programs to encourage breastfeeding. Brazil, one such country, has used a four-pronged approach to encourage breastfeeding: living-in at maternity hospitals; antenatal care; supervision and advice; and training of doctors, nurses, and midwives in the theory and techniques of breastfeeding (Applebaum 1970). Material advertising infant formulas and samples should be strictly controlled and company nurses prohibited from hospital or clinic prem-

ises. Health professionals must come to recognize the dangers of becoming financially dependent on formula companies. With the help of experienced organizations such as La Leche International, support groups for mothers are being formed. Not only do mothers acquire confidence and learn about practical breastfeeding from experienced mothers, but through women's networks the mothers become involved with others (Helsing and King 1982; Jelliffe 1974). Health professionals should also be able to diagnose and counsel mothers if problems arise. First and foremost, it is most important to determine the attitude of the mother to breastfeeding, as she is the provider.

Improved weaning also leads to optimal feeding practices. The infant is often removed from the breast abruptly, and bitter substances (such as aloe) applied to the nipples as a deterrent, or the child is sent away to a relative. *Weaning* means "to accustom" and begins when breastfeeding is no longer exclusive; it ends when the child is eating a full adult diet. At the time of weaning, appetite may be severely reduced, exposure to infection increased, and inappropriate and inadequate foods given infrequently, with serious resulting problems. At this time, the infant is most vulnerable to disease, and the downward spiral of malnutrition and infection is initiated (Jelliffe 1984*b*).

Attention to both the quality and quantity of the diet is of utmost importance. Infants should be fed frequently—five to six times a day—because their stomach capacity is small. They should be fed separately with high-density and freshly prepared foods or protected foods to avoid contamination. Utensils such as cups and spoons are less easily contaminated than are bottles. Where possible, hygienic preparation should be encouraged (Baumslag 1978).

In addition to the child's needs for growth and development, extra calories, sometimes called "sickness preparedness calories," are also required to ensure a safety margin. Another important consideration is that foods have to be calorie dense and easily digestible. Caloric density can be increased by adding sugar or oil to the diet (30 milliliters of cooking oil daily can provide 25 percent of the infant's caloric needs) and by including compact calorie foods, where possible (Jelliffe 1990b) or by using the ancient process of malting (Gopaldas et al. 1982). If a staple of low caloric density is used and not properly prepared, the child has to ingest an incredibly large volume to obtain enough calories.

It is best to use local foods, and a variety of mixes are available or can be devised (Jelliffe and Jelliffe 1984b). Commercial weaning foods are costly and for many reasons have been unsuccessful. In Malawi, Lukeni Phale (groundnuts, beans, and maize) was taken off the market because of the aflatoxin in the ground nuts. Benimix (groundnuts, sesame seed, rice) production in Sierra Leone was hampered by lack of electricity, and mothers were suddenly left without a product they had become accustomed to. Incaparina (corn flour and cottonseed flour), a Guatemalan food, is not very pleasant tasting and is also relatively costly. In Tanzania, soybeans, which normally do not grow in the country, were introduced, while the equally nutritious and more familiar cowpeas were ignored.

Cow's milk is a useful weaning food when available and can also be mixed with porridge. Formerly, the American Academy of Pediatrics was against its use for infants for fear it caused iron-deficiency anemia. However, in August 1983, in view of new evidence, the Committee on Nutrition of the American Academy of Pediatrics revised its decision and gave its blessing to the use of cow's milk (an age-old excellent weaning food) for infants over 6 months of age but suggested that supplementary feeds be given as well (Committee on Nutrition 1983). Between 1980 and 1987, the cost of infant formula doubled and was six times more expensive than cow's milk (the major ingredient).

Every health professional should develop a weaning checklist in their locality (Table 8.4). It is far better to establish the weaning patterns first and then, if there is a problem, find a local solution (Brown and Brown 1977).

Providing nutrition rehabilitation is another important practice. The case fatality of severely malnourished children is often 40 percent or more (Cook 1971). Early detection can prevent this waste of life. There is evidence that when children can be treated at home rather than in wards, they are less liable to severe hospital cross-infections (Cook 1971).

Initially, medical care is required and an intensive diet therapy, based as much as possible on local food mixtures (Hay and Whitehead 1976; Jelliffe and Jelliffe 1984b). Mothers should be admitted with the children for observation, as well as to assist with the nursing. Hospital diets should be carefully supervised, and regular follow-up by health professionals and home care services should be organized from the hospitals after discharge. Some hospitals have rehabilitation units where nutrition education is stressed and home gardens and small livestock raising demonstrated. The tendency, however, is to integrate rehabilitation at the village level. Health aides, primary health care workers, and nutritionists are recognizing the importance of ascertaining problems and constraints in the home and, with the mother, solving them. It has become apparent that the rest of the family also needs attention and that the process of recovery is often long.

Rehabilitation units can be very expensive, isolate the mother from her family and community. When interventions can be implemented in the home and followed up regularly, they prove cheaper and more successful (Shingwekar et al. 1977). It is important that health workers be given the time, tools, and transportation necessary to make home visits.

Table 8.4. Health Workers' Weaning Checklist

Who:	Who feeds the child? (an interested or disinterested party? mother/grandmother/sibling?)
What:	What foods and preparation methods are used? (e.g., watered staples, multimix, local/purchased, calorie dense, is breastmilk supplementary?) What local foods are available to provide needed nutrients? What foods are available during different seasons? What shortages occur, and how are they handled? What utensils are used? (a bottle/a cup) What are the beliefs and practices?
When:	When is the child fed? (how often?) When is the child sick? When is the child weaned? (when mother is pregnant? when the child has teeth?)
Why:	Why do certain beliefs and practices exist? (reasons for cultural customs, taste preferences, fears, past and present experience.)
Whether:	Whether the mother holds her infant in her lap when feeding. Whether the mother's attitude is positive or negligent. Whether breastmilk is still given. Whether the diet is balanced. Whether extra calories are given during illness. Whether the diet and environment are marginal or safe. Whether the food is freshly prepared. Whether the child is getting enough food.

Health centers and home visiting organizations should concentrate on nutrition education. There should be regular and frequent supervision of the infant's growth by serial weighing or measuring arm circumference, use of growth charts, and nutrition education for mothers. Special attention should be paid to high-risk groups such as weanlings and to proper feeding during and after illness, since these are the most likely times that a child may slip off the road to health and into overt malnutrition. When necessary, community health workers should be able to provide supplements if no locally available sources are identifiable.

Doctors, nurses, and midwives need to be better trained in practical nutrition and in management of conditions leading to nutritional disorders by better basic training. By provision of short-term refresher courses, increasing the numbers of medical and auxiliary staff, and improvement in supervision, distribution, and conditions of service, we might be able to abolish most cases of malnutrition. Education—above all, education at the individual level—is more important than supplementary feeding.

Nutrition must be integrated into primary care. Complex relationships exist between different aspects of poverty and health interventions—for example, child spacing and family planning. Interventions that seek only to improve nutrition or health often fail to have the desired effect because other aspects of problems are not addressed. When supplementary feeding is given without paying attention to health problems, such as diarrhea or worms, nutrients are lost, and deterioration continues, while the health worker continues to believe, mistakenly, that something is being done.

Primary health care services, including nutrition, make a difference (ICN 1992;

Baumslag and Sabin 1978). When a number of primary health care programs were reviewed, it was found that infant and child mortality was reduced by as much as 40 percent within one to five years at a cost equivalent to 2 percent of the per capita income (Gwatkin et al 1980). This has been achieved in part through community health workers who provide a whole host of activities (WHO 1981):

- Get to know the community and develop a work plan.
   Establish rapport with the villagers.
   Determine felt needs and nutrition-related problems.
- Motivate and organize the community; involve community groups in nutritional activities.
- Provide nutrition monitoring.
   Ascertain age and weight, record on growth chart, and interpret for necessary action.
   Use field techniques for detecting severe malnutrition, including arm and chest circumference.
   Provide nutrition education.
   Educate on nutrition in growth and development.
   Encourage breastfeeding; help mothers understand breastfeeding, the value of colostrum, and the importance of frequent feeding; impress on mothers the high risk of bottle feeding.
   Determine existing feeding practices in the community, and advise on sources and practices to improve feeding of infants.
- Identify and manage nutritional deficiencies.
   Recognize children in the community suffering from malnutrition, anemia, and those at risk for nutritional blindness.
   Manage and treat.
   Recognize cases that require referral.

- Control and manage infections.
   Diagnose diarrhea and dehydration; take appropriate measures.
   Organize immunizations in the community.
   Prepare educational messages for the prevention and management of infectious diseases.
- Improve water supply, disposal of excreta and refuse.
- Collaborate with other workers for nutrition promotion.

Results indicated that home visiting and continuity of care were critical.

Although dietary therapy is usually the major treatment of severely malnourished children, dietary supplementation is not the only answer in dealing with malnutrition in a community. Economic planning, immunization programs, provision of improved water, new roads, higher crop yields, food ration stores for times of want, price fixing of staple foods, provision of day care centers, knowledge of child feeding practices suitable for the weanling, and breast feeding are some of the many protection and support areas that have to be considered.

REFERENCES

Akesode, F. A., and Ajibode, I. A. (1983). Prevalence of obesity among Nigerian school children. *Soc. Sci. Med.* **17**, 107.

Alleyne, G. A. O.; Hay, R. W.; Picou, D. I.; Stanfield, J. P.; and Whitehead, R. G. (1977a). The ecology and pathogenesis of protein-energy malnutrition. In *Protein-Energy Malnutrition*, pp. 9–24. Edward Arnold, London.

Alleyne, G. A. O.; Hay, R. W.; Picou, D. I.; Stanfield, J. P.; and Whitehead, R. G. (1977b). Prevention and rehabilitation of protein-energy malnutrition. In *Protein-Energy Malnutrition*, pp. 168–95. Edward Arnold, London.

Applebaum, R. M. (1970). The modern management of successful breast feeding. *Pediat Clin. N. Amer.* **17**, 203.

Baumslag, N. (1978). *Perspectives in Maternal*

Infant Nutrition. U.S. Department of Health, Education and Welfare, Office of International Health, Rockville, Md.

Baumslag, N. (1979). *Nutrition Education in Medical Schools.* Testimony for the Subcommittee on Agriculture Nutrition and Forestry, U.S. Senate, Current Status, Impediments and Potential Solutions, pt. 1, U.S. Government Printing Office, Washington, D.C.

Baumslag, N. (1989). *Passport to Life.* NGO Committee on Nutrition, UNICEF, New York.

Baumslag, N. (1992). *Do Infants Under Six Months of Age Need Extra Iron? A Probe.* Working Paper 12. Mother Care, Arlington, Va.

Baumslag, N., and Sabin, E. (1978). *AID Integrated Low Cost Delivery System Projects.* U.S. Department of Health Education and Welfare, Office of International Health, Rockville, Md.

Beaton, G. H. (1983). Energy in Human Nutrition. W. O. Atwater Memorial Lecture, Western Hemisphere Nutrition Congress, Miami Beach.

Beaton, G. H., and Bengoa, J. M. (1976). *Nutrition in Preventive Medicine.* World Health Organization, Geneva.

Booyens, J., and McCance, R. A. (1957). Individual variations in expenditure of energy. *Lancet* i, 225.

Brown, J. E., and Brown, R. C. (1977). Finding the causes of protein-calorie malnutrition in a community, Part III: The causes of malnutrition, Zaire. *Envtl. Child. Hlth.*, p. 254.

Brown, R. E., and Sandhu, T. S. (1966). Autopsy survey of perinatal deaths in Uganda. *Trop. Geogr. Med.* 18, 292.

Cameron, M., and Hofvander, Y. (1983). *Manual on Feeding Infants and Young Children.* Oxford University Press, Delhi, Nairobi.

Chandra, R. K. (1983). Nutrition, immunity and infection: Present knowledge and future directions. *Lancet* i, 688.

Chetley, A. (1979). *The Baby Killer Scandal.* War on Want, London.

Committee on Nutrition (1983). Whole cow's milk for older infants. *Pediatrics* 72, 253.

Cook, R. (1971). Is the hospital the place for treatment of malnourished children. *Trop. Pediat.*, 17 15.

Daulaire et al. (1992). Childhood mortality after a high dose of Vitamin A in a high risk population. *Brit. Med. J.* 304, 207.

DeMaeyer, E. M. (1976). Protein-energy mal-nutrition. In *Nutrition in Preventive Medicine*, pp. 23–55. Ed. G. H. Beaton and J. M. Bengoa. World Health Organization, Geneva.

Ending Hidden Hunger (1991). Policy conference on micronutrient malnutrition, October 10–12, Montreal, Quebec, held by Task Force for Child Survival and Development, Atlanta.

Golden, B. E. and Golden, H. N. (1981). Plasma zinc, rate of weight gain, and the energy cost of tissue deposition in children recovering from severe malnutrition on a cow's milk or soya based diet. *Amer. J. Clin. Nutr.* 34, 892.

Gopalan, C., and Naidu, A. N. (1972). Mortality under five. Effect of malnutrition on fertility. *Lancet* ii, 1077.

Gopaldas, T., et al. (1982). Studies in the reduction of the viscosity of thick rice gruels. *Fd. Nutr. Bull.* 8, 42.

Grant, J. (1984). *The State of the World's Children.* Oxford University Press, New York.

Gwatkin, D. R.; Wilcox, J. R.; and Wray, J. D. (1980). *Can Health and Nutrition Interventions Make a Difference?* Overseas Development Council Monograph no. 13. Washington, D.C.

Hay, R. W., and Whitehead, R. G. (1976). *The Therapy of the Severely Malnourished Child: A Practical Manual.* National Food and Nutrition Council of Uganda with MRC Child Nutrition Unit, Kampala.

Helsing, E., and King, F. S. (1992). *Breastfeeding Practice: A Manual for Health Workers.* Oxford University Press, Oxford.

Hendrickse, R. G. (1988). Kwashiorkor and aflotoxins (editorial). *J. Ped. Gastroenteral Nutr.* 7, 33–636.

Hetzel, B. S. (1989). *The Story of Iodine Deficiency: An International Challenge in Nutrition*, Oxford University Press, Delhi.

Howie, P. W., et al. (1990). Protective effects of breastfeeding against infection. *Br. Med. J.* 300, 11–16.

ICN (1992). *Nutrition and Development—A Global Assessment.* International Conference on Nutrition, FAO/WHO, Geneva.

Jacobsen, O. (1978). *Economic and Geographical Factors Influencing Child Malnutrition. A Study from the Southern Highlands, Tanzania.* BRALUP Paper no. 52. University of Dar es Salaam.

Jelliffe, D. B. (1968). Health problems in pre-school children, II. General review. The pre-school child as a bio-cultural transitional. *J. Trop. Pediat.* **14**, 217.

Jelliffe, D. B. (1974). Protein-calorie malnutrition of early childhood. In *Medicine in the Tropics.* Ed. A. W. Woodruff. Churchill Livingstone, London.

Jelliffe, D. B., ed. (1992). *Child Health in the Tropics.* 6th ed. Arnold, London.

Jelliffe, D. B., and Jelliffe, E. F. P. (1984a). Nutritional assessment at village level. *J. Trop. Pediat.* **30**, 290.

Jelliffe, D. B., and Jelliffe, E. F. P. (1984b). The principle of multimixes. In *Advances in International Maternal and Child Health,* vol. 4. Ed. D. B. Jelliffe and E. F. P. Jelliffe. Oxford University Press, Oxford.

Jelliffe, D. B., and Jelliffe, E. F. P. (1985). The key role of breastfeeding in GOBI-FF. *J. Trop. Pediat.* **31** (2).

Jelliffe, D. B., and Jelliffe, E. F. P. (1990a). *Community Nutritional Assessment.* Oxford University Press, Oxford.

Jelliffe, E. F. P., and Jelliffe, D. B. (1990b). Improving dietary density. *J. Trop. Pediat.* **36**, 210.

Keen, H.; Thomas, B. J.; Jarrett, R. J.; and Fuller, J. H. (1979). Nutrient intake, adiposity, and diabetes. *Br. Med. J.* **1**, 655.

Kielman, A. A., and McCord, C. (1978). Weight for-age as an index of risk of death in children. *Lancet* **i**, 1247.

Lappe, F. M., and Collins, J. (1979). *Food First: Beyond the Myth of Scarcity.* Ballantine Books, New York.

Lauber, E., and Reinhardt, M. C. (1981). Prolonged lactation performance in a rural community in the Ivory Coast. *J. Trop. Pediat.* **27.**.

Lucas, A., et al. (1992). Breast milk and subsequent intelligence quotient in children born preterm. *Lancet* **339**, 261–64.

McDowell, J. (1978). Appropriate technologies for tackling malnourishment. *Contact* **45**, 1–9.

McLaren, D. S. (1963). *Malnutrition and the Eye.* Academic Press, New York.

McLaren, D. S. (1966). A fresh look at protein calorie malnutrition. *Lancet* **ii**, 485.

MARHIA (1991). Institute for Social Studies and Action (ISSA). IV(1).

Mata, L. (1978). *Nutrition and Health in Societies in Transition: Proceedings of the West-*ern Hemisphere Nutrition Congress V. American Medical Association, Chicago.

Meneghello, J.; Rosselot, J.; Aguila, C.; Monkberg, F.; Undurraga, O.; and Ferreiro, N. (1960). Infantile diarrhoea and dehydration: Ambulatory treatment in a hydration centre. *Adv. Pediat.* **11**, 183.

Narayanan, I.; Prakash, K.; and Gujral, V. V. (1981). The value of human milk in the prevention of infection in high risk low birth weight infants. *J. Pediat.* **99**, 496.

Pirie, A. (1983). Vitamin A deficiency and child blindness in the developing world. *Proc. Nutr. Soc.* **42**, 53.

Roberts, I. F. (1979). Malnutrition in infants receiving cult diets. *Brit. Med. J.* **1**, 296.

Schaefer, O. (1971). When the Eskimo comes to town. *Nutr. Today* **6**, 8.

Shaumburg, H.; Kaplan, J.; Windebank, A.; Vick, N.; Rasmus, S.; Pleasure, D.; and Brown, M. (1983). Sensory neuropathy from pyridoxine abuse. *New Engl. Med. J.* **309**, 446.

Shingwekar, A. G.; Gopaldas, T.; Srinivasan, N.; Bhargava, V.; and Seth, R. (1977). Nutritional rehabilitation at the hut level: Educational impact. *J. Trop. Pediatr. Envtl. Child Hlth.* **23**, 97.

Shingwekar, A. G.; Mohonram, M.; and Reddy, V. (1979). Effect of zinc supplementation on plasma levels of vitamin A and retinol blinding protein in malnourished children. *Clin. Chim. Acta.* **93**, 97.

Solomons, N. W., and Torun, B. (1982). Infantile malnutrition in the tropics. *Pediat. Annals* **11**, 991.

Sommer, A., et al. (1986). Impact of vitamin A supplementation on childhood mortality: A randomized community trial. *Lancet* **1**, 1169–73.

Tomkins, A., and Watkins, F. (1989). *Malnutrition and Infection: A Review ACSCNN.* FAO/WHO/UNICEF, Rome.

Torem, S. (1990). Covert multiple personality underlying eating disorders. *Am. J. Psychotherapy* **44**, (3), 356.

Trowell, H. C.; Davies, J. W. P.; and Dean, R. F. A. (1982). *Kwashiorkor: A Nutrition Foundation Report of Kwashiorkor.* Edward Arnold and Academic Press, London.

UNICEF (1990). *Strategy for Improved Nutrition of Women and Children in Developing Countries.* UNICEF Policy Review 1990–1. United Nations, New York.

USAID (1992). *Child Survival.* Report to Congress, Washington D.C.

USAID (1979). *Iron Deficiency in Infancy and Childhood.* Report of the International Nutritional Anemia Consultative Group (INACG), Washington, D.C.

Victora, C. G. (1987). Evidence for protection by breast-feeding against infant deaths from infectious diseases in Brazil. *Lancet* 2, 319–22.

Vis, H. L., and Hennart, P. H. (1978). Decline in breast feeding: About some of its causes. *Acta Paediat. Belg.* 31, 197.

Waterlow, J. C. (1972). Classification and definition of PCM. *Brit. Med. J.* 2, 566.

Whitehead, R. G. (1977). Infection and the development of kwashiorkor and marasmus in Africa. *Am. J. Clin. Nutr.* 30, 1281.

Williams, C. D. (1933). Nutritional disease of childhood associated with a maize diet. *Arch. Dis. Childhd.* 8, 423.

Williams, C. D. (1938a). Child health in the Gold Coast. *Lancet* i, 97.

Williams, C. D. (1938b). Common diseases of children in Singapore. *J. Malaya Brit. Med. Asso.* 2, 113.

Williams, C. D. (1946). Rickets in Singapore. *Arch. Dis. Childhd.* 21, 37.

Williams, C. D. (1957). World nutrition. *Roy. Soc. Hlth. J.* 77, 47.

Williams, C. D. (1962). Malnutrition. *Lancet* ii(84), 342.

Williams, C. D. (1963). The story of kwashiorkor. *Courier* 13, 361.

Williams, C. D. (1980). An outsider's view of disease prevention. In *Optimal Nutrition and Disease Prevention*, pp. 242–56. Proceedings of Public Health Nutrition Update. Ed. J. B. Anderson. School of Public Health, Chapel Hill, N.C.

Wiseman, G. (1964). *Absorption from the Intestine.* Academic Press, London.

WHO (1968). Nutrition in maternal and child health with special reference to the Western Pacific. *J. Trop. Pediat. Monogr.* 5, 149.

WHO (1973). *Trace Elements in Human Nutrition.* Wld. Hlth. Org. Rep. Ser., no. 532.

WHO (1981). *Guidelines for Training Community Health Workers in Nutrition.* WHO offset publication no. 59. World Health Organization, Geneva.

WHO (1991). *Child Health and Development: Health of the Newborn.* EB89/26. World Health Organization, Geneva.

Wright, V.; Hopkins, R.; and Burton, K. E. (1979). What shall we teach undergraduates. *Brit. Med. J.* 1, 805.

9

Measurements
of Health

*Ethical values cannot be measured . . . but that there is a
relationship between the revelations of vital statistics and human
responsibility in a modern society we can scarcely dispute.*
JOHN RYLE, 1947

Medicine is a combination of a science, an art, and a craft. Using both the natural and the social sciences, health professionals try to obtain exact measurements of the condition, the progress, and the needs of patients, both individuals and groups.

In addition to exact measurements, practitioners learn to depend on imponderables or unmeasurables—in fact, the same type of information that ancient physicians depended on. They notice that "the patient seems better today," "the mother is still very worried," or "feels drowsy," or is "delighted with the new nurse." Through observation, health professionals learn to assess progress and to measure the value of services (Emery and Irvine 1958; Falkner 1966).

With respect to individuals, health workers give numerical measures to age, height, weight, pulse, temperature, respiration, bowel movements, and so forth. They try to measure accurately the hemoglobin, blood sugar, white cells, and a number of other factors that may reflect the condition of the patient. Health workers must be aware that hemodilution or hemoconcentration may be influencing the numerical data, or that the weight may be affected by the presence of edema or an enlarged liver, and that even the best laboratories can make mistakes. A constant watch must be kept on the efficiency and accuracy of people, methods, and machines.

The physician must know the disorders to expect. Tuberculosis, for example, is more common in the United Kingdom in unskilled workers than in professional and managerial employees; ascariasis is exceedingly probable in children from certain areas of the world but would be a medical curiosity in other areas. So although health care workers must always be prepared to encounter rare conditions, they will be wasting valuable time for the patient and for themselves unless they know what conditions are likely to occur within a certain context and the range of variations within normal limits.

Health professionals must constantly review their own and other people's work to judge the results of treatment and improve the quality of the service. They must be alert to changing patterns of disease, and prevention and therapy. Examples include the resurgence of malaria in many parts of the world, drug-resistant tuberculosis in recent years in the United States, and the AIDS epidemic. Good public health is based on good clinical judgment, and vice versa (Glass and Eversley 1965; UN 1955; WHO 1950). With respect to groups, it is desirable for clinical and administrative health workers to obtain reliable figures for births and deaths and mortality and morbidity. As well as these vital statistics and health statistics, accurate and timely numerical information should be available on a wide range of subjects: environmental sanitation, housing, education, food supply, transport, industries, meteorology, shopping facilities, and wages. An enormous number of factors may affect human health and well-being. Health care workers must select those that are significant in a particular context.

SOCIAL ASPECTS OF STATISTICS

Before one attempts to collect statistics, or before one places too much faith in them, it is necessary to become familiar with some of the local traditions and attitudes, the standards of education, and responsibility, all of which may interfere with the collection of data or may modify the relevance and accuracy of reports, as well as almost universal logistical and social difficulty in collecting such personal, often socially sensitive, data (Fig. 9.1) (Horwitz 1968; Huxtable 1967).

The propagation and care of children are highly important functions in every community. Birth and death, sickness and health, and hunger are surrounded by emotional and cultural factors. They vary from place to place, and the variations may be extreme. In communities where child mortality is high, people believe that it is unlucky to speak of dead chil-

dren or even to enumerate the living: "If I count them today, tomorrow they will die." In a small, well-run maternity hospital in East Africa, the records showed that 100 mothers admitted for confinement had 296 children, of whom 294 were reported to be still alive. In fact, in the previous year, there had been nearly 100 funerals of children under the age of 2 years.

In a study in Uganda, Welbourn (1956) found that in 1950, 5 percent of the mothers reported that their children had died; in 1955, in spite of improvements in health and living conditions, the reported figure was 13 percent. Welbourn postulated that "the figure obtained in 1950 was probably inaccurate" because "mothers do not like answering questions about dead children. It is only in recent years that we have had confidence to pursue our inquiries sufficiently relentlessly."

The process of collecting data requires confidence on both sides. This is established only when there is continuity of personnel and of policy.

In some countries, boys are much preferred to girls. If a man is asked the number of children he has, he may not mention the girls. Even in a relatively sophisticated community in the Middle East, it was found that the infant mortality rate for boys was less than two-thirds that for girls; boys who were ill were taken to hospitals and doctors, and girls were not. Even though the women are hard working, girls are looked upon as a liability (Glass and Eversley 1965; Powers 1955).

In other areas, especially in equatorial Africa, girls may be preferred to boys for cultural and economic reasons. In traditional cultures, men do the hunting and fighting, while women bear and rear the children, grow and prepare the foodstuffs, carry the wood and water, and in some areas even build the houses. Now that there is little hunting and, in good times, less fighting, many of the men are

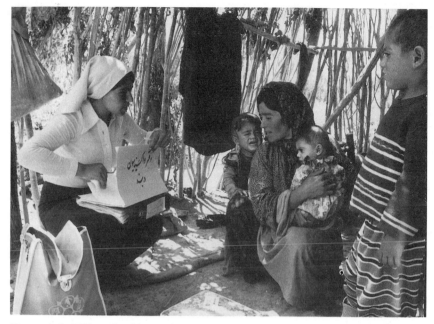

Figure 9.1. Village health worker collecting statistics. A village health worker records growth information and other health data as part of a child health survey in the Mansehra district, Bangladesh. UNICEF photograph by Akil Kahn.

relatively idle unless they become mechanics, or industrial, clerical, professional, or political workers. A large family of daughters, therefore, provides many workers and many candidates for the bride-price, enriching the father's property by several head of cattle. In a polygamous society, a man's prestige may be related to the number of wives he possesses. Women are therefore always in demand, and if there is any alternative, more trouble will be taken to ensure the survival of a girl than of a boy. In some areas, twins and multiple births are looked upon as particularly lucky; in other regions, the opposite is true.

In many parts of the world, fertility is much desired. A woman's prestige depends on the number of pregnancies she has undergone as much as on the number of surviving children, and when asked about her children, she may or may not count abortions and miscarriages. Anxiety about producing children, however, may give rise to cases of pseudocyesis.

These factors must be considered in any retrospective survey.

Among many communities, efforts are now being made to register births and deaths. Some of the individual community or village leaders are interested, and the records may be accurate; others may show little interest and fail to understand the value of such figures. On one occasion, it was found that births were being entered in the deaths book. In another area, it was found that the infant mortality rate appeared to be high because deaths were regularly registered to obtain a burial permit and because of the traditional funeral ceremonies, while births were not routinely reported. A few families were prosecuted for failure to register births, which resulted in a considerable reduction in the reported infant mortality rate.

Less developed areas have less accurate statistics. Even so, figures should not be ignored. Only by persistent care and emphasis can they be made accurate, or the reason for inaccuracies understood and improvements in collection made, sometimes initially in a trial area. The first point to stress is the need for reporting births and deaths and the sex and age at death. The cause of death specified is often unreliable unless the report is made by a qualified and conscientious medical practitioner, and preferably after a postmortem examination has been performed. Even in the more advanced countries, it is often impossible to give a confident and definitive diagnosis without an autopsy. It is true that in many countries one is told that "these people will not allow autopsies." But when the people have confidence and the doctor makes the time and takes the trouble to explain their importance, often autopsies will be permitted. Even in a Muslim population this is true. The Koran directs that a dead body must be treated with respect, but some followers of Islam are convinced that a postmortem does not infringe this injunction. In fact, postmortems are vital for a clearer understanding of child deaths and their prevention.

The fact of death is relatively easy to ascertain; the cause of death is much more difficult. Medical students are always taught to beware of a double diagnosis, but in developing countries it is by no means unusual to have children admitted to hospital suffering from many conditions simultaneously—for example, diarrhea, bronchitis, scabies, ascariasis, malnutrition, and malaria. Each of these conditions must be identified and treated and, if possible, subsequent attacks prevented. Which of these conditions is regarded as the major cause of ill health, or possibly of death, will depend on the judgment, interest, and training of the health care worker.

If the sick child dies, the immediate cause of death may well be a terminal bronchopneumonia, but practically every baby who dies can be found to have some autopsy indication of pneumonia since it is a pathological terminal event rather than a cause of death. It is therefore necessary not only to record the terminal condition but to search for all the factors that have led to this outcome. Numbers of children labeled as cases of malnutrition are, in fact, the outcome of maldigestion and diarrhea—acute, chronic, and recurrent. What may be needed for prevention and therapy is not only a better diet but also better hygiene in the home.

There are many areas in which there are only a few qualified doctors, and the inhabitants still prefer indigenous forms of treatment. In one area in Malaysia, deaths were reported to the local police station, and if there was no suspicion of foul play, a burial permit would be issued. The police were given some training in this subject, and there was a list of about fifty diseases from which they could select the most appropriate diagnosis. In fact, the diagnoses that were frequently recorded were "convulsions" and "crying convulsions" for children under 5 years and "fever" and "hot fever" for persons between the ages of 5 and 30. After age 30, the usual finding was senility. The inclusion of these figures in the official summary seriously compromised the accuracy of the whole report (Williams 1942).

If, in a developed country, parents have three children, they can look forward with considerable confidence to rearing three children. But there are still many regions where the life of the baby is regarded as so insecure that no preparations are made for the birth and no name is given for several months as these actions would indicate foolhardiness. The result sometimes is that there is a reluctance to become emotionally involved with a creature whose life may be so short. An elderly woman in Karamoja, Uganda, was asked how many children she had. The reply was, "Oh, I can't remember a thing like that. I know I've only got one now."

Registration is frequently omitted for babies who die very young: "He was so small when he died, that I did not trouble the government to register him." Babies who die after a few days may not be registered as either births or as deaths, and these omissions seriously distort the infant mortality rate.

The search for reliable information is sometimes met with fear of bad luck, of conscription, or of taxation increases and usually with indifference because the objectives are not understood. Occasionally governmental authorities fear to reveal conditions that are unflattering to their administration. A doctor was once informed that all his blood samples sent for a Widal test were found to be negative because he "could not have more than twelve cases of typhoid in one year." It is only gradually that the need for absolute honesty rather than prestige in reporting can be appreciated by all the people concerned—at governmental, health worker, and patient levels. Such honesty is usually taken for granted in more technically developed countries, but it is by no means easy to achieve. A maternity hospital must be careful to report a baby as a live birth and not as a stillbirth if he or she shows any sign of movement (respiratory, cardiac, or voluntary) after delivery. If such cases are not reported correctly, as well as those associated with maternal mortality, the figures will not be valid for estimating progress or assessing health care.

The doctor may be doubtful in cases of multiple diagnosis and may not know what to give as the primary or secondary cause or causes of death. But sometimes the doctor's own lack of interest or knowledge is responsible for misinformation. One doctor, going to a district in Africa for the first time, was informed by his predecessor and others in the neighborhood that there were no cases remotely resembling kwashiorkor. This new doctor was interested in nutrition and in pediatrics. Within five years he had recognized and treated over 400 cases

with varying but obvious evidence of severe nutritional deficiency.

To give a further example, an exhaustive search through the medical records of the Gold Coast (Ghana) showed that no cases of pellagra had been reported up to 1931. Shortly after this, a controversy arose as to the nature of "kwashiorkor." Various authorities (some of them without seeing the cases) decided that this disorder was "infantile pellagra." After this, "pellagra" was diagnosed on a number of occasions. We can see that a confusion in nomenclature may thus lead to unreliable records. Doctors who have had little training or interest in pediatrics may completely fail to recognize blatant cases of scurvy, beriberi, or mongolism. Moreover, failure to look for and to recognize early xerophthalmia in babies may be one of the most important causes of preventable blindness in the world.

In many areas of the world, children are not brought to hospitals or dispensaries because the parents do not recognize that they are sick or that anything can be done. They take it for granted that though the baby of 6 months is chubby and cheerful, the toddler and weanling is invariably potbellied, spindle-legged, and miserable, with frequent attacks of diarrhea, worms, or respiratory disorders. Often when MCH services are started, child mortality and morbidity figures increase rather than decrease, for the effect of the new services will be first to stimulate an interest, which may lead to more accurate records, and then to demonstrate what can be done in this area of medical care and supervision.

VITAL STATISTICS

A seventeenth-century definition of *statistiks* is "political arithmetic." Certain vital statistics reflect in particular the health of women and children in a community. To collect and interpret these, it is imperative to use definitions and classifications laid down by international agreement so that valid comparisons can be made. *Breastfeeding* is an example of a term that is poorly defined; thus, wrong conclusions can be drawn and incorrect actions taken. Breastfeeding may be defined as once a day (the definition currently used in the WIC program) or fully or partial, but for optimal effects, breastfeeding should be exclusive. Exclusive breastfeeding is defined as:

Breast milk only

Nursing within an hour of birth

Demand feeding

Colostrum

Frequent feeding in twenty-four hours (plus night feeds)

Duration of four to six months

When the effect of breastfeeding was measured in a study in a Lahore slum in Pakistan, it was erroneously found not to be protective against diarrhea. When practices were examined, researchers found that breastfeeding did not start until three to five days after birth. In that period, various polluted concoctions were given to the baby. When those who breastfed exclusively were followed, the protective effect of exclusive breastfeeding was found. In India, when exclusive breastfeeding rates were separated from nonexclusive rates, the duration of breastfeeding was very different. Measurement of exclusive breastfeeding determined the duration of breastfeeding (Fig. 9.2) (Baumslag 1989).

Definitions

Birthrate: The number of live births in one year per 1,000 population. This will vary with the average age of the population and with the male-to-female ratio, as well as with other factors.

A live birth is the complete expulsion or extraction of a product of conception, irrespective of the duration of pregnancy, which after separation breathes or shows any evidence of life, such as beating of the heart, pulsation of the umbilical cord, or definite movements of the voluntary muscles, whether or not the umbilical cord has been cut or the placenta is attached.

Death rate: The number of deaths registered per 1,000 population. This crude death rate may be adjusted in various ways. For instance, in a hospital, there may be many deaths occurring in people from other areas. Moreover, deaths may be further analyzed by age, sex, occupation, social class, disease, district, and

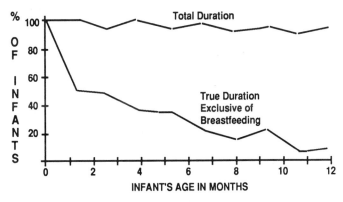

Figure 9.2. Health planners can be lulled into complacency when imprecise measures are used. Source: Modified from Gopujkar in India, Baumslag (1989).

various other relevant factors. Death rates by age groups may be calculated per 1,000 of population or per 1,000 of that particular age group.

Growth rate to natural rate of increase: The difference between birth and death rates.

Fertility rate: The number of total births per year per 1,000 women between ages 15 and 45. This gives a more accurate indication of the rate of reproduction than does the birthrate.

Stillbirth rate (also termed *late fetal death rate*): The number of stillbirths per year per 1,000 births (live and still) with a gestation period of twenty-eight weeks or more. It is often difficult to be certain that every stillbirth has been registered.

Perinatal mortality rate: Total number of stillbirths plus the number of deaths under 1 week old, per 1,000 births (live and still), or the sum of late fetal deaths and early neonatal deaths.

Infant mortality rate: The number of infants under 1 year of age dying per 1,000 live births. The younger the child at death and the greater the distance from the registration center, the less likely it is to be registered, as either a birth or a death. Infant mortality is the sum of neonatal and postnatal deaths.

Neonatal mortality rate: The number of deaths under 28 days of age per 1,000 live births.

Postneonatal mortality rate: The number of deaths over 28 days but under 1 year of age per 1,000 live births.

Under-5 mortality rate (U5MR): The number of children who die before the age of 5 for every 1,000 live births. It is one of UNICEF's principal indicators to measure levels of and changes in the well-being of children, and is highly correlated with the infant and child mortality rate. The U5MR is the way countries are ordered for comparison in the *State of the*

Table 9.1. Under-5 Mortality Rates, 1990, Selected Countries

Very high U5MR (over 140)	
Mozambique	297
Malawi	284
Cambodia	193
Nepal	189
Bolivia	160
India	142
High U5MR (71–140)	
Haiti	130
Peru	116
Kenya	108
Middle U5MR (21–70)	
Philippines	69
Jordan	52
Mexico	49
Costa Rica	22
Rumania	34
Low U5MR (20 and under)	
Jamaica	20
Poland	18
Greece	11
United States	11
United Kingdom	9
Hong Kong	7
Japan	6

Source: UNICEF (1992).

The U5 MR is one of the principal indicators used by UNICEF to measure level of and changes in the well-being of children. When rates fall below 150/1,000 live births (e.g., India) and move toward and through the 100 barrier, the strong consistent patterns of fertility change begin to emerge.

World's Children report (Table 9.1). Note that this data is a result of extrapolating 1980 or earlier trends and may differ from individual (and possibly) more recent national estimates (UNICEF 1992).

Child mortality rate: The number of deaths between ages 1 to 4 years in a year per 1,000 children. This rate reflects the main environmental factors affecting the child's health, such as nutrition, sanitation, communicable diseases, and accidents around the home. It is a sensitive indicator of socioeconomic development in a community and may be twenty-five times higher in developing countries compared with the so-called developed countries. This information is often not readily available.

Maternal mortality rate: Usually stated as deaths of mothers per 100,000 live births. This rate is more significant when related to live and stillbirths. Maternal mortality and infant, neonatal, and perinatal mortality rates are all reduced by good antenatal care, as well as by good care at delivery.

Measurement of women's health has focused primarily on maternal mortality rates. The importance of this information globally is illustrated in Table 9.2. Although a maternal mortality rate of 630 per 100,000 live births or about 1 in 200 for Africa would appear relatively small, the lifetime risk of such women, taking into account the high fertility rate is 1 in 23. In West Africa, the risk is 1 in 18, or more than 5 percent. These women die as payment for bearing their children—a price too high. Further, there was no improvement in these rates from 1983 to 1988.

At the community level, where perhaps each year some thirty births occur yearly, even one pregnancy-related maternal death should be cause for concern. Indeed, some communities conduct an audit to help them understand preventive measures in the future. Hence, the measurement of one event is sufficient, provided action is taken.

Where maternal mortality rate is not readily available, a simple methodology has been developed: the **Sisterhood Mortality Method.** Women are interviewed to determine what happened to their sisters during childbirth (Graham and Campbell 1991).

HEALTH STATISTICS

Morbidity can be assessed by mortality statistics to a certain extent. But particularly for the more chronic disorders, analyzing figures from hospitals, health centers, and private practitioners is necessary. Morbidity and health statistics may be more accurate in regions where most of the health facilities are provided by the state than where there are large numbers of private practitioners (Wootton 1956; WHO 1969). Other indicators are also available that can measure health policy, social and economic factors, health care provision, and health status (Table 9.3).

Health statistics can be obtained from a variety of sources:

- Vital events registers
- Censuses (population and household)
- Routine health service records (hospital, clinic, practitioners)
- Epidemiological surveillance data
- Sample surveys
- Disease registers and special studies
- Other sectors, such as labor, agriculture, or commerce
- Religious authorities

Table 9.2. Estimates of Maternal Mortality (per 100,000 live births)

	Maternal mortality	Lifetime risk	Total fertility
Developed countries	26	1 in 1,825	1.9
Developing countries	420	1 in 57	3.8
Africa	630	1 in 23	6.1
Oceania	600	1 in 32	4.8
Asia	380	1 in 71	3.4
Latin America	200	1 in 131	3.4

Source: Adapted from Graham (1991).

Table 9.3. Types of Health Indicators

Health policy indicators	Political commitment to health for all
	Health resource allocation and priorities
	Community involvement in attaining health for all
	Degree of equity of distribution of health resources
	Organizational framework and managerial process
Social and economic indicators of health care	Rate of population increase
	Gross national product or gross domestic product
	Income distribution
	Work conditions
	Adult literacy rates
	Housing
	Food availability
	Water supply
	Environmental sanitation and waste disposal
Indicators of health care provision	Coverage by primary health care
	Coverage by the referral system
	New facilities installed
Health status indicators	Nutritional status and psychosocial development of children
	Infant mortality rate
	Child mortality rate (ages 1–4 years, inclusive)
	Life expectancy at birth or at other specific ages
	Maternal mortality rate
	Birthweight

Source: WHO (1981).

In villages there is always someone who knows about who died and who was born. This invaluable information often is not used.

For the selection of sources of data for health status and service indicators, see Table 9.4.

Certain diseases—for example, yellow fever, cholera, and plague—are notifiable under international law. Others, such as typhoid, poliomyelitis, and tuberculosis, are notifiable in certain countries. The efficiency of notification will depend on the understanding of the local population and even more on the prevalence of conscientious and reliable health workers.

Hospitals, health centers, and individual practitioners should make regular analyses of local mortality and morbidity statistics. Their compliance can be ensured by means of legislation requiring annual reports. All records should be organized to make annual reports possible and to facilitate special investigations when indicated. By this means, the changing frequency and pattern of disease can be studied to assess incidence and prevalence and the demand for and results of treatment. These data can be compared with results from other methods and other institutions and used to improve services. In order to improve the accuracy of records, the total number of births may be cross-checked with the proportion of women attending for antenatal supervision and with the total number of babies under supervision in health centers. The total number of deaths recorded in children of various age groups should, if possible, be compared with the number of death certificates signed by doctors in other age groups and the deaths by age groups of babies born.

Every effort must be made to ensure good diagnosis and efficient follow-up. Even an overcrowded clinic should have a microscope available, and a voluntary worker or auxiliary health aide can be trained to prepare slides from blood, urine, feces, and sputum. In this way, the phy-

Table 9.4. Sources of Data for Health Status and Service Indicators

Indicators	Vital events registers	Population and household censuses	Routine health service records	Epidemiological surveillance data	Sample surveys	Disease registers	Other
Health status indicators							
Birthweight	P				A		
Weight and height			P	A	A		
Arm circumference			P	A	A		
Infant mortality	P	P		A			
Child mortality	P	P			A		
Under-5 mortality	P	P			A		
Under-5 proportionate mortality	P				A		
Life expectancy at given age	P	P			A		
Maternal mortality	P	P	P			A	
Crude birthrate	P	P			A		
Disease-specific death rates	P		P	P	A	A	
Proportionate mortality from specific disease	P		P	P	A	A	
Morbidity							
Incidence rate			P	P	A	P	
Prevalence rate			P	P	A	P	
Prevalence of long-term disability			P		A		P
Indicators of the provision of health care							
Physical accessibility		P	P	A	A		
Percentage of population served		P	P	P	A		
Water and sanitation		P			P		P
Immunization coverage			P	P	A		
Population/health personnel ratio		P	P		A		P

Source: WHO (1981).

Note: P = primary, A = alternative.

sician can identify an unexpected sickling; acute diarrhea due to strongyloides, amoebae, or giardia, hematuria due to schistosomiasis, and so forth. Postmortem examinations must be carried out wherever possible. It may also be necessary to find out what is meant by a postmortem. In some contexts, this means simply an inspection of the body; there is no autopsy unless there is some indication of foul play. On one occasion, a doctor was called in to examine the body of a child of 7 who had died after a few hours' illness. He carried out an autopsy and then wrote on the death certificate "cyanogenetic glucoside poisoning." He explained that this was the answer he invariably received when specimens were sent to the laboratory and therefore there was no point in sending another.

Avoid drawing conclusions from vital statistics until there is some idea of their accuracy, including those published by international bodies. These vital statistics will never be accurate until good MCH services are achieved; conversely, good MCH services are dependent on accurate vital statistics. The two are thus interdependent. Regular analysis and good follow-up will help to guide policies and ensure the best use of hospitals and other facilities. The work of Puffer and Griffiths (1967) illustrates the differences that may exist in health records in different cities. In Bristol, England, the death rate among adults (aged 15 to 75) was 4.4 and in Mexico City 37. The differences would have been far greater if children had been counted.

VITAL STATISTICS AND MCH SERVICES

Vital statistics are valued as overall indicators of MCH—indeed, of health conditions as a whole. Perinatal mortality rates are now being studied intensively in countries that provide an advanced type of health service. The control of preventable diseases has reduced the infant, toddler, school-age, and maternal mortality rates to marked degrees, but the perinatal mortality rate has proved more resistant. The two aspects involved—late fetal mortality and mortality under 7 days—are now receiving much attention, especially where the majority of births take place in hospitals. Low-birthweight infants have a higher perinatal death rate. Many of these infants are immature or small for gestational age. The signs of immaturity and the duration of pregnancy must therefore be taken into account, as well as the birthweight. Duration of gestation may be very difficult to estimate in less developed areas—hence, the need for careful observation and accuracy.

Statistical information should be collected on patterns of disease, to complement vital statistics health resources, services and their effects. Some of the tables and figures in this chapter that follow

were compiled at national levels and some from small village observations. They illustrate a few examples of how figures of many sorts may be used to reflect the biological and social status of a community or may be employed to guide policy and programs and measure progress.

Patterns of Disease

The causes of death in adults (Table 9.5) and infants in the United States in 1900 and in 1989 (Table 9.6) show that patterns of disease and death have changed (Hanlon 1960; NCHS 1992). During those years, the overall death rate in the United States was reduced by half, from 1,719 to 866 per 100,000 population. Moreover, the pattern of disease showed considerable changes as a result of many factors: improvements in education, health services, economic production, food and living patterns, medical supervision and treatment. Despite the technological advances in the United States by 1979, the IMR for whites was 11.8 (for 1,000 live births) while the figure for nonwhites was nearly double—23.9. The difference still exists, although the proportion of deaths from diseases of early infancy has decreased.

In many developing countries the proportion of diseases of early infancy is still very high, a reflection of the lack of services for infants (Fig. 9.3). Rohde, et al. in 1978, suggested that a handful of existing primary health care technologies could reduce the annual infant and child deaths from 17 million to 10 million worldwide (Rohde et al. 1978). Indeed, during 1990, 13 million children died from preventable diseases (USAID 1990). Unless there is continuity of care, the effect will, however, not be appreciable.

Perinatal Mortality Rate

A Viennese study in 1920 found that good antenatal care and rest reduced per-

Table 9.5. Causes of Death in Adults in the United States, 1900, 1989

1900	Death rate per 100,000	% of deaths	1989	Death rate per 100,000	% of deaths
All causes	1719	100.0	All causes	866.3	100.0
Pneumonia and influenza	202	11.8	Diseases of the heart	295.6	34.1
Tuberculosis	194	11.3	Malignant neoplasms	199.9	23.1
Diarrhea and enteritis	143	8.3	Cerebrovascular disease	58.6	6.8
Heart disease	137	8.0	Accidents	38.3	4.4
Cerebral vascular lesions	107	6.2	Chronic obstructive pulmonary		
Chronic nephritis	81	4.7	diseases	34.0	3.9
Accidents	72	4.2	Pneumonia and influenza	30.8	3.6
Cancer	64	3.7	Diabetes mellitus	18.9	2.2
Certain diseases of early infancy	63	3.6	Suicide	12.2	1.4
Diphtheria	40	2.3	Chronic liver disease and		
			cirrhosis	10.8	1.2
			Atherosclerosis	7.8	0.9
			Certain conditions originating		
			in the perinatal period	17.6	0.9
			All other causes	117.5	13.6

Source: National Center for Health Statistics (1992).

inatal mortality rates. This outcome was even more evident in unmarried mothers, who carried greater risks (Table 9.7).

The causes of perinatal mortality are generally attributed to trauma and stress of labor, toxemia, antepartum hemorrhage, maternal disease (particularly malaria and malnutrition), congenital anomalies, infections, and induced abortions.

The perinatal mortality rate in Africa is high—81 per 1,000; in Asia it is 58 and in Latin America 54 per 1,000. In absolute numbers globally, Asia has the largest percentage of infants dying: 63 percent (WHO 1991). Approximately half

of the perinatal deaths occur in the neonatal period. In Mauritius it is just over 30 per 1,000; in Sweden and Japan, it is much lower. Improvements in prenatal and delivery care appear to affect the decline in perinatal mortality.

Rates and causes of perinatal mortality are less well documented in developing areas. Available data indicate that in some areas like Addis Ababa, Ethiopia, the perinatal mortality rate was as high as 66 per 1,000 live births (Tafari 1978) and that amniotic fluid infection syndrome was a significant cause. The associated finding of low zinc and absent antibac-

Table 9.6. Changes in Causes of Infant Mortality, United States, 1900–1989

	1900	1954	1989
Death rate per 1,000 live births	150.0	26.6	—
Causes of death			
Infective and parasitic diseases	7.9%	1.15%	0.9%
Diarrhea and enteritis	24.7	2.97	0.2
Pneumonia and influenza	14.7	6.93	3.2
Congenital malformations	6.4	12.54	20.5
Certain diseases in early infancy (including prematurity)	34.5	52.1	46.8
All other causes	11.8	11.6	37.9

Sources: NCHS (1982); Hanlon (1960); NCHS (1992).

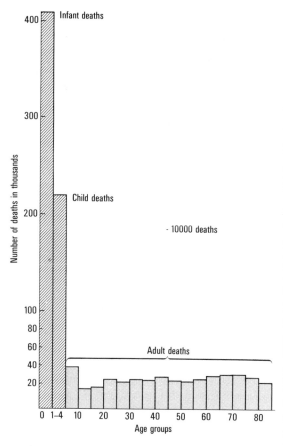

Figure 9.3. Number of deaths in Java, by age. Source: Rohde et al. (1978).

Table 9.7. Effect on Perinatal Mortality Rate of Good Antenatal Care, Vienna, 1920

Antenatal maternity homes Days in home before delivery	0–7	8–28	29–56
Perinatal mortality rate			
Legitimate	88	30	16
Illegitimate	102	43	32

Source: Czermsk and Hansluwka (1962).

terial effect of amniotic fluid in these cases suggests that zinc may play an important part in the etiology of this syndrome.

Care of the Premature

Care of the premature has become highly specialized and is often associated with expensive equipment, complicated biochemistry, and a large and highly trained staff. An example of how accurate measurement can support promising initiatives in the care of premature or low-birthweight infants follows. Dr. Sam Wayburne developed a simple and extremely successful method of care for premature infants at Baragwanath Hospital, Johannesburg, South Africa, where mothers were always admitted with their babies, and there were no incubators in the ward. The newly admitted mothers were assisted by other mothers, as well as nurses. Each was taught how to express her own milk and feed it to the baby. The temperature and humidity of the ward was regulated by the nurses, and hypothermia was treated with carefully protected hot water bottles. Nasogastric feed tubes were used for infants below 1,500 grams. After discharge, supervision was maintained by municipal health nurses and doctors, as 50 percent of the mothers were illiterate. A 93 percent survival rate was achieved for babies with a birthweight between 1,500 and 2,500 grams (Table 9.8).

This pattern of care is suitable for many countries, particularly where breastfeeding is encouraged, and has been used in a modified form in Uganda. The results at Baragwanath compare favorably with many services that are far more complicated and expensive and far less educational for the mother.

Life Expectancy

One hundred and eighty years ago in Europe, life expectancy was 20 to 40 years; in the more technologically advanced industrial countries, it is now over 70 years. In countries where there is balanced progress in the establishment of law and order, health and education, and economic progress (including food availability), there is increased survival and longevity and improved quality of life. Disease control and assistance programs

Table 9.8. Survival Rates of Premature Babies, Baragwanath Hospital

	Number of babies	Percentage of total cases	Percentage of survivals
Birthweight			
Below 1,000 g	87	9	16
1,001–1,500 g	335	34.9	69.3
1,501–2,000 g	476	49.5	93.1
2,001–2,500 g	62	6.3	93.8
Fully breastfed on discharge		74.4	
Partially breastfed on discharge		19.5	

Source: Kahn et al. (1954).

result in increased survival and longevity, although they do not automatically improve standards of education and responsibility.

Death Rates by Sex

In Sri Lanka (Ceylon) in 1950, the maternal mortality rate in one area was being investigated, but it was recorded as being remarkably small; at that time, however, deaths were classified by age groups and by sex (Table 9.9). It would appear from these figures that there was a higher mortality in women than in men and that it was confined to the childbearing years. This example shows that careful attention to age and sex differences in mortality rates can identify groups in need of special services.

Effects of Progress and War

In Singapore, the birthrate in 1925 was found to be only 25 because the population was 75 percent male. During the Japanese occupation of 1942–1945, the mortality rate rose and the birthrate decreased; after the war, there was a baby boom because many men brought their wives to live in Singapore. Family planning clinics were started, associated with the already well-patronized MCH clinics. In 1968, the birthrate was reduced to 24 and the IMR to 23. In 1980, the birthrate dropped to 17 and the IMR to 12 (Table 9.10). In 1990, the birthrate had dropped to 17 and the infant mortality to 8 per 1,000 live births.

The Netherlands has developed excellent MCH services. By 1940 its vital statistics were among the best in the world. The effect of the German occupation was to increase death rates (especially among children) and lower the birth rate. After the war, there was an increase in the birth rate. Today, family planning is being widely employed, and the vital statistics are among the world's best (Table 9.11).

Prevalence of Doctors

Where countries have sufficient doctors, nurses and midwives per population, the infant mortality is low because services can be extended to reach rural areas. Poor standards of health are sometimes attributed to the scarcity of doctors; the

Table 9.9. Differences in Age and Sex Mortality Rates, Ceylon (Sri Lanka), 1950

	Age group							
	0–4	5–9	10–14	15–19	20–24	25–39	40+	Total
Males	70	6.5	3.3	4.4	6.5	7.7	11.3	19.5
Females	69	7.5	3.5	5.8	10.8	12.5	12.9	21.4

Table 9.10. Vital Statistics in Singapore, 1928–1990

Date	Birthrate	Maternal mortality rate	Infant mortality rate	(1–4) Mortality rate
1928	—	—	280	60
1939	25	160	130	20
1944[a]	35	140	300	20
1950	25	100	100	—
1955	50	70	50	—
1966	40	15	25	5
1980	17	5	12	1
1990	17	10	8	9

Source: WHO (1982); UNICEF (1992).

Note: Birthrates are based on 1,000 population; maternal mortality rates are based on 100,000 live births; infant mortality rates are based on 1,000 live born; 1–4 mortality rates based on 1,000 age group at the midpoint of year.

[a]The rise in infant mortality in 1944 was due to the Japanese occupation of Singapore (1942–1945).

organization and distribution of services and the way in which medical and other health staff are utilized also affect the results of health care (Table 9.12).

Effect of Direct Interventions for Maternal and Child Care

In 1840, there was little major epidemic disease in the United Kingdom—little or no malaria, cholera, plague, smallpox, or typhus—yet when organized registration of births and deaths was begun in 1840, the IMR was recorded as 149. Sixty years later, in 1900, the IMR was 150. During that time, the country had enjoyed economic prosperity and spectacular advances in general education and literacy. The training of doctors had been improved; Florence Nightingale had organized nursing, home visiting, and midwifery training. The work of Pasteur and Lister and the development of anesthetics had transformed hospitals from refuges for the destitute into centers of medical care.

On the other hand, England in 1840 was much more rural than in 1900. The period 1840–1900 saw the growth, in the Midlands, of the cotton and woolen industrial towns from villages to some-

Table 9.11. Vital Statistics in the Netherlands, 1870–1990

Date	Birthrate	Death rate	Infant mortality rate	1–4 years mortality rate	Life expectancy
1870	40	25	148	33.1	39
1900	32	16	173	17	50
1940	21	9	37	3	—
1945	30	15	79	8	—
1950	23	7.5	25	1.6	70
1960	20	8	17	1	70
1964	14	8	14.8	0.7	73
1968	18.6	8.3	13.6	0.9	73.5[a]
1978	12.6	8.2	9.5	0.6	75
1980	12.8	8.1	8.6	0.5	76 (1977)
1989	12.6	8.5	7.3		80.5

Sources: NCHS (1968); UN (1979); WHO (1980, 1982); World Bank (1991).

[a]Estimated from averages of male and female life expectancy rates.

thing a little less than their size today, and the laws of 1860 and 1890 concerning environmental sanitation, conditions of labor, and municipal housing did not exert their full effect until after 1900. The rural population also suffered much, for the period saw the enclosure of virtually all remaining common land and the final subjugation of former yeomen to become badly paid agricultural laborers entirely at the mercy of landowners. Economic prosperity was unevenly distributed. The introduction in the 1870s of universal compulsory school attendance could not be expected to be effective until the generation profiting by it reached maturity. Nor did the regulations ending the Dickensian "Sairey Gamp" age of unsupervised, dangerous midwifery come into effect until the early 1900s. Finally, as many mothers went to work in the factories, bottle feeding became common and was carried out in as unhygienic and haphazard a manner as it is today in cities in developing countries.

Around the 1900s infant welfare centers were started in an attempt to lower infant mortality and by 1912 were rapidly being taken over by local authority governments from the voluntary societies that had established them. Between 1913 and 1917, over 100 were established in London alone. The fall in the IMR that started in 1900 has never looked back (Fig. 9.4).

The establishment of infant welfare centers and, later, antenatal clinics was the first, and perhaps the most important, of a succession of waves of health developments that, added to the delayed effects of legislative measures, carried the IMR down from 150 in 1900 to 18 in 1968, and the mortality rate of the age group 1–4 years from more than 20 to less than 1. The IMR has continued to fall; in 1990, it was reported as 8 per 1,000, with the under-5 mortality rate at 9 (UNICEF 1992).

No one can state with certainty how great a part each of these health service developments played, but the following list is a reasonable interpretation, although it does not include advances in education and economics:

1900–1930	Establishment of infant welfare clinics and later, antenatal clinics.
1920–1940	Establishment of pediatrics and increase in children's wards.
1910–1940	Mainly through the infant welfare clinics, attention to feeding patterns and timing.
1930–1950	Immunization against diptheria.
1935–1950	A natural decline in the severity of scarlet fever.
1945–1955	Advent of antibiotics, with decline in importance of many killing diseases, including tuberculosis.
1950–1960	Immunization against pertussis and poliomyelitis.

Table 9.12. Doctors, Nurses, and Midwives per Population in Three European Countries, 1990

Countries	Population per doctor	Population per nurse	Infant mortality rate	Birthrate
Netherlands	450	168	7.3	12.6
United Kingdom	611	120	8.7	13.7
Austria	388	184	8.6	11.5

Source: World Bank (1991).

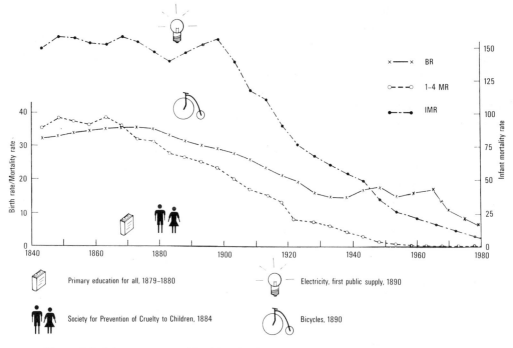

Figure 9.4. Measurements of health. The decline in birthrate in England and Wales was associated with a decline in the child death rate, 1840–1980. Source: Gossling (1970).

1948–1968 National Health Service (U.K.): Financial considerations no longer impede access to ordinary medical care.

1950–1968 Improved care for premature babies.

1967–1980 Immunization against measles, hepatitis.

1970s Improved antenatal care and introduction of new fetal diagnostic tests.

1979–1993 Primary Health Care and Health for All; Child Survival programs.

As the child and infant mortality rate fell, so did the birthrate. There was no campaign for birth control at any time, and it is only since 1950 that there has been anything like generalized access to family planning clinics.

It is worthy of note that the most spectacular improvement occurred between 1900 and 1930. The rate of improvement in the figures has not accelerated with improvements in technology. Possibly the effectiveness of environmental, economic, and educational improvements was in large measure extended through the establishment of MCH services and an improved standard of child care in the homes that is now taken for granted.

Distribution of Services

The distribution and the effects of services can be assessed by examining vital and health statistics. In a rural area, it is particularly valuable to have some statistics before any health work is started. These can then be used to measure the effect of programs (Gamble 1952; Nhonoli 1954).

The maldistribution of services in Jamaica was demonstrated by figures of Kingston and Lower St. Andrew, where 7,102 births (of a total of 8,497) had taken place in a hospital, or similar institution, while on the rest of the island, only 2,137 (of a total of 37,874) births had been in hospitals (approximately 83 percent compared to 6 percent) (Williams 1954).

In most Middle Eastern and some other countries, boys are considered highly desirable, while girls are not. Powers (1955) found that in certain rural areas in Lebanon, the infant mortality rate of males was 82, while of girls it was 162. The fact that parents were willing to pay for medical care for their sons was reflected in the pediatric wards of the American University Hospital in Beirut, where a few spot counts revealed that about 70 percent of the patients were boys. This report also showed that the availability of medical care was a major factor in survival. Villages with good communications in areas with asphalt roads had an IMR of 120, compared to villages with dirt roads, where the IMR was 247, and areas with no roads at all, where the IMR was 375.

Clinics for Under-5s

In Western Nigeria, Morley (1963) demonstrated that child health services based on the under-5s clinic reduced both the IMR (from 295 to 72) and the 1- to 4-year morality rate (from 70 to 31) at a remarkably low cost between 1957 and

1962. These clinics were run mainly by nurses and emphasized regular supervision, especially by serial weighing, prevention, early detection, effective treatment of major local problems (such as diarrhea, scabies, and pneumonia), and appropriate immunizations and antimalarials. This work was linked to hospital and children's wards.

Second-Year Mortality

The particular risks of the second year of life are often due to a combination of malnutrition and infectious disease (Gordon et al. 1967; Jelliffe 1969). Where practical, it is desirable to analyze mortality data for young children in one-year age groups (Cook 1969). When statistics from the West Indian island of St. Vincent were compared with figures from Barbados (Table 9.13), it was found that the IMR in less economically developed St. Vincent was one to three times as great as that of Barbados, while the mortality of children ages 1 to 4 years was more than five times as high. In St. Vincent the postneonatal mortality rate was twice as high as in Barbados, and the second-year mortality rate was eight times as high (Gordon et al. 1967; Jelliffe 1969) in St. Vincent compared with Barbados.

Vital Statistics as a Measure of Progress

Table 9.14 gives details of vital statistics in six Western hemisphere countries.

The percentage of deaths under the age of 5 years to total deaths is a sensitive index of health and progress. Registra-

Table 9.13. Analysis of Young Child Mortality Rates, Barbados and St. Vincent

	IMR (1966)	1–4-year MR (1960–64)	Postneonate IMR (1–11 months) (1966)	Secotrant MR (second year)
Barbados	50	3.6	25	6.0
St. Vincent	65	19.6	52	50.2
	1.3x	5.4x	2.1x	8.4x

Source: Jelliffe (1969).

Table 9.14. Vital Statistics of Some Western Countries, 1990

Country	BR	DR	MMR	IMR	U5MR	Per capita GNP (US$)
United States	16	9	8	9	13	21,700
Canada	15	7	4	7	8	20,450
El Salvador	36	8	70	55	84	1,100
Ecuador	31	7	160	57	87	960
Jamaica	25	5	110	17	22	1,510
Guatemala	39	7	76	61	99	900

Sources: UN (1990); UNICEF (1990); Pop. Ref. Bur. (1992).

Note: BR = birthrate; DR = death rate; MMR = maternal mortality rate; IMR = infant mortality rate; U5MR = under-5 mortality rate; GNP = gross national product.

tion of births and of deaths in infancy is often still incomplete. Much work has been done recently in the United States using vital and health statistics in order to identify various subgroups of "disadvantaged" communities and the conditions that produce the disadvantages. These figures are also used for making policy. The United States is financially the richest country in the world and yet ranks only seventeenth among those countries whose vital statistics are considered relatively reliable. The mortality rate among black infants is higher than among whites (NIH 1989). Infant mortality rates vary even in different parts of the same city; adjacent counties in a single state have significantly different rates. Clearly there is a need to examine not only the aggregate figures but the disparities and the causes.

Too much emphasis has been given to average per capita income and nutrient intake and too little to the inequitable distribution of the total world income and resources for good health and nutrition (20 percent of the population has 83 percent of the total world income). Measurements must pay attention to the distribution of amenities and resources in establishing causes of deprivation.

CENSUSES

Most of the so-called sophisticated countries have their population enumerated at least every ten years, a highly specialized undertaking that calls for good organization and a large, trained staff. It is the only means by which movements of population can be ascertained and suitable plans made for roads, schools, housing, industrial enterprises, hospitals, and environmental amenities. In a developing country, a census is a serious expense; if suitable personnel are available for training, it can supply useful information that may not be otherwise available because of faulty or absent registration. A census may be taken over the whole country or over selected communities.

Whatever the extent of the census or the stage of development, it is essential to aim at the highest degree of cooperation and understanding of the population. Even so, as with all other community statistical data, difficulties occur in practical enumeration of human communities; for example, the 1990 census in the United States was estimated to be 5 million below the actual total.

SURVEYS AND LONGITUDINAL STUDIES

Cross-sectional Surveys

There has been a tendency recently to perform short-term surveys when an answer is required to any question. With greatly increased speed in communications and with greater availability and mobility of medical personnel and equipment, there is a temptation to call for these surveys irrespective of cost and without sufficient relation to the validity of their findings or to the possibility of these being implemented or followed up. Yet such surveys are valuable when they can supply essential information lacking from vital or biological statistics (Abramson 1979; Jelliffe and Jelliffe 1990). This is particularly so when work can be started on the basis of their findings, and "before" and "after" figures are available for comparison. However, if the planned survey is expensive in terms of money, time, equipment, and personnel, it may be preferable to spend these resources to develop a long-term plan for medical care and supervision, with teaching and training facilities, based on existing observations and information, even if they are incomplete.

Certain answers can profitably be sought in a short-term survey, such as the prevalence of leprosy, blindness, or xerophthalmia. Others answers, such as attitudes and the incidence of acute diseases, can be found only by long-term observation. When considering a survey, the following aspects should not be forgotten:

1. Surveys may be expensive in money, transport, equipment, and personnel. If statistically sound, uncomplicated sampling techniques are used, the survey may yield valuable results at reasonable cost. Recent advances have highlighted the potential of low-cost laptop computers for quickly entering and analyzing data.

2. A short-term prevalence survey can identify chronic conditions but not acute disorders. The mathematical chances of encountering acute gastroenteritis, pneumonia, or beriberi, all of which may kill in a few days or hours, are minute compared with the chances of finding pellagra, blindness, or schistosomiasis, each of which may last for many years.

3. It may be difficult to appreciate the importance of seasonal variations.

4. Retrospective questions may not be accurately answered, from failure of either memory or cooperation.

5. Identifying the signs and symptoms of disease, such as those associated with some forms of malnutrition, may be easy, but many of these have a multiple and complicated etiology. The causes that lie behind these signs and symptoms are more difficult to identify in rapid surveys.

6. Surveys are often conducted by medical or statistical specialists, but they should also include personnel with a broad perspective.

7. Cross-sectional surveys may produce antagonism among the population if they are repeated or not followed by constructive action.

8. In any survey that expects the population to attend at specified centers, it may be found that only selected groups comply. Subsequent house-to-house visiting may show that those who are sick or uncooperative have been left at home.

9. The figures produced by a survey can identify what is average for that area. This must not be confused with what is optimal or satisfactory.

10. Observer differences may account for a great many variations in results.

Longitudinal Studies

Physical, mental, and social factors affect growth and development. Without examining these factors, the study of growth and development becomes a mere academic exercise. Watching families through the crises of birth, death, and marriage and through episodes of sickness and health is the best way to learn about the conditions under which people live and their reactions and changing attitudes and behavior.

Family care, including supervision, treatment, and support, is the best way to measure health and to check on the accuracy of statistics. How detailed the observation and care are may well depend on the area, the number of patients, the personnel available, and their skill. However intensive or diluted, or skillful or amateur, this care may be, the operation will alter both the observers and the observed. The more frequent or detailed the efforts at follow-up are, the more selected the subjects observed. The more prolonged the study, the more dropouts of subjects and examiners there will be. All such surveys are likely to be expensive and very time-consuming.

The most historic, and perhaps still the best, example of longitudinal studies in children is *A Thousand Families in Newcastle upon Tyne* (Spence 1954) and the sequel, *Growing Up in Newcastle upon Tyne*. The work of Dr. Jamal Harfouche (1966) in Beirut contains some excellent detailed observations, though it covered only pregnancy plus 18 months of life. Ideally, cross-sectional studies need to be complemented by longitudinal studies.

The size of the groups studied and the frequency and detail of the investigations will depend on a number of factors, and guidance in this area is needed from a statistician with practical experience. In fact, a well-run health center with reasonably good treatment and follow-up facilities can provide an enormous amount of information that will repay analysis, quite apart from any specific research project.

Observation

The value of any measurement depends on the capacity for observation of the people who conduct the investigations. Statistics are misleading unless they are reliably collected, and many experienced workers depend on their own general impressions rather than on statistics. But it is always infinitely preferable to combine observation with facts and figures that can be checked and compared.

In areas where health services are in the early stages and little confidence can be placed in available statistics, it may be possible to start simply by reporting births, deaths, and ages at death. Reports on cause of death may be quite unreliable, but analyses of death by sex and age groups will give a valuable indication of health status.

The following report is taken from a 1930 unpublished memorandum of Dr. C. D. Williams:

The village consisted of about 2700 people. The village elders were approached and agreed to keep records of births and deaths. There were one or two younger men who could read and write, and one of them agreed to help with the records. We found four women who were most usually called in to act as midwives, and they agreed to report any births or deaths that came to their knowledge. An occasional visit from the doctor from 50 miles away, who came to hold a clinic once a month, encouraged them to keep their records up-to-date. At the end of the year, it was found that there had been 120 live births and a total of 63 deaths distributed as [shown in Table 9.15].

The ages were largely a matter of guesswork. However, from these figures the following was deduced:

1. There was a high infant and child mortality, over 50 percent of the total deaths were in the under-fives.
2. A high death rate in women of childbearing age—probably due to a high maternal mortality.
3. A high birth rate of about 50 per 1000. Six stillbirths were said to have taken place during this period, but whether these were over 28 weeks' gestation was not known.

No attempt was made to ascertain causes of death except in a few cases seen by the doctor on his monthly visits. At least two were due to accidents, an adult who fell out of a tree (collecting honey) and a child who was drowned in the river. Many of the other deaths were attributed to "fever" or "witchcraft" or both.

In addition to patterns of death and

Table 9.15. Number of Age-Specific Deaths

	Ages									
	0–1	1–4	5–9	10–14	15–19	20–29	30–39	40–49	Over 50	Total
Male	11	7	3	1	0	1	1	1	5	30
Female	10	6	2	1	2	3	3	1	5	33
Total	21	13	5	2	2	4	4	2	10	63

Note: Health workers can be mobilized at the village level to collect simple statistics. Analysis of age-specific deaths can be a valuable indicator of health status. In this village of 2700, 41 of 63 deaths were of children under 15 years old.

disease, patterns of growth and development can be discerned by collecting and analyzing heights, weights, and arm circumferences of children or pregnant women attending a clinic. At the same time, it is important to examine the various factors that affect growth. In making use of the data collected, it must be borne in mind that:

1. A selected group of the population may be the ones most willing to attend the clinic.
2. The "average" results may not be equivalent to the "normal." In a country with a high child mortality, the "average" child may be suffering, or have suffered, from worms, malnutrition, or malaria. None of these should be considered normal. Internationally recognized and available standards may be reasonably used instead.
3. Attendance at a clinic or a visit in the home by a doctor or nurse, quite apart from any medication specific or otherwise, may change the attitude and the attention given to a child and influence his or her progress, but it is also influenced by distance and the mother's work load and how accessible the clinic or home is.

Observation Visits

A health worker sometimes has to assess a situation without any of the staff, preparation, or equipment that most "scientific" workers would deem minimal. Whenever possible, wander about a town or a slum or an encampment for half an hour, and get an impression of the types of people, their attitudes, housing, environment, sanitation, food, education, the position of their women and their children. If there is an interpreter, so much the better, but all babies speak the same language, so the pediatrician is at an advantage. An isolated village may take a little longer to observe if people are traditionally shy of strangers. The health worker may have to sit around and drink a few quarts of coconut water or eat a few yards of sugar cane but before long some of the children will come sidling up. Providing you are not foolish enough to make advances or to look at them, some will squat on their heels and gaze fixedly at you. Keep quite still; don't look hard; go on talking but keep the voice ordinary. A few bolder spirits will gradually approach and start feeling your skin, especially if the pigmentation is unusual; children seem to have no instinctive color prejudice. Soon there are small fingers stroking your forearms. As long as you make no attempt to rush the adjusting process, you may within a short time be able to obtain a rough picture of the state of nutrition, the muscular development, skin diseases, cleanliness, clothing, the attitudes, and a good deal else of at least some of the children in the neighborhood. The observer will then be able to assess the condition of the spleen, liver, anemia, ears, eyes, and oral hygiene before the child realizes that he or she has been examined. During the process, some of the elders come to exchange greetings and will ask innumerable questions. They are followed by the different age groups, largely depending on the time of day. The health worker will then probably be in-

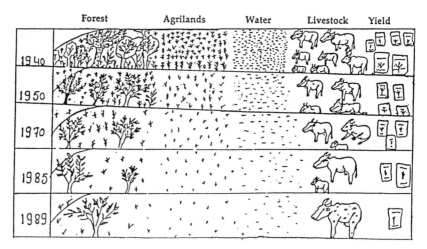

Figure 9.5. History of resources by villagers of Ardanarypura, India. Source: Mothers and Children (1991).

vited into some houses, which may reveal horrific conditions, and it may take even longer to escape from social acceptability than it has taken to achieve it. If health workers can produce some ointment for scabies and a few aspirins, they are probably welcome forever more.

Participatory Measurement

The need for community involvement in measurement and action has spurred the development of measures that facilitate rapid assessment, analysis, and action of and by the community—the "triple A" approach. The rapid assessment procedure (RAP) is used to obtain information on subgroups not covered adequately in national samples in a fairly rapid and relaxed manner. Analyses put less emphasis on numbers and more on descriptive data, which can be used to explain community dynamics. This procedure can also be used to generate interaction between researchers and the community.

In India, several groups have developed innovative and unique methods for collecting and analyzing information. A nongovernmental organization, MYRDA, in South India has found rural people's knowledge and experience to be an untapped and valuable resource. MYRDA uses the term PALM (participatory learning methods) to describe this approach. The uniqueness of the approach can be seen in Fig. 9.5, which shows how an Indian community depicted changes in agricultural production and through this was able to analyze the situation and make plans for change.

Program Information

The decision as to what information should be collected in a MCH program for use in planning and evaluation of services is important. Often too many data are collected, or data collection is not properly planned so that the results cannot be easily summarized and used. Many hospitals, clinics, and health centers have long lists of statistics that have been recorded since the beginning of the program but are never used at any level of decision making. When too much information is collected, the accuracy of the data often suffers, and data that might be useful become unreliable (Bennett 1979; McMahon et al. 1980).

In assessing the adequacy and usefulness of the MCH service information system, the following questions might be asked:

Table 9.16. Measures for Monitoring Evaluation

Topic	Indicator	Group	Goal by the year 2000
Under-5 mortality (R)	U.S. mortality rate/1,000 live births	0–5 years	Reduce by one-third, or to 70
Maternal mortality (R)	Maternal mortality rate	14–45 years	Reduce by half
Severe/moderate malnutrition (R)	Underweight/age	0–5 years	Reduce by half
Safe water	Protected supply	Households	All
Safe sanitation	Protected affluent	Households	All
Basic education of children	Attending school	5+ years	All
Complete primary education	Completing school	5+ years	80 percent
Adult illiteracy rate (R)	Can't read or write	Over 15 years	Reduce by half
Equal educational opportunity/sex	Percentage attending	Over 15 years	Female or male 1:1
Protection for children in especially difficult circumstances	1990 Convention on Rights of the Child	0–14 years	All counties observe

Source: Adapted from UNICEF (1992).

Note: (R) = reduction goal; all others require increase.

1. *Are the MCH program goals well enough specified so that its strengths and weaknesses can be identified?* Without well-defined service objectives, determining what information will provide the best measures of success may be difficult. Goals must include indicators that can be readily measured and interpreted (Table 9.16).

2. *How will the information collected be used in the program, and at what level?* Data needed by the national MCH director will be collected and tabulated differently from information useful primarily to individual caregivers. If no use for a particular item is foreseen, such as the number of injections given daily by each nurse in a clinic, it probably should be eliminated.

3. *Do the data show what is really happening in the program?* One important measure of the effectiveness of MCH care is coverage, or the proportion of the population in need reached by the services. Immunizations, for example, might be recorded as both the number and type of immunizations given and the estimated coverage of the under-5 population attained at that time. If certain groups of women or children are not being served, the reasons can be investigated and corrected.

4. *How can those who collect the information be given the quickest and most helpful feedback about their work?* An auxiliary midwife who provides prenatal care, for example, may want to know how many complicated cases she referred to the hospital compared with the program average. Routine data collection can be a less tiresome task if it is known that a summary and interpretation of the results are shared with those doing the work.

CONCLUSION

Measurements of health for both individual patients and groups are indispensable for the following reasons:

1. They provide basic information about health status, patterns of disease, and the factors that affect health.
2. They help solve technical and operational problems and help create relevant policies and programs.
3. They provide information for the health education of politicians and the public. However, epidemiologists, economists, and politicians should not make use of figures without first assuring themselves of their accuracy.
4. They measure progress by evaluating to what extent set goals are achieved.

5. They help MCH services to remain flexible, adapted to the changing needs and the resources of the community. For these services in particular, it is necessary to take measurements of health for guidance of policies and for assessing progress.

Vital and health statistics will never be accurate without good MCH services. The reverse is equally true. Both areas of service must go forward together.

All health personnel need to become measurement minded; and descriptive observation must be complemented by the language of figures (Bennett 1979; Horwitz 1968; Wootton 1956) but not complicated by unintelligible mathematical abstraction. Health data need to be collected. These data are almost always imperfect but nevertheless helpful as long as their imperfection is recognized.

REFERENCES

Abramson, J. (1979). *Survey Methods in Community Medicine.* Churchill Livingstone, Edinburgh.

Baumslag, N. (1989). *Breastfeeding: The Passport to Life.* NGO Committee on UNICEF (Working Group on Nutrition), New York.

Bennett, F. (1979). *Community Diagnosis and Health Action: A Manual for Tropical and Rural Areas.* Macmillan, London.

Blanc, A. (1991). *Demographic and Health Surveys: World Conference Executive Summary.* IRD/Macro International, Columbia, Md.

Chambers, R. (1990). *Rapid But Relaxed Participatory Rural Appraisal Towards Application in Health and Nutrition.* International Conference Rapid Assessment Technologies for Planning and Evaluation of Health Related Programs, Nov. 12–15. Washington, D.C.

Cook, R. (1969). Nutrition and mortality under five years in the Caribbean area. *J. Trop. Pediat.* **15**, 109.

Czermsk, H., and Hansluwka, H. (1962). Infant mortality in Austria. *Brit. J. Prev. Soc. Med.* **16**, 196.

Emery, J. L., and Irvine, K. A. (1958) . Death certification of children. *Brit. Med. J.* **2**, 1510.

Falkner, F., ed. (1966). *Key Issues in Infant Mortality.* U.S. Government Printing Office, Washington, D.C.

Falkner, F. (1970). Infant mortality—an urgent national problem. *Children* **17**, 83.

Gamble, D. P. (1952). Infant mortality rates in rural areas in Gambia Protectorate. *J. Trop. Med. Hyg.* **55**, 145.

Glass, D. V., and Eversley, D. E. C., eds. (1965). *Population in History: Essays in Historical Demography.* Edward Arnold, London/Aldine, Chicago.

Gordon, J. E.; Wyon, J. B.; and Ascoli, W. (1967). The second year death rate in less developed countries. *Am. J. Med. Sci.* **254**, 357.

Gossling, W. (1970). *A Time Chart of Social History.* Butterworth Press, London.

Graham, W. J. and Cambell, O. M. R. (1991). *Measuring Maternal Health: Defining the Issues.* Maternal and Child Epidemiology Unit. London School of Hygiene and Tropical Medicine, London.

Hanlon, J. J. (1960). *Principles of Public Health Administration.* 3d ed. C. V. Mosby, St. Louis, Mo.

Harfouche, J. K. (1966). *Illness and Growth Patterns of Lebanese Infants.* 4 vols. Khayat Press, Beirut.

Horwitz, A. (1968). *Balance Sheet of Accomplishments, 1967.* Pan American Health Organization, Washington, D.C.

Huxtable, D. L. (1967). Vital statistics aid in developing nations. *Am. J. Publ. Hlth.* **57**, 504.

Jelliffe, D. B. (1969). The secotrant—a possible new age category in early childhood? *J. Pediat.* **74**, 808.

Jelliffe, D. B., and Jelliffe, E. F. P. (1990). *Community Nutritional Assessment.* Oxford University Press, Oxford.

Kahn, E.; Wayburne, S.; and Fouche, M. (1954). The Baragwanath Premature Baby Unit—An analysis of the case records of 1000 consecutive admissions. *S. Afr. Med. J.* **28**, 453.

McMahon, R.; Barton, E.; and Piot, M. (1980). *On Being in Charge.* World Health Organization, Geneva.

Krasovec, K., and Anderson, M. A. (1991). Monitoring pregnancy. *Mothers and Children* **10**, 2.

Morley, D. (1963). A medical service for children under five years of age in West Africa. *Trans. Roy. Soc. Trop. Med. Hyg.* **57**, 79.

Mothers and Children (1991). Research for action: participatory rural appraisal in nutrition. *Mothers and Children* **10**, 2.

NCHS (1968) *Infant Loss in the Netherlands.* National Center for Health Statistics, U.S. Public Health Service, Hyattsville, Md.

NCHS (1982). Death rates and percent of total deaths for the 15 leading causes of death, US 1979. *Monthly Vital Statistics Report.* **31** (Suppl. 6), 4.

NCHS (1992). Monthly vital statistics report, Jan. 7. *National Center for Health Statistics,* **40** (8), Supp. 2, 5.

Nhonoli, A. M. M. (1954). An enquiry into the infant mortality rate in rural areas of Unyamwezi. *E. Afr. Med. J.* **31**, 1.

PAHO (1967). *Health Conditions in the Americas.* Pan American Health Organization, Washington, D. C.

PAHO (1982). *Health Conditions in the Americas, 1980.* Pan American Health Organization, Washington, D.C.

Pop. Ref. Bur. (1982). *World's Children Data Sheet.* Population Reference Bureau, Washington, D.C.

Pop. Ref. Bur. (1992). *World Population Data Sheet.* Population Reference Bureau, Washington, D.C.

Powers, L. E. (1955). *Infant Mortality in Rural Lebanon.* Proceedings of the Fifth Middle East Medical Assembly.

Puffer, R., and Griffiths, W. (1967). *Patterns of Urban Mortality, Scientific Publications,* no. 151. Pan American Health Organization, Washington, D.C.

Rohde, J. E.; Hull, T. H.; and Hendrata, L. (1978). *Who Dies of What and Why.* Prisma.

Scrimshaw, S. C. M., and Hurtado, E. (1987). *Rapid Assessment Technologies.* PAHO, Washington, D.C.

Spence, J. C.; Walton, W. S.; Miller, F. J. W.; and Court, S. D. M. (1954). *A Thousand Families in New Castle upon Tyne.* Oxford University Press, London.

Tafari, N. (1978). Prime causes of perinatal mortality. In *Birth Weight Distribution—An Indicator of Social Development.* Ed. G. Sterky and L. Mellander. SAREC Report no. R:2. Stockholm.

UN (1955). *Handbook of Vital Statistics Methods.* UN Publications, New York.

UN (1979). *Demographic Yearbook.* UN Publications, New York.

UN (1980). *Selected Demographic Indicators by Country, 1950–2000.* UN Publications, New York.

UNICEF (1992). *State of the World's Children.* UNICEF, New York.

USAID (1992). *Seventh Child Survival Report.* U.S. Agency for International Development, Washington, D.C.

Welbourn, H. F. (1956). A comparison between children attending child welfare clinics in 1950 and 1955. *E. Afr. Med. J.* **34**, 47.

Williams, C. D. (1942). Health work in Trengganu. *Indian Med. Gaz.* **77**, 552, 689.

Williams, C. D. (1954). *Vomiting Sickness Report: Jamaica.* Government Printers, Kingston, Jamaica.

Williams, C. D. (1976). Nutrition in the community. Foreword to *A Text for Public Health Workers,* pp. xi–xxi. Ed. D. S. McLaren. John Wiley, London.

Wootton, I. D. P. (1956). International biochemical trail, 1954. *Clin. Chem.* **2**, 296.

World Bank (1991). *Social Indicators of Development.* Johns Hopkins University Press, Baltimore.

WHO (1950). *Expert Committee on Health Statistics: Report on the Second Session.* Wld. Hlth. Org. Tech. Rep. Ser., no. 25.

WHO (1969). *Statistics of Health Services and Their Activities.* Wld. Hlth. Org. Tech. Rep. Ser., no. 429.

WHO (1980). *World Health Statistics.* World Health Organization, Geneva.

WHO (1981). *Development of Indicators for Monitoring Progress Towards Health for All by the Year 2000.* Health for All Series, no. 4. World Health Organization, Geneva.

WHO (1982). *World Health Statistics.* World Health Organization, Geneva.

10

Health Education

All of the problems of maternal and child health can be improved in some degree by health education—that is, by motivating and persuading people to make vital but quite often minor modifications in their life (Bennett 1966; Bennett and Letlhaku 1966). The incidence of diarrhea, for example, can be reduced when mothers are convinced of the need to boil drinking water for their babies and have the fuel and/or wash their hands; the mortality from measles could be reduced by better nutrition and home nursing. In most parts of the world, malnutrition would be much less common if parents could be persuaded to feed their infants nutritious foods already available in the village. Even more clearly, tetanus neonatorum, a totally preventable disease, would disappear if effective health education on care of the umbilical cord could be undertaken for TBAs and for mothers. Health education should be aimed at updating information for consumers as well as health care workers, rectifying misinformation, modifying harmful behavior, and reinforcing beneficial practices.

The process of changing behavior through education requires awakening or enhancing an awareness that a problem exists, creating an interest and desire for more information, convincing people that there is a practical solution, and helping people to make the needed change in behavior. Changes will be successful only if the community is directly involved. In order to create a desire for change, health professionals must listen to the people and find out what interests them. What are they talking about? What do they fear? What do they consider their health priorities? What would they like to see happening in their community? It is important not to introduce subjects that people consider boring, irrelevant, or useless (Siceloff 1982).

In Peru women's organizations have worked with illiterate women to improve their lives (Quality 1992). Through interactive focus groups they have worked to determine the knowledge, attitudes, and practices of the women. Wife beating was identified as a serious problem. Through drawings underscored with health messages, they produced health education materials. The women were given color-

Table 10.1. Media for Health Education: A Comparison

	Advantages	Limitations
Radio	Suitable for mass messages, can reach illiterate audience, ususally low cost	Needs face-to-face follow-up. Must be understandable to community. Difficult to reach areas with poor reception
Television	Can reach mass audience, if public access available	Expensive, usually limited to urban, high-income audience; lack of resourcs for producing local programs
Newspapers	Can reach mass audience, inexpensively; good for simple messages, stories in comic strip form	Limited to literate, mostly urban audiences
Films, slides,	Effective for groups; variety of possible teaching techniques	Usually require electricity, equipment maintenance; difficult to produce locally; usually costly
Posters	Good for mass, group, or individual audiences; can use local materials; low cost	Must be simple message; pretest and evaluate effectiveness
Flannel boards, growth charts, food charts, chalk boards	Low cost, portable, easy to use; audience can respond and participate	Pictures and messages must be appropriate for local culture (pretest); limited only by creativity of user
Skits, puppets, games, songs, poems, stories, role playing, dances	Low cost, good for groups; can be spontaneous; use local materials; excellent audience involvement	Subjects and stories should be of interest locally, developed locally
Demonstrations (focus groups)	Good for groups if audience participates in activity; low cost; can be simple and practical if local foods and real babies are used	Demonstrator must be familiar with environs and culture; activities are not always replicable

Note: For a discussion of low-cost, locally produced teaching aids, see Werner and Bower (1992) and Aaron et al. (1979).

ing books and colored pencils, which they took home with care and pride. The women have responded positively to this form of health education. They talked about their enjoyable "painting classes." Evaluation of the project found that family planning had increased and large numbers of women had enrolled in literacy classes.

Health education as a philosophy and a practice must permeate all types of MCH programs and must be carried out by all health professionals (Ritchie 1967; WHO 1969, 1980a). Topics for health education need not be limited strictly to health (or illness) issues; they should address subjects that indirectly affect health, such as food preservation, insect control, and the family budget. Educational messages should involve other sectors—for example, agriculture, general education, and community development—and should be reinforced by parallel efforts on the part of other extension services. Educational activities should not be limited to the clinic setting but should take place in schools, at the market, in the workplace, at meetings and festivals, and throughout the community, directly or through mass media. Methods should be adapted to local resources and levels of literacy (WHO 1980b ; Zeitlin and Formacion 1981) (Table 10.1).

Periodic in-service education of the

health staff and other extension workers is essential to ensure that updated messages reaching the community are consistent. Messages will be much more effective if educators from different sectors work together, coordinating their efforts (Jelliffe 1982).

ATTITUDES

Any educational process depends on the attitudes of the health professionals (Fig. 10.1). They must speak the same language, empathize with, and respect those they are trying to educate. The tone of voice or the way in which a question is asked can erect barriers or effect a rewarding exchange of information. For example, a visitor to a rural health center was interested in the prevalence of pica (eating inedible material, such as earth or stones) in that area. The nurse, who

thought that it was no longer prevalent, asked the women, "None of you here eat dirt, do you?" and everyone responded emphatically, "No!" When the visitor explained to the group that women in many parts of the world eat dirt and clay when pregnant due to a shortage of iron (thin blood), three-quarters of the women in the group indicated they ate dirt or clay.

The personal example set by the educator and the environment of the clinic or teaching setting are also of primary importance. For example, a lesson on how to protect the water supply should take place in an area where the well or water jars are covered, and a male community health worker should not lecture to mothers on the merits of breastfeeding while his wife sits in the background bottle-feeding their baby (Fig. 10.2).

Health education is a logical and economical method of disease prevention in the community. It is concerned with

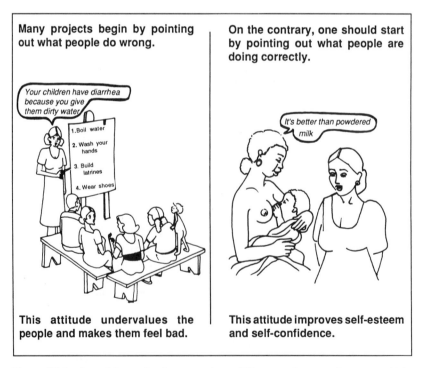

Figure 10.1. A positive attitude can make a difference. Source: Contact (1988).

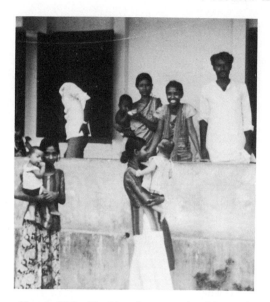

Figure 10.2. Health educators should set the example. This health educator in Bangladesh is teaching mothers about breastfeeding while his wife bottle-feeds their baby.

TEACHING METHODS AND AIDES

Teaching methods that actively involve people get the message across through role playing and discussion groups (Werner and Bower 1992). Paulo Freire, the controversial Brazilian educator who influenced education for health and community action in the 1960s and 1970s, distinguished between two concepts of education: the "banking" approach and the "problem-posing" approach. In the banking approach, a predetermined body of information is pumped into students, like water going into an empty jug. This approach does not teach methods or comprehension but instead memorization, leaving the students with only the knowledge passed on to them by those in authority. In the problem-posing or awareness-raising approach, the facilitator meets the learners as equals, helps them value and analyze their own experience, and creates plans of action to meet their needs. They learn to think for themselves.

Demonstrations can be effective if appropriate materials are used and if mothers can participate in the activity. For example, a lesson on bathing babies should involve a baby, not a doll. Materials used in demonstrations should be only those items standard in the majority of homes. In a nutrition rehabilitation program in Zimbabwe, mothers were asked to bring something from home for the food demonstration. In this way they contributed and were involved (Baumslag 1980).

Pamphlets, posters, charts, and other visual aids are most effective when they are written, designed, and produced by members of the local community and pretested in the community before general use. An outside consultant might be needed for technical expertise in photography or printing processes, but the ideas and stories should come from the community. Many countries have developed

working with people, informing them of the benefits of different concepts of disease, food, and child rearing, and motivating them to make appropriate changes. The best method is to gain confidence with medical care and to give individual demonstrations, particularly in the homes (Byrne 1962). Patterns of behavior are always involved in the slow process of change, and health education is also concerned with guiding people more rapidly toward learning how to make beneficial changes in their traditional way of life. The key words are *simplification, understanding* (on both sides), and *common sense.* Unfortunately, success is not often automatic or even easy. The relative failure of health education directed toward smoking in industrialized countries is an obvious example. Ill-health education (health misinformation) may be widespread in the form of advertisements in the press, radio, and television for inappropriate medicines or unaffordable, dangerous infant formula.

their own health education materials and techniques (APHA 1982a; Bennett 1966; Intl. Nutr. Comm. Service 1981).

TYPES OF HEALTH EDUCATION

Health education can be considered on two main levels. In the first place, there is a continuing need for health care workers to understand and to explain each idea and procedure to the individual patient and mother. In the second place, there is a need for certain ideas and procedures to be presented to individuals and small groups of people in talks and demonstrations and by means of the press, radio, and television to large audiences— for example, a talk and exhibit at an agricultural show, a lecture to a teacher-training college or a group of scouts, a newspaper article on water conservation, or a radio broadcast on polio immunization or AIDS prevention video. (APHA 1982b; Restrepo 1981) (Fig. 10.3).

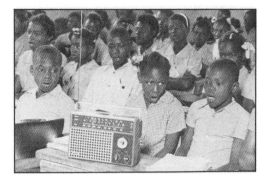

	Number of People Radio
Afghanistan	20.5
Australia	2.5
Brazil	2.0
France	2.9
Ghana	5.5
Mexico	4.2
Singapore	4.3
USSR (former)	3.4
USA	0.5
Venezuela	5.5

Figure 10.3. Radio is the cheapest and easiest way of educating mass audiences. Source: UNICEF (1982); Hunter (1991).

One-to-One Interaction

The first type of health education—at the individual level—must be inculcated into all health workers during the course of their training—both formal teaching and informal and service experience. This is particularly necessary in developing areas and for certain individuals, where health workers are introducing new ideas and attempting to change behavior. When patients see the good results of treatment or of diet, they have confidence in the health worker and will accept advice.

At the personal level, information must be practical, realistic, and, above all, appropriate to the problem that concerns the individual. A mother can learn by actual participation. She beats the egg into the cornmeal porridge, or the powdered milk or beans into the soup, and then feeds it to the child and holds him or watches to see that he does not refuse

it or vomit half an hour later. This type of teaching can be done in a hospital ward, a health center, or a mud hut. It takes time and understanding but is rewarding. The convinced mother may pass on the information to others in the community and serve as an agent of change.

It is often said that doctors and nurses are too busy to spend time on health education. Once medical workers are persuaded of the need, they will always find the time. While the nurse is dressing burns, for example, she will point out the benefit of having the paraffin lamp on a bracket rather than on the floor. While the doctor is writing out a prescription for scabies, the nurse can advise the mother to bring her other children for examination and treatment or to clean out her hut and sun all the clothing and furnishings. Very brief but specific suggestions are often more effective than long lectures. All health staff should observe and practice health education as part of their training. To help the mother give a bed bath to a sick child or to clean the cockroaches out of the cupboard is not just material assistance; it is a priceless opportunity for communication.

Group Teaching

A trained health educator can be helpful by identifying all the opportunities for delivering health education—at schools and training colleges, at meetings of parent-teacher associations, voluntary societies, trade unions, or agricultural societies, and opportunities for speakers and writers on all the available mass media—and should have the resources for obtaining or for creating audiovisual aids and for using them to advantage.

Professional health educators can be of great service in showing health workers and volunteers how to teach, helping to supply them with teaching aids, and helping them to prepare posters, pamphlets, and books, which often have to be adapted for local problems and resources. The poster shown in Figure 10.4 used health messages to motivate the community to reduce lymphatic filariasis risk (Holmes 1964; Jelliffe 1960; Ritchie 1967).

Health educators can contribute to the practical value of a health program by helping to analyze priorities (Jelliffe and Jelliffe 1982; WHO 1969). They must be aware of the leading health problems, which of these can be prevented or modified by health education, and whether this education can be delivered on a mass basis or needs more attention at the individual level. For instance, in Scotland, it was decided that smoking, alcoholism, and dental care should receive special emphasis. Other areas might reveal a very different list of priorities. In Uganda, kwashiorkor, hookworm infection, malaria, and AIDS would be selected.

Between the opportunities for individual advice and the more organized groups

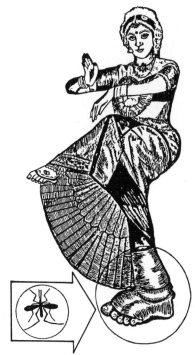

"Should tender feet meant for dancing become deformed? We must destroy mosquitos that deform beautiful damsels."

Figure 10.4. Motivating the community. Source: TDR News (1990).

are numerous occasions that may be converted into learning situations. A group will collect around a child who is being treated in a casualty department; during a home visit in a village, the health visitor is often the center of a following, and it may be far more difficult to leave than it ever was to be accepted in an area. The type of health teaching to be given on these occasions cannot be prescribed beforehand, but a great deal can be accomplished by using appropriate opportunities once the principle of adaptation has been accepted and a certain amount of experience has been achieved.

Health education messages are more effective when a good relationship has been established between educator and patients. The educator must first find out what people want to know. Question-and-answer sessions in which nurses and experienced mothers share experience and knowledge can be very productive. The following topics are possible for health education discussions:

Keeping healthy—how our bodies work.

Having a baby— what to expect.

Live babies and healthy mothers.

How the clinic can help you.

Danger signs in pregnancy.

"New mother" groups (special subjects).

Diarrhea prevention and treatment.

Hygiene (protecting your water, latrines).

Looking after yourself during pregnancy and after.

Family spacing.

The toddler.

Why your baby needs injections.

Making sure you have enough food for the dry season (food budgeting, storage, gardens).

First aid.

Preventing accidents and burns.

What to do about insects and pests.

Tuberculosis, venereal disease, AIDS.

Helping your baby grow (understanding growth charts).

Health news of the week.

Talk time (skits, talks, e.g. "advertisements—what can you believe?")

At the most informal level are focus group discussions, with much learning by both health professionals and mothers as a result of ongoing dialogue by all present (Scrimshaw and Hurtado 1987).

Health and nutrition education can be combined with literacy classes. In a nutrition program in Tunis, a physician discovered that the women most wanted to learn how to write their names in order to eliminate the socially degrading practice of using fingerprints. After learning to write their names, sessions continued with such subjects as interpreting growth charts and reading labels and prices of foods (personal communication, Dr. S. Khadrahyi, Tunis).

Antenatal clinics, family planning clinics, sick child care in wards and outpatient departments, and maternity wards all provide opportunities for health education. This is even more true where there is rooming-in for mothers and babies in the maternity ward or where the mother is admitted with the sick child, as in many parts of Africa. Mulago Hospital in Kampala, Uganda, was one of the first hospitals to initiate an extensive mother-child health education program. Too often an overcrowded ward or outpatient department is used simply for physical treatment or check-ups, and opportunities for teaching and discussion are missed. Where a home care service has been organized, this again gives valuable opportunities for health education.

Many professionals and books recommend teaching to groups in clinics. This sounds easy but in fact is rarely practiced successfully except when groups are small and informal. While mothers are waiting, they often talk with each other, they may give each other hints on health matters. Interruptions are frequent; some patients or mothers have been many times before and may be bored unless they themselves are asked to do the talking. It is sometimes possible to collect a group—of primiparas (mothers with their first babies) at their first clinic attendance, couples who want to learn about family planning, or schoolchildren who want to become health workers— and give a useful and informative talk. But when people come to a clinic, they usually do not take kindly to a health lecture. Group discussion with interactive exchange of ideas and information is more effective (Johnston 1987).

HEALTH CAMPAIGNS

Health education techniques can be usefully employed when a special campaign or project is being launched. Whether this is for measles vaccinations in Liverpool or oral rehydration in India, the methods used and the subject matter must be geared to the type of work, the length of time it will last, and the existing local conditions. It is always advisable to identify the leaders in a community and get their support. If there are political or communal divisions, care must be taken that all the recognizable groups are approached and that the campaign is for the benefit of every person, not for the leading groups only.

An example of a successful implementation of a health campaign was that carried out in the People's Republic of China against schistosomiasis. The program was designed to enlist the help of the people in the physical work of eliminating contaminated water reservoirs that harbor the schistosome snail and also to mobilize their energy and enthusiasm in fighting the disease through mass case finding and treatment. The campaign's success has been attributed to the effective communication of the importance of the identified problems to the entire community and their active involvement in the planning and implementation of solutions in group discussions at all levels (Sidel and Sidel 1982).

Sometimes the efforts of a health department or hospital can be facilitated by the formation of local committees. If it is feared that these may be merely critical and nonconstructive, it may be advisable to organize individual consultations at various levels. A small subcommittee will sometimes achieve action where a large committee may not.

Too often, health education is all mouth and no hands because the health professional is isolated from the local culture. In the past, health education has been ineffective because doctors and nurses have been trained exclusively within institutions, hospitals, and laboratories and have been unable to visualize the correlation between a disease and the environment that produces it or may modify its treat-

ment. To gain acceptance and to devise culturally appropriate solutions to problems, personal experience with the lifestyle and beliefs of the community is essential. If health professionals never go to homes, they cannot appreciate what the community health worker is describing—if indeed they ever see a community health worker—and equally impossible for them to direct the health worker in what should be observed, supported, and advised.

It is, above all, impossible for institution-bound doctors or nurses to give instructions to patients or parents on what care or treatment or diet should be given in the home. This failure to appreciate the need for health education, in both content and form, has led to a great deal of unnecessary and expensive inpatient treatment, unnecessary readmissions, and wasted opportunities at every level. One doctor, for example, gave a mother a detailed demonstration and instruction on how to express her milk for a baby with thrush and how to feed the baby with a teaspoon. On visiting the house the next day, he found there was not a single teaspoon in the village. Health education must be a two-way process.

In a health project in Bangladesh, women were advised to see that all family members washed their hands before eating, to reduce the risk of infection. Instead of simply giving advice, soap and water containers were provided, with some guidelines about washing hands and clothes. Without any attention to cooking food or boiling water, transmission of shigella dysentery among household contacts was reduced by 67 percent (Khan 1982).

Health education is an essential element of supervision and of continuity and is a recognized aspect of mother and child care. It is just as necessary to the community as a whole as schools. For example, in a group of four villages in Egypt, 131 wells were constructed and 2,771 latrines. After seven years, only 37 wells were still serviceable and only 636 of the latrines (Shipman et al. 1958). Both the wells and the latrines were a felt need, but care and maintenance for them were not provided. If there is a lack of continuity in care and lack of continuing education, a large number of admirable and well-intentioned enterprises will be found to have had the same results: ultimate failure.

In some circumstances, health education may borrow from advertising techniques and sell its "goods" by means of attractive displays or by emphasizing the desirability, the cheapness, or the modernity of what is offered (Manoff 1985). For social occasions, the entertainment value can be stressed. One early antimalarial campaign, for example, was greatly assisted by an item at a concert: a large and popular health inspector, dressed as a mosquito, performed a dance, not unlike that of the Dying Swan, which demonstrated his feelings at the approach of a DDT residual spray campaign. In Latin America *fotonovelas* (short picture-stories) and comic books have been successfully used for health education, as they were already widely used as popular forms of entertainment. (Parlato et al. 1980). The message is usually more effective if it is repeated through other media and promoted on an individual basis by health workers.

Testing of Materials

Whether an educational campaign, posters, or other visual aids are aimed at the mass, group, or individual level, pretests can determine whether they will be interpreted by the target population as intended. It is also important to post-test to find out whether the situation has been improved by the activity.

Ideally, local people should be involved in designing their own materials, to ensure understanding and acceptability (Ritchie 1967; Werner and Bower 1992). Figure 10.5 is an example from Pakistan of a goiter poster that depicted

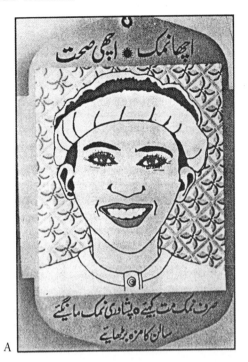

A

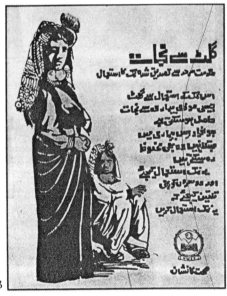

B

Figure 10.5. Posters as an educational tool. The original posters (A) showed only women goiter victims, which carried a negative image and offended traditional ideas of female modesty. Pleasing pictures of a healthy young man (B) elicited a much better response. Source: Mason and Azhar (1982).

an unveiled woman; it was torn down because it was offensive to the Muslim community. Another problem with this poster was the use of too much writing in an area of low literacy (Mason and Azhar 1982). Figure 10.6 is an example from the Republic of South Africa of a breastfeeding promotion poster that contains useful information for mothers and not the usual pretty but uninformative picture of a mom breastfeeding.

Pictorial literacy must also be tested. Figure 10.7 shows an example from a study in Nepal in which pictures were interpreted in a variety of ways (UNICEF and Nat. Dev. Ser. 1976). If pictures are not drawn in a local style and do not use familiar symbols, observers might have no idea what is being depicted. A drawing of a stylized fish might be interpreted as a cooking utensil, a river bank, or a scorpion.

Familiarity with local mythologies and storytelling traditions can be useful in developing educational materials. In West Africa, the belief that spirits inhabit certain trees is not uncommon. Therefore, the portrayal of malaria as a mosquito-like evil spirit in a tree may be a vivid and appropriate teaching tool (Fig. 10.8) (Ministry of Health Mali 1982)

The method for testing a picture is to ask people in the target group open-ended questions to find out what they can perceive in it. For post-testing, questions can be asked to test comprehension of the ideas that were intended to be taught.

Planning and Evaluation

Any health education campaign should have a built-in evaluation method. For planning and evaluation, task analysis can be an effective tool when used in combination with testing. It can sensitize an educator to local conditions and can help in devising a plan for educational goals, community action, and follow-up (Abbatt 1980; Werner and Bower 1992).

Figure 10.9 shows an example of task analysis.

Special Problems

In the case of certain diseases, such as tuberculosis, epilepsy, leprosy, diabetes, deafness, spastic paraplegia, and mental retardation, families, and particularly the mother, may require special health education and support. Some conditions respond to special care, but for others the health problem is insolvable. All that can be done to help the family in a tragic situation is to keep the child as comfortable as possible. Whatever the problem is, the health nurse or community health worker who can home visit and help the parents with practical assistance and encouragement can be invaluable.

Personnel

Some areas enjoy a multiplicity of personnel, all willing to give advice to parents. The doctor, health nurse, social worker, community development worker, nutritionist, and schoolteacher may all be anxious and willing to give advice on, say, diet. Under these circumstances, it is wise to ensure that their efforts are complementary and reinforcing. If the advice is conflicting or has gaps, it will be an unpardonable waste of time for both patients and staff and may bring confusion and even tragedy.

Research

How can training of health professionals be improved to move health education out of the arena of lip-service? How can we reach rural or widely dispersed populations or the urban poor? How might current marketing techniques be used to influence people in a positive way? How can educators make use of common sense that comes from practical experience? Recent experience suggests that a combined approach yields best results: indi-

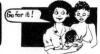
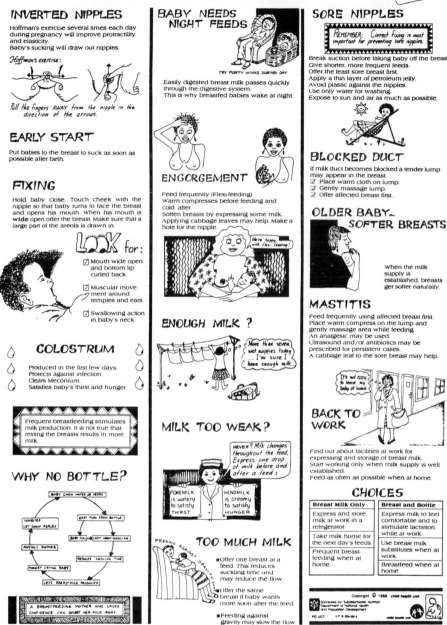

Figure 10.6 Educational materials should provide information in an attractive manner. Source: The Child Health Unit, University of Cape Town, South Africa, in 1981.

Artist's intention: DEATH (funeral pyre)

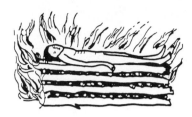

Question 1: What is this?

Responses: Person   79%
            Don't know   11%

  For flames:
            Plants (trees,
            grass, jungle,
            flowers)   18%
            Birds   2%

Question 2: (If first answer was "person")
             What kind of person?

Responses: Sleeping,
            lying down   33%
            Dead   32%
            Sick   11%

Figure 10.7. Pictorial literacy. Source: UNICEF and Nat. Dev. Ser. (1976).

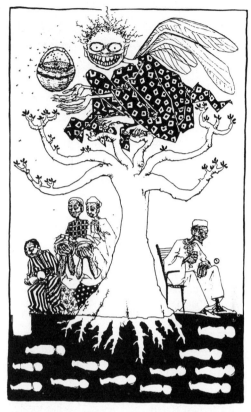

Figure 10.8. Using stories for teaching. This illustration is from a story about malaria in the *Manual for Traditional Birth Attendants*, Mali. The story tells of the Great Malaria Monster, an enormous red giant with orange wings and yellow eyes that throw flames. He flies across the country as soon as the planting season begins, sowing fever and death. Source: Ministry of Health (1982).

vidual or small group face-to-face demonstration discussions plus reinforcement through mass media, principally the radio.

CONCLUSION

In providing health education one should keep in mind the following principles:

Education begins with listening.

Create awareness of the problem and solution.

Involve the community.

Set the example—not all mouth and no hands.

Decide the priority of objectives and set goals.

Provide support, supervision, and continuity.

Give a consistent message.

Repeat messages in different media and settings.

Have a positive attitude. Behavior change takes time and understanding.

Be aware of cultural practices.

Develop local educational materials.

Use local artists, actors, and "big shots" to deliver and design messages.

Combine health education with literacy.

Remember that health education is a method of disease prevention.

TASK ANALYSIS SHEET		
The Task: Introducing latrines		
Stages of the Task Actions (A) Decisions (D) Communications (C)	Knowledge and Skills Needed	Ways to Learn
1. Find out community interest. (C)	ability to explain and listen	talk with experienced health workers; role plays; group dialogue
2. Decide if latrine project is possible at this time. (D)	understanding of people and customs	community dynamics; discussions about traditions & behavior
3. Help people learn importance of latrines to health. (C)	knowledge of how disease spreads; teaching skills	from observation, books, and discussions; practice teaching
4. Decide where latrines will be built. (D)	knowledge of safety factors	books and discussions; thinking it through with local people
5. Get materials needed. (A)	what local materials can be used; what else is needed; where to buy at low cost, etc.	talk with local mason; trip to market
6. Help people build the latrines. (A)	dimensions of pit and platform; how to mix, cast, reinforce, and cure cement; how to build outhouse & lid	have students take part in actually making latrines
7. Encourage people to use latrines and to keep them covered and clean. (C)	home visits; art of giving suggestions in a friendly way	practice, role plays, and discussion

To collect the information you need to do a complete task analysis, you can use these sources:

- your own knowledge and experience
- books and information sheets
- observation of health workers in action
- discussion with other instructors or persons with the skills and experience required
- discussion with health workers

Figure 10.9. Sample task analysis. This example is not intended to apply to all communities. Source: Werner and Bower (1992).

The word *doctor* comes from the Latin *doceo*—"I teach." It is wise to remember that teaching is the basis of health work.

REFERENCES

Aaron, A.; Hawes, H.; and Gayton, J. (1979). *Child to Child*. Macmillan, London.

Abbatt, F. (1980). *Teaching for Better Learning: A Guide for Teachers of Primary Health Care Staff*. AMREF, Nairobi, Kenya.

APHA (1982*a*). Educational aids and training. In *Primary Health Care Bibliography and Resource Directory*. American Public Health Association, Washington, D.C.

APHA (1982*b*). Using radio for primary health care *Primary Health Care Issues*, ser. 1, no. 1. American Public Health Association, Washington, D.C.

Baumslag, N. (1980). *Mothers and Children—Nutrition and Health Care in Kenya, Zimbabwe, Mozambique, and Botswana*. Ford Foundation, New York.

Bennett, F. J. (1966). Health education. In *Medical Care in Developing Countries*. Ed. M. H. King. Oxford University Press, Nairobi.

Bennett, F. J. and Letlhaku, L. (1966). Organization of MCH services in developing regions: Health education. *J. Trop. Pediat.*, **12**, 32.

Byrne, M. (1962). Nutrition education in the home. *J. Trop. Pediat.* **8**, 22.

Cameron, M., and Hofvander, Y. (1983). *Manual on Feeding Infants and Young Children*. Oxford University Press, Delhi, Nairobi.

Contact (1988). Community-based or oriented: The vital difference. *Contact* **106**, 17.

Holmes, A. C. (1964). *Health Education in Developing Countries*. Nelson, London.

Hunter, B. (1991). *The Statesman's Yearbook 1991–92*. 12th ed. St. Martin's Press, New York.

Intl. Nutr. Comm. Service (1981). *Nutrition Training Manual Catalogue for Health Professionals, Trainers, and Field Workers in Developing Countries*. Ed. R. Israel and P. Lamptey. Educational Development Center, International Nutrition Communication Service, Newton, Mass.

Jelliffe, E. F. P. (1982). Nutrition education in a changing world. In *Advances in International Maternal and Child Nutrition*, 2: 133–47. Ed. D. B. Jelliffe and E. F. P. Jelliffe. Oxford University Press, Oxford.

Jelliffe, D. B. and Bennett, F. J. (1960). Nutrition education in tropical child health centres (some practical guidelines). *Courier*, **10**, 569.

Johnston, M. P., and Rifkin, S. B. (1987). *Health Care Together* (training exercises for health workers in community based programmes). Macmillan, St. Albans, U.K.

Khan, M. U. (1982). Interruption of shigellosis by hand washing. *Trans. Roy. Soc. Trop. Med. Hyg.* **76**, 1964.

Manoff, R. (1985). *Social Marketing*. Praeger Press, New York.

Mason, D. and Azhar, K. (1982). Don't just say "salt." *UNICEF News* **114**, 12.

Minett, N. (1978). *Health and Nutrition Education—Developing "Small Talks,"* CARE, Freetown, Sierra Leone.

Ministry of Health, Mali (1982). *Manuel pour les acco ucheuses traditionelles*. U.S. Agency for International Development, Washington, D.C.

Parlato, R.; Parlato, M. B.; and Cain, B. J. (1980). *Fotonovelas and Comic Books*. Development Support Bureau, U.S. Agency for International Development, Washington, D.C.

Quality (1992). *Adding Color to Life: Illustrated Health Materials for Women in Peru*, no. 4, p. 13. The Population Council.

Restrepo, S. (1981). A multi-media strategy for a breast-feeding campaign in Colombia. *Mothers and Children* **1** (3).

Ritchie, J. A. S. (1967). *Learning Better Nutrition*. FAO Nutrition Studies 20. Food and Agriculture Organization, Rome.

Scrimshaw, S., and Hurtado, E. (1987). *Rapid Assessment Procedures*. UN University, Tokyo.

Shipman, H.; Agamieh, M.; Ibrahim, M. R.; Mawla, A.; and Mawla, M. A. (1958). Report on a survey of water—supplies and latrines in certain Egyptian villages. *Bull. Wld. Hlth. Org.* **18**, 477

Siceloff, J. (1982). Villagers teaching us to teach them. *UNICEF News* **114**, 18.

Sidel, R., and Sidel, V. (1982). *The Health of China*. Beacon Press, Boston.

TDR News (1990). *TDR News*, November 24.

UNICEF (1982). Communications: The facts. *UNICEF News* **114**, 18.

UNICEF and Nat. Dev. Ser. (1976). *Commu-*

nicating with pictures in Nepal. Report of a Study by the National Development Service and UNICEF. UNICEF, Kathmandu, Nepal.

Werner, D., and Bower, B. (1992). *Helping Health Workers Learn*. 2d Hesperian Foundation, Palo Alto, Calif.

WHO (1969). *Planning and Evaluation of Education services*. World Health Organization Tech. Rep. Ser., no. 409.

WHO (1980a). *Sixth Report on the World Health Situation 1973–1977*, Pt. 1: *Global Analysis*. World Health Organization, Geneva.

WHO (1980b). *Towards a Better Future, Maternal and Child Health*. World Health Organization, Geneva.

WHO/UNICEF (1989). *Facts of Life*. World Health Organization, United Nations International Child Educational Fund, Geneva/New York.

Zeitlin, M. F., and Formacion, C. S. (1981). Nutrition education. In *Nutrition Intervention in Developing Countries*, pp. 49–72. Harvard Institute for International Development, Cambridge, Mass.

11

Health Services for Mothers and Women

Newton's discovery of the law of falling bodies is all very fine, but that doesn't mean that a mother's discovery of how to hold her baby isn't important too.
JEAN RENOIR

The word *underprivileged* has sometimes been used to describe certain communities. However, this is not a satisfactory connotation. Many people consider themselves proud, rich, healthy, and fulfilled, even if they recognize that they are unfortunately vulnerable in some respects. This outlook may be changing with the worldwide revolution in expectations, especially regarding modern goods and amenities that are highly advertised in the mass media.

The term *underdeveloped* has been used in this book to refer to communities that have not been exposed to the relatively recent mechanical, scientific, and economic developments typical of the more technologically sophisticated societies, with all the advantages and immense problems that have accompanied such changes.

A main factor that divides societies is facility in communication. Where people have been isolated in small groups, they tend to be static in their culture, and the factor that divides this static outlook from others was, until recently, the ability to read and write and so to communicate with the outside world and to make contact with a variety of ideas. To this has now been added, for better or (too often) for worse, the worldwide stimulus of the mass media, particularly the transistor radio, and other commercial pressures.

Preliterate societies are hampered by a heavy burden of preventable disease, and they are excessively anxious to have better health. As we have seen, education and health go together. In the modern world, one cannot be enjoyed without the other, whether the well-being is physical, mental, or social. Nothing but the most repressive totalitarianism can prevent people from seeking to know what is happening in other parts of the world.

PREPARATION FOR CHILDBEARING

Childbearing is a natural process but nonetheless associated with risks. Mod-

Table 11.1. Maternal Mortality Rates for Selected Countries, 1976–1990

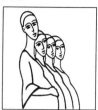

	1976	1980	1990
Costa Rica	59	—	36
Philippines	142	—	100
Hong Kong	18	5	6
Sri Lanka	98	—	80
The Netherlands	5	9	10
Rumania	130	132	150
Singapore	14	5	10
United Kingdom	13	11	8
Sweden	4	8	5

Source: WHO (1982).

Note: Rates per 100,000 live births.

ern medicine has done much to improve on nature, and this is particularly true in the fields of midwifery and obstetrics (Lawson and Stewart 1967). In Europe, maternal mortality varies from 4 per 100,000 live births in Sweden to 180 in Rumania (Table 11.1). The statistics for both countries are probably accurate, but the numbers would be higher if they were calculated for live births and stillbirths together. In many countries, it is difficult to get accurate statistics, but it is known that in parts of South America, the maternal mortality rate is estimated at over 200 per 100,000 live births. This is in addition to a high mortality due to procured abortions. Rates in Africa are much higher: (160 to 1,100 per 100,000 live births (Rosenfield and Maine 1985).

Traditional preparation for motherhood is often more appropriate in preliterate villages than in a sophisticated urban context. The little girl in a preliterate type of home shares fully in the family life, and her behavior is generally governed by fairly strict rules. Both of these elements of her upbringing give her security. Almost as soon as she can walk,

she begins to share the responsibility of looking after her juniors, performing household chores, and learning about practical motherhood by personal observation, practice, and involvement. As she grows older, she has more hard work to do and greater responsibilities. At or about the age of puberty, she may have to undergo forms of initiation, some of which are educational, while others may be hideously painful and dangerous (such as the practice of pharaonic circumcision—now more aptly termed "genital mutilation"—in parts of Africa), but she may consider herself incomplete without them. She enters her matrimonial responsibilities knowing well what they entail. In one area of Africa, it was said that the Roman Catholic church was embarrassed by its large numbers of postulant nuns; the local women had decided that the religious life was preferable to matrimony. However, in most traditional societies, the woman accepts her lot of marriage, pregnancy, hard work, child care, and, often, child mortality. She is desperately unhappy if she has failed in either producing children or any other of her responsibilities, but she often has the physical and emotional support of her extended family.

The girl from an "advanced" culture, on the other hand, may belong to a small nuclear family. While young, she may be protected from the facts of life, but at a very early age she is exposed to advertisements, fantastic romanticism, "tele-glamour," "telehorror," and "televiolence." She tends to run with her own age group. At school, she learns about history, geography, world achievements, art, and science, but she may learn relatively little about her own personal life and that of her neighbors. She may not even have held a small baby, let alone seen one breastfed, until she has her own. Apart from her own physiological and developmental urges, which may or may not be considerable, she may be subjected to peer pressure. She may have episodes of disturbed behavior when it is said she is seeking for her identity.

More and more young people are marrying in Europe and North America. The younger the age at marriage, the higher is the divorce rate. At the same time, teenage pregnancy is increasing in all social groups, even where religious sanctions provide a disciplined way of life as well as a philosophy. All this tends to show that our advanced type of education does relatively little for family life apart from reducing mortality and morbidity rates and now, possibly, the birthrate.

Polygamy is accepted in many parts of the world. The Koran allows a man four wives at one time but stipulates that each must be treated fairly. It goes on to say, "Of course it is impossible to treat four wives equally well," and many followers of Islam take this as an injunction against plurality of wives. In polygamous marriages, some of the wives may be deprived of funds and access to health care. Most damaging is the extreme ease of divorce; the husband has only to repeat one word three times *(talak, talak, talak)*, and the divorce is completed. The divorced woman has little security, and this is often reflected adversely in care of the children. Difficulties are greatly increased where women are kept in purdah.

Many emerging or newly independent nations are gradually introducing legislation to protect women and children from the worst types of hardship and exploitation within the framework of their own cultures. This is particularly necessary where the women are excessively dependent on the men of the family. In Yemen, for example, the problem of child marriage has been solved by Family Law (1978), which deals with fundamentals and conditions of marriage, bride-price, and dissolution of marriage. One article states that the marriage of a minor is valid provided she gives consent at the time of the wedding, "unless she is not less than 16 and is apt [fit], for intercourse." The penalty is one to three years' imprisonment for violation of this law (Baasher et al. 1982).

One of the merits of the formerly communist countries was that they actively discouraged early marriage, multiple sexual partners, and the rearing of large families. They paid a great deal attention to the care and education of children, with considerable emphasis on political conditioning.

The parents' circumstances—geographical, cultural, and educational—make a great difference in the type and amount of care and supervision mothers require, especially during the childbearing and child-rearing years. During pregnancy, delivery, and the postdelivery period, including lactation, the mother needs special consideration. Each woman needs:

1. Medical care for herself, as and when necessary.
2. Education for marriage, childbearing, and child care.
3. Supervision, counseling, and, if necessary, referral during pregnancy.
4. Skilled care at delivery.

5. Postnatal care for herself and the child.
6. Supervision, advice, and support for offspring, especially in cases of hardship or disabilities.
7. Access to advice and resources with respect to family planning, nutrition, and other problems.

The services must be flexible, not merely to provide routine supervision and adequate facilities but to identify individuals and families with special disadvantages, special hazards, and special problems and to ensure that disadvantages are redressed, hazards avoided, and problems mitigated as far as is possible (Fig. 11.1).

Health education and sex education in schools are efficient only where there is good parent-teacher cooperation. Moreover, there must be good medical-educational and agricultural-educational cooperation. It has been found advisable for parents to be invited to attend sex education classes before they are held for the children; it is distressing for a father to learn from his 10-year-old son all about the seminiferous tubules and risks of AIDS.

Home economics and nutrition teaching must be related to local conditions and family life. Too often, the only households that are "demonstration worthy" are those without children.

Whenever available, children should be able to take courses in first aid, home nursing, child care, and nutrition through youth groups. They should learn from school meals and school gardens, as well as through the regular curriculum. The nutritional needs and stresses of adolescence need consideration. Health care and education are attained through various channels, and this should be a continuing process. Some schools in Israel, for instance, organize their boys and girls in groups every day to devise, discuss, purchase, cook, and present the school lunch to the others. Nutritional balance, cost in money and time, and acceptability are all noted.

Children should be allowed to help at school, clinics, hospitals, health centers, children's homes, day care centers, nurseries, and orphanages. During an outbreak of influenza in England, scouts looked after babies in an orphanage because the regular staff was incapacitated. Children can pay visits to houses and provide domestic and social help for handicapped and geriatric cases, for acute as well as chronic cases. When offered in moderation and when the children feel they are of real use, such activities can provide important opportunities for understanding and experience. Young people should have a chance to learn of the risks, the skills, the hard work, and the responsibilities of family life.

The health of children and their families depends on the routine management of food, cleanliness, exercise, and behavior far more than on immunization, supplementary vitamins, and hospital facilities. It is helpful if girls and boys get practical experience in the routine handling of babies (including breastfeeding) and children and have some realistic idea of both the drudgeries and the rewards of parenthood. For too long, domestic work has been regarded as shameful and degrading, and children have been deprived of opportunities for learning and gaining immensely valuable experience. Ideally, marriage counseling should be available through schools, youth clubs, and religious groups. Many young people feel that to consult a stranger about their problems is less embarrassing than to go to a member of their own family. Voluntary agencies, such as the Salvation Army, provide admirable services in some countries.

Traditional societies have methods of regulating fertility, including a period of abstinence in some societies. Most of these, such as prolonged lactation, are not infallible. Some of the abortifacients used are dangerous or damaging, and one of the great needs is to find methods of

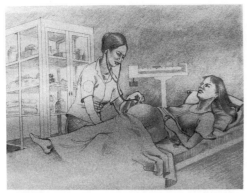

Prenatal Care
identifies women at high risk of pregnancy complications
so they can be referred to a doctor in time.

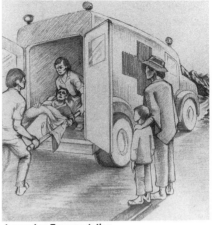

Improving Transportation
speeds evacuation to the hospital when complications occur during labor.

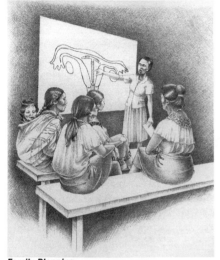

Family Planning
helps women space births and avoid high-risk pregnancies.

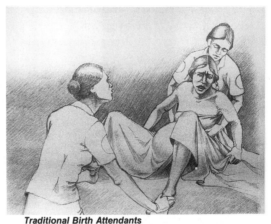

Traditional Birth Attendants
can learn to refer women at high risk and to give first aid
when emergencies occur.

Figure 11.1 Comprehensive care. Source: Produced by Family Health International
(P.O. Box 13950, Research Triangle Park, N.C. 27709).

fertility control that are dependable, acceptable, and safe. Whether family planning advice should be freely available to
the unmarried, as well as to the married
or about-to-be married, is a matter of
dispute. Most medical people, however,
agree that it is advisable, provided it includes mature family planning and counseling rather than merely handing out
birth control devices (Population Bulletin
1969).

For many women, young and old, a

baby is attractive as a baby and as a
possession and overshadows social and
economic problems that its production
may involve. Only if they are given opportunities for discussion and consideration will young women be able to count
the long-term cost to themselves and to
the child and arrive at important decisions in this highly emotional field. Education and demonstration, too, can do
much to counteract the fatalism, the fear
of witchcraft, and the dependence on

damaging aspects of tradition that in the past have done much to endanger child health and family well-being.

SUPERVISION DURING PREGNANCY

Antenatal care, through clinics and home visiting, should not be regarded in isolation or aimed merely at diminishing the risks of childbearing but as a part of total family care (PAHO 1970; Population Bulletin 1969; Rosa 1970). The objectives are:

1. To supervise the health of the mother and provide treatment and advice for disorders, whether or not these are associated with the pregnancy.
2. To ensure that the baby has a good start in life.
3. To provide opportunities for health education of both parents with respect to their own and their children's well-being, including preparation for breastfeeding.

The mother's attitude toward her pregnancy is the most important factor in the life of the child. Pregnancy is usually a cause for congratulations, but sometimes it demands consolation. The first antenatal attendance is usually the best time to introduce the idea of family size, child spacing, or some type of fertility control. The parents then have time to examine, discuss, and decide these before the term of the current pregnancy.

The health of the deposed baby (i.e., one taken off the breast to allow a younger child to feed) has been one of the most serious and one of the most documented problems in the field of child health and nutrition (Williams 1938). For generations, certain communities have regarded small, whining, potbellied, spindle-legged toddlers as the norm for that age group. The mother will bring her youngest baby to the clinic at the first sign of diarrhea, fever, skin blemish, or cough, but she has

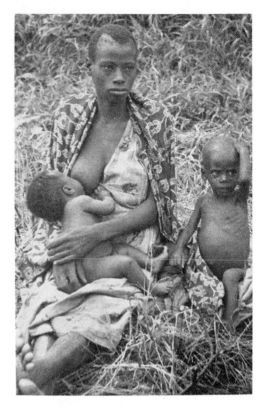

Figure 11.2. Care of the "deposed infant" is critical. The breast-fed baby is beautiful; the deposed child suffers from severe malnutrition, due to an inadequate diet, infections, and the psychological trauma of separation from intimate contact with the mother (Western Uganda).

less time and interest for the older child no longer being breastfed (Fig. 11.2) (Gyorgy and Burgess 1965; Williams 1938).

One invaluable way of combating health hazards is to encourage the mother to bring the youngest child with her to the antenatal clinic; this is no undue hardship in the early months of pregnancy. Where the mother expects to be working and carrying loads irrespective of pregnancy, there is a strong argument for having frequent, small, well-distributed clinics rather than large, central, overcrowded centers. This will foster a continuing interest in the "about-to-be-deposed" child and provide an unsurpassable opportunity for nutritional assessment and dietary advice, together with treatment, as and when necessary. When this pattern is accepted, the mother who is advanced in pregnancy will often find that the father or other relative will carry the toddler to the clinic with her. The major problem usually lies in getting the doctors, nurses, and midwives to accept this family care program instead of the more easily organized, orthodox, assembly-line mechanical type of antenatal session.

Nutrition

Women are often at a disadvantage nutritionally (Harrison 1979; Jelliffe and Jelliffe 1989; PAHO 1970; WHO Organization 1965), especially in pregnancy, because of ill-advised, often restrictive food customs, diseases, and heavy manual work.

Health education must aim at encouraging the mother to take an adequate diet based as far as possible on local foods and with regard to the most prevalent dietary defects (Jelliffe 1968). Anemia is common all over the world (PAHO 1969). Lack of thiamine, vitamin A, iodine, or protein may require special attention, but usually a low caloric intake is the main problem.

At the first attendance, all antenatal patients should have their height recorded, as mothers under 5 feet tall are usually at risk. Their weight or arm circumference should be recorded at every subsequent attendance. A single weight alone does not provide the height-weight ratio that is important for evaluating high-risk patients, but serial weights act as a guide to nutritional status and progress and also to the development of edema. The height-weight ratios of antenatal patients can provide a rough idea of the extent of food shortage in the community.

Nutrition education must include emphasis on the use of local foods, preparation for breastfeeding, and the care and supervision of existing children. Nutrition supplements may be advisable in different regions (PAHO 1969, 1970; WHO 1965), including iron, folic acid tablets, or protein in the form of dried skimmed milk, legumes, fish flour, and so on (Baumslag et al. 1970). But it is preferable to identify individuals truly in need than to provide mass supplements.

High-Risk Patients

Antenatal clinics provide an opportunity for identifying patients for the following high-risk factors:

Obstetrical/medical history
> Age—under 16 and over 40 primipara
> Unmarried woman or unwanted pregnancy
> History of abortions, stillbirths, prematurity, abnormality
> History of long, obstructed labor, abnormal presentation
> Too long or too short intervals between pregnancies
> Excessive number of pregnancies (four to six)
> Rubella or other infections
> Reproductive tract infections
> Mental illness or instability
> Headaches, giddiness
> Overwork

Examination
> Short stature (under 5 feet tall)
> Breast examination (especially for inverted nipples)
> Pelvic abnormalities, disproportion, poor vaginal outlet (from trauma or infibulation)
> Multiple pregnancy
> Hypertension (blood pressure 140/90 or higher)
> Edema, albuminuria, vomiting
> Overweight, diabetes, rapid weight gain
> Underweight (for height), serial weight measurements (if feasible)

Table 11.2. Antenatal Health Services for Possible Maternal, Fetal, and Neonatal Conditions

Condition	Management—test or treatment
Malnutrition	Initial height and weight measurements Serial weight measurements during pregnancy Examination for signs of malnutrition Examination of eyes for xerosis Food supplement *only* when indicated Child spacing advice Advice to adolescents on nutrition and family planning Examination of breasts and advice on breast feeding
Anemia	Routine examination of conjunctiva, and hemoglobin estimation Advice on diet, especially local sources of iron, folic acid, and protein Diet supplements of iron and/or folic acid Treatment of helminths, malaria, etc., where appropriate
Malaria	Routine antimalaria therapy through pregnancy
Intestinal helminths	Routine stool examination and deworming
Dysentery	Prompt investigation, including microscopy, and appropriate treatment; investigate possible food poisoning
Tuberculosis	Investigate chronic cough, loss of weight Treat active cases and contacts
Obstetric	Detection of pelvic deformities, including rickets and osteomalacia Antenatal supervision and referral of cases at risk Education concerning dangers of oxytoxic herbs Appropriate arrangements for midwifery
Peripartum hemorrhage	Prevention of anemia Emergency methods for management and referral
Puerperal infection	Avoidance of contamination of birth canal Instruction of traditional birth attendants
Toxemia	Routine antenatal tests (urine for albumin, blood pressure, pitting edema, sudden weight gain) Advice on adequate diet
Infection	Serological screening for syphilis Microbiological screening for gonorrhea Screening for bacteria
Primary prevention of infection	Tetanus immunization in pregnancy for women of childbearing age

Uterine abnormalities (such as fibroids)

Intestinal parasites, tuberculosis, malaria, pyelitis, vaginitis

Heart disease, asthma, chronic bronchitis

Rh sensitization (Caucasians—15 percent, Africans—6 percent)

Anxiety

Fistula

Activities in the antenatal clinic should be carefully planned to ensure the most effective use of time, to exclude meaningless routines, and to include examinations designed to detect major problems, especially those of local importance (Table 11.2).

Screening Programs

Overcrowded antenatal clinics offer few services of sufficient quality to be worthwhile. Furthermore, it is estimated that among the 20 percent who have access to such services, the number of visits averages one antenatal visit throughout pregnancy. This is not surprising; in many cultures, women do not talk about pregnancy until it is well established. Accessibility, fragmentation of services, money for transport or clinic fee, and lack of empathy between staff and patients constitute major obstacles to health care.

Women have long been accused by health professionals of neglect and ignorance and have been blamed for infant mortality (Dyhouse 1981). An understanding of their life-styles and living conditions, however, would go a long way to adapting the services to the women who need them. Emphasis should be placed on teaching women about their bodies and how to stay healthy, as well as on home economics. Women could be taught to screen themselves for specific conditions, such as self-examinations for breast cancer. In pregnancy, for example, Neldham (1980) suggested a method for identifying fetal distress based on counting fetal movements. Although rates of movement vary, a change in rate or a low rate may be significant. This method could prove to be a powerful strategy for preventing intrauterine deaths. Pearson (1979) has suggested an hourly "kick count." If there are more than ten kicks, the mother stops counting even though the hour is not over. If the count is less, referral is required. Of course, a clock or hourglass is also required. Results depend not only on identification of the fetus at risk but also on prompt delivery. Measures like these need to be verified and, where suitable, applied.

In many parts of the world, the village-level health worker has to decide which pregnant women to refer to health centers or hospitals. Several screening tests are in use in different regions (Shah 1980); for example, in India, arm circumference measurements are made with a Shakir tape (Fig. 11.3) (Tibrewala and Shah 1978). Through the use of this color-coded tape measure, the patient is classified as normal or malnourished. In Guatemala, the 3H (head circumference,

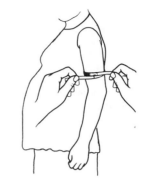

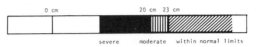

Figure 11.3. Arm circumference, a useful method for screening for maternal malnutrition. Screening for malnutrition in adult women can be done even by nonliterate health workers using a color-coded Shakir tape.

height, and home score) score is used (Gibbons 1981). In Latin America, fundal height is measured by village-level workers using a color-coded tape measure (Villar et al. 1979). Such methods are not precise but can categorize and refer those needing urgent attention.

Simple screening methods for anemia have also been devised for use by community health workers and other health professionals where no laboratory facilities exist for hemoglobin determinations, such as pictures of anemic and nonanemic tongues and use of a color swatch that matches the conjunctival colors by those of different red shades in the chart (Ghosh and Mohan 1978). Failing this, eliciting a history of pica may be helpful in deciding whether iron supplements are needed. The World Health Organization has recommended that iron not be given routinely to all pregnant women. A history of malaria or a folate-deficient diet will suggest folic acid deficiency.

Health workers also have to be aware of warning symptoms that require referral (Kloosterman 1978):

- Vaginal bleeding
- Sudden onset of edema

- Epigastric pain or headache
- Reduced fetal movements
- Anemia
- Obstructed labor
- Vaginal discharge (water, bloody, or malodorous)
- Fever
- Retained placenta
- Malpresentation
- Hypertension
- Albuminuria

Prompt attention to warning symptoms and signs may avert serious sequelae. Methods of screening, referral, and management depend on local conditions and resources.

Adaptive Antenatal Clinics

As with any other health services, the activities must be adapted to resources of staff, funds, equipment, and supplies, to such geographical factors as distance and communications, to pressure of work, to local disease patterns, to traditional behavior in pregnancy and during labor, to the puerperium and lactation, and to the effect of maternal health on the offspring (Ampofo 1969; Fleming et al. 1969; Haroon 1967; Maitland 1966). Anemia in the mother may lead to poor fetal stores of iron, predisposing to anemia in infancy. It also seems likely that an inadequate or unbalanced diet, especially in late pregnancy, will produce permanent mental impairment in the offspring (Jelliffe 1968; Jelliffe and Jelliffe 1992).

The causes of maternal morbidity and mortality (Jelliffe and Jelliffe 1989; Mootoo 1967) need to be analyzed for the particular region. Obstetric facilities and transportation must be taken into consideration. Anemia, malnutrition (undernutrition, overnutrition, and imbalances such as osteomalacia), intestinal helminths, tuberculosis, dysentery (including ame-biasis), and, often, malaria and too-frequent childbearing are important. Puerperal deaths result from obstructed labor, infection, peripartum hemorrhage (often with a background of anemia), ruptured uterus, eclampsia, and abortions. High perinatal mortality rates will also be found, mainly due to low birthweight, birth injuries, neonatal infections, including umbilical tetanus, and congenital abnormalities (Brown and Sandhu 1969). Many of these are closely associated with the maternal disorders.

Each area has its own particular problems. Cephalopelvic disproportion and inefficient uterine action are two of the biggest obstetric problems in African primiparas. The high incidence of vesicovaginal fistulas, ruptured uteri, and maternal mortality bear testimony to this. TBAs help to reduce tetanus and other infections by adopting hygienic measures. They cannot do anything themselves about obstructed labor and malpresentations, but they can be trained to recognize complications early and refer promptly. Diagnosis must be competent, and much can be done with clinical observation, experience, and any appropriate laboratory assistance available, such as a microscope (King 1972). Treatment must be prompt and efficacious and as inexpensive and uncomplicated as possible. A clinic can do little good unless essential drugs are kept in stock and are dispensed carefully and conscientiously. If injections are necessary, they should be available and given promptly. If the patient is told to "come back on Thursday to the VD clinic" or "go to the dispensary" three miles away, she probably will not go and will lose confidence in the health system.

Much of the burden of maternal, fetal, and neonatal illness can be prevented by basic prenatal supervision, uncomplicated treatment, advice, and simple but experienced care at delivery and during the puerperium (Measham 1992). It is worthwhile to make these services well known, acceptable, and effective. The management of a patient will depend on an evaluation of the general situation, the family, the attitudes, the home condition, and the physical and mental states of the patient (Baird 1970).

Research is vital at the country's main centers into the prevalence, importance, epidemiology, pathology, causes of abnormalities, and scientifically based but practicable, methods of prevention or treatment (Ampofo 1969; Fleming et al. 1969 Haroon 1967; Lawson and Stewart 1967; WHO 1980). A knowledge of the local causes of iron-deficiency anemia and the roles played by poor absorption, dietary intake, and intestinal helminths will help in determining the need for screening tests. Unless a deficiency is known to be widespread, iron should be given only once a diagnosis is made. In the same way, a high prevalence of tetanus in the newborn indicates a special need for training of TBAs and possibly for maternal immunization. In hyperendemic malarial areas, chloroquine or other appropriate antimalarials may be given routinely throughout pregnancy to reduce the incidence of maternal anemia and low-birthweight infants (Jelliffe 1968). Procedures at clinics should be geared to the management of local problems. Clear instructions, usually in the form of a manual, are needed to record and test, for referrals and emergencies, and for advice and treatment. Special procedures can be recommended for transport and rapid communications and for blood supplies in cases of hemorrhage.

Attendance

It appears that at least one antenatal visit is essential, and eight to ten attendances are generally encouraged for the normal pregnancy. More visits may be needed for high-risk cases and for special education or support. This number of visits, however, is often not feasible, and even one visit (commonly the case in developing countries) is much better than none. If the patient is to be delivered at home by a relative or TBA, this individual should be asked to come to the antenatal clinic and be given simple instructions. Primigravidas, especially among very young women, need extra care and education.

Some authorities have found it helpful, and quite feasible, to set up a "maternity village" or hostel where women, as well as some of the younger children and the grandmother, can come and stay for some days or even weeks before the onset of labor. This is also useful for postnatal care and will relieve the strain on beds in a maternity ward. It provides superb opportunities for health education and can most usefully form part of a "mother-craft" or "rehabilitation and nutrition center." It should be conveniently close to the hospital so as to ensure ready supervision and admission.

The first examination should be carried out by a health professional. Nurse practitioners, medical officers, and health professionals do much of the routine care and follow-up; doctors, when available, see problem cases and provide highly specialized treatment. In some areas, village-level health workers provide the bulk of the routine care.

Special risks are common in certain areas—for instance, anemia in some urban areas, premature deliveries in rural regions, ruptured uteri in East Africa, and undernutrition or osteomalacia in parts of the Middle East and Indo-Pakistan.

Home visits by nurses, midwives, and community health workers should provide home care and supervision of environmental conditions, such as sanitation, water supply, cleanliness, and bed bugs and should enable them to ascertain the numbers, state of health and education, and attitudes of other members of the household and to decide if home delivery is suitable.

Analysis of antenatal records can supply information on:

1. Fertility and marriage customs.
2. Infant and child mortality and morbidity.
3. Maternal nutrition and diseases.
4. Attitudes and customs related to childbearing and child rearing.

These matters are always important; they are particularly valuable in areas that lack accurate vital statistics for the population as a whole.

CARE AT DELIVERY

The place of delivery and the kind of birth attendant vary over the world. Most births in most developing areas still take place in homes under the supervision of TBAs. Philpott (1972) has devised a chart, called a partograph, to help semiskilled health workers define cases requiring transfer for specialized care. The chart (Fig. 11.4) uses "alert" and "action" lines based on the progression of cervical dilation and advancement of the head. By using the chart, midwives and nurses in isolated villages are able to refer cases

earlier, allowing enough time for transportation to the hospital (Fig. 11.5). This chart still needs to be tested in other areas and requires supervision.

Rapid referral provides an opportunity for lifesaving measures, and rapid referral of women who are bleeding can also reduce maternal mortality. Harrison (1979) found in Nigeria that exsanguinated late arrivals require sixty units of blood per bed-year compared with only eight units of blood per bed-year in the United Kingdom—a difference of more than seven times the amount. Avoidance of all but the most necessary blood transfusions has been made imperative by the risk of HIV infection.

It has been suggested that the person best qualified in a community should be trained to do whatever needs to be done regardless of the person's educational attainment. In Natal, South Africa, nurse-midwives in small rural hospitals are being trained to perform forceps deliveries and cesarean sections (Ross 1992, personal communication). In areas where there are not enough obstetricians, such as Mozambique, surgical assistants are being

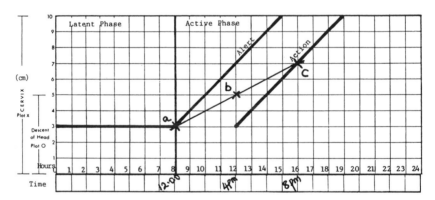

a At 12 noon, the woman, in established labor with 3 centimeters (cm) cervical dilation, is admitted to the health center.
b At 4PM, the cervix is 5cm dilated, showing that labor is progressing slower than normal making referral from the health center to hospital necessary.
c At 8PM, the woman reaches the hospital when the cervix is 7cm dilated. With her graph now having reached the "Action line," a decision must be made on the medical attention required.

Figure 11.4. A partograph that provides warning guidelines. Source: WHO (1988).

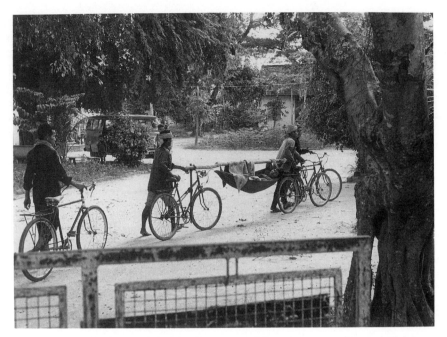

Figure 11.5. Improvised transportation for a woman in labor requiring emergency hospital care. Source: ICEF 8462/Cambodia UNICEF.

trained to perform lifesaving procedures (including manual removal of the placenta), so that mothers do not die in childbirth (Safe Motherhood News 1993).

Hospital deliveries are generally preferred for pregnancies most at risk, where maternity beds are available in sufficient numbers. Good antenatal supervision will identify most of the cases that are likely to need referral. The antenatal card (record of blood pressure etc.) must always be available at the place of delivery. An emergency squad and ambulance service can be invaluable, although expense, distance, and poor communications usually make such service impossible. At an innovative maternity clinic in Uganda, a flag was flown whenever an endangered mother was in need of transport to hospital. People in the community then marshaled whatever transport was available to aid the mother. This service not only kept expenses at a minimum but involved the community.

Rural health centers should have a few beds available for maternity cases for observation and emergencies. Trained and experienced midwives can provide an excellent and inexpensive domiciliary service. With good antenatal care and good transport, this sort of service can be admirable. The Sudan Medical Service has long shown that training illiterate women in the rudiments of midwifery and home care reduce the incidence of tetanus neonatorum and fatalities due to obstructed labor. The secret to success seems to lie in a thoroughly practical training and in good supervision and referral. Gravitational drainage of placental blood into the newly delivered baby before cutting the cord may be important prophylaxis against subsequent iron-deficiency anemia (Yao and Lind 1969).

Breastfeeding is highly recommended; indeed, anything else may be a sentence of death for the infant. Breastfeeding is taken for granted in rural areas in most of the developing countries, but it is tending to die out where imported misconceptions concerning social status demand bottle feeding. In particular, mixed milk feeding—breast and bottle—is increasing (Baumslag 1989). When doctors and nurses from highly industrialized countries do not appreciate the importance of breastfeeding and are ignorant of its management, the situation is increasingly serious, especially when combined with commercial pressures to bottle-feed by formula companies and gifts of formula.

Nurseries in maternity hospitals should be abolished; instead, the baby should be kept with the mother in her bed or in a crib next to the mother's bed. It is remarkable how soon mother and baby come to some arrangement when this pattern is followed, and there are fewer screaming babies and fewer cracked nipples or engorged breasts. Four-hourly feeding routines and nurseries down the corridor have done as much to discourage breastfeeding as have commercial advertisements for human milk substitutes (Jelliffe 1968; Jelliffe and Jelliffe 1978). Breastmilk is the most valuable, the cheapest, and the most neglected source of nutrients. Some observers have found that it is easier to establish breastfeeding after home deliveries than after hospital deliveries. La Leche League is doing much to encourage this valuable method of feeding among educated American women (La Leche League International 1987). Breastfeeding mother support groups have developed with special modifications for local circumstances in many countries, including Brazil. Wellstart is training doctors and nurses worldwide to be more knowledgeable about breastfeeding and counseling so that breastfeeding can be protected, promoted, and supported, especially in maternities. They are also developing mother support groups.

A slow revolution in perinatal care is taking place in the Philippines. The program was started by Dr. Clavano in the Bagiou General Hospital in 1974 by making breastfeeding and rooming in the norm and, by closing the nursery for well newborns, she was able to show a sharp decrease in the rate of neonatal sepsis and diarrhea. At the Dr. Jose Fabella Memorial Hospital 100 deliveries (40 percent abnormal) take place per day, and all infants are given breastmilk including low-birthweight infants who are given expressed breastmilk. No bottles are used. Lactation assistants provide practical and psychological support to new mothers. No mother is discharged until breastfeeding is well established. The program saves the hospital $290,000 a year by not purchasing feeding bottles, formula, and intravenous fluids. Neonatal sepsis and diarrhea are nonexistent in these wards. Dr. Gonzalez, the medical director of the hospital, believes it is essential to provide mothers with comfort, dignity, and safety. This hospital serving poor women is a unique example of how MCH services can be improved even when resources are very limited. The wards are immaculate and mothers handle their infants from the moment of birth.

After delivery, whether at home or in hospital, the baby and mother must be carefully examined for any sign of abnormality. Premature infants must receive special care, preferably with the mother involved in the care, and using the breastmilk of the mother (Khan et al. 1954; King 1966; Jelliffe and Jelliffe 1978). The mother, especially the primipara, who handles, observes, and attends to her baby from birth has much more skill and confidence in baby care when she leaves the hospital and returns to her home (BMJ 1970; Brown and Sandhu 1969; Connor 1970).

In the Netherlands, where the infant mortality rate is less than 7 per 1,000 live births (UNICEF 1992), the maternal mortality rate is very low, and yet only about half the births take place in hospitals. There is also a high incidence of breastfeeding, and many of the cases that are admitted stay in hospital for less than twenty-four hours. The home care service, however, is well organized and excellent.

Some maternity hospitals in the past delayed feeding the baby until twenty-four hours or even longer after birth. This practice is now much less frequent. Wards where the baby is handed to the mother soon after birth have been successful in establishing the practice of breastfeeding and good mother–child relationships. It also has a marked effect on development and neuromuscular control in the baby. It is found that the sucking reflex may be active soon after birth but may be reduced if there is a long waiting period. For the mother, the early suckling stimulates uterine contractions; the earlier the breasts are stimulated, the sooner lactation is established.

The practice of episiotomy, almost universal in some hospitals, may also have helped to diminish breastfeeding. Some mothers suffer severe pain from this procedure and are so occupied with the pain that they scarcely want to see the baby, much less nurse him or her. It is claimed that this operation has done much to reduce immediate risks to the mother and the baby and also to reduce long-term risks of urinary incontinence, but this is a subject that requires research and evaluation.

Table 11.3 lists barriers to breastfeeding and some suggestions of how these can be modified.

POSTNATAL CARE

The puerperium is an important period and recognized as such by most cultures. A wide variety of practices and customs exist throughout the world. Many are beneficial, such as a period of seclusion or a more generous diet; others can be harmful, for example, not giving the baby colostrum or severe dietary restriction of the mother. In Yemen, TBAs apply antimony and tumeric to the perineum to hasten healing; they insert alum and sweet-smelling herbs into the vagina to improve the tone of vaginal walls and narrow the orifice, and women sit in the squatting position over smoking herbs that they believe will heal the perineum. Worrying about breastmilk production without considering the perineum is senseless; a torn perineum will affect the mother's ability to concentrate on breastfeeding. In some cultures, sexual intercourse is taboo for forty days after birth. Special high calorie foods and high protein are given to pregnant women—for example, eggs in China. In parts of China, mothers confined or "doing the month" may not be allowed to go to health services (Baasher et al. 1982). Thus, it is imperative that the health services go to the mothers at home to correct anemia, infections, tears, and other problems, including providing support of breastfeeding and care of the infant.

When mother and child return home from the hospital, information, such as a copy of the notification of birth form, should be sent to the health authorities (the ministry of health or a health center) in the area from which the mother comes. On the back of the form should be a list of the usual conditions noted in hospitals that must receive special attention: family history of mental disorder, social problems, prenatal history of rubella, toxemia, vomiting, peri- and postnatal conditions such as jaundice, low birthweight, feeding difficulties, convulsions, or any other abnormalities. The doctor should mark the conditions that need to be observed. The ministry of health or director of the health center can then maintain a list of babies at risk, and the health nurse will visit in the home and ensure continuing supervision. Once it is certain that the child is developing normally, he or she will be removed from the list of those at risk. Many handicaps are not apparent at birth, so risk awareness should be continued and reviewed from time to time. The establishment of assessment centers (specialized centers for evaluating the de-

Table 11.3. Health Services to Promote Breastfeeding

Barriers	Modifications
Lack of knowledge among health professionals and families	Sensitize and educate health professionals and community, including the avoidance of financial involvement with formula companies Prenatal preparation of mothers for labor and breastfeeding (especially correct inverted nipples) Advice on management and positioning (in urban groups)
Poor practices in antenatal, labor and delivery, and postnatal care	Avoid pre- and postlacteal feeds Promote demand feeding morning, noon, and night (night feeds account for a third of the infant's intake) Rooming in Give colostrum to all newborns Use fresh expressed milk for premature or low-birthweight infants whenever possible.
Advertising infant formula	Stop free samples and handouts of formula feeding literature Promote and protect breastfeeding
Unnecessary interference	Avoid unnecessary separation of mother and infant Avoid and underemphasize test weighing Avoid routine episiotomies and unnecessary sedation
Lack of support	Assist mother with cesarean section or episiotomy in positioning while breastfeeding Maintain contact between mother and infant, including sick or low-birthweight infants Establish support groups (La Leche League, local experienced mothers) with linkages in hospital, clinic, and home Home visit all newborns, especially primiparas and low-birthweight infants

Some mothers persevere despite institutional disincentives.

fects and needs of the child) has proved to be useful in some areas.

Locally appropriate simplified modifications of this approach can be devised for less sophisticated circumstances. The list should reflect local indicators of high risk, such as previous infant with malnutrition, current difficulties with breastfeeding, or low birthweight. The principles are the same: identification and communication of information to ensure continuity of care.

Home visits should be paid by the midwife or the health nurse soon after the mother's discharge from the hospital. In some cases at risk, it is ideal for the mother to be escorted home by the health nurse. The process is relatively useless if the visit is delayed. Some authorities will claim that "all newborns are visited in the home," but then it is discovered that visits may not take place until two, three, or four weeks after births. By this time, one mother has become distraught, another has already started her low-birthweight child on dilute, contaminated bottle-feeds or, in a sophisticated setting, on tins of meat and vegetables—with disastrous results. For the continuation of successful breastfeeding, especially in urban areas, a visit during the first week has been shown to be critical.

Some obstetric wards are so overcrowded that the mother is discharged from the hospital within eleven hours, or even less, of delivery. It should, however, be the aim to provide long-stay facilities for the very young mother and for others at risk, provided this includes rooming in. The plan may prove valuable for both treatment and prevention of disorders and a special opportunity for health education and the initiation of successful lactation.

Most health workers agree on the advantages of hospital deliveries for high-risk mothers, provided the rapid turnover does not lead to increased overload, perfunctory services, or unintelligent routines. Hospital deliveries should not be used simply to ensure obstetric facilities, such as the availability of blood transfusions. They should also provide a valuable opportunity for identifying many of the risks and disorders that beset childbearing and childrearing and for health education (Dyhouse 1981; Lawson and Stewart 1967). Postnatal care of the mother must be emphasized, as examinations are always advised but often avoided. Some mothers are so immersed in their household chores and so absorbed in and fascinated by the new baby that they tend to ignore their own health. Others feel that the baby is getting altogether too much attention, considering it was they who had to do all the work. A balanced point of view must be maintained. Other members of the household, particularly the father, may need advice, help, and encouragement in the process of adaptation. The whole affair is a learning situation.

HEALTH SERVICES FOR WOMEN

Relatively little information can be found on women's health because the primary concern has been on women only as mothers and childbearers, with the main focus on navigation of the birth canal (and even here information is lacking). Most scientific studies on females in the reproductive ages are concerned with low birth weight; few with the health of women. This situation exists because women's health has never been considered important. One only has to look at national health budgets to see how little is spent on services and research into women's health.

Women have unique health problems throughout their life cycle, beginning with menstrual iregularity and hygiene. A UNICEF study in Zimbabwe showed that menstruating girls missed three or four days of school per month as they had no sanitary hygienic measures available to them. In China (personal observation in 1986) menstruating women can purchase low cost sanitized paper and this has reduced urinary and vaginal infections, decreasing the time women and girls lose from work and study.

Statistics as well as services for women's health are practically nonexistent in developing countries. The incidence of heart disease is not known. In the United States it has recently been recognized that heart disease is a significant killer of women as well as men. But doctors have failed to make the diagnosis because heart disease among men only has been well documented. Cancer is another leading cause of death in women. In developing countries cancer of the cervix is the commonest cancer and if seen early, treatment carries a good prognosis. Breast cancer is the commonest cancer in women in developed countries (WHO 1992c).

The incidence of malaria, hepatitis, and tuberculosis in women is not documented although the impact on mothers and working women is immense. Efforts to obtain gender-specific data are only now beginning. Problems perceived by health providers differ from those of the women. When women are asked what their commonest problem is, beating by the husband is the most frequent answer (Heise 1989). In the United States, every 15 seconds a woman is beaten in her own home. Women are twice as likely to be injured by violence as to be diagnosed with cancer.

In developing countries women who suffer from mental disease remain undiagnosed but depression is prevalent. Even in the United States women suffer twice the rate of clinical depression as men. Three quarters of all American women who experience clinical symptoms of depression never receive treatment and an overwhelming percentage (90%) of eating disorders occur in women.

Services for older women are rare in developing countries. Of late, however, the medical fraternity and drug companies have displayed a great interest in the menopause. This attention has turned menopause, a natural phase in a woman's life cycle, into a disease requiring hormone replacement therapy (HRT). HRT is now credited with preventing heart disease, aging of the skin, osteoporosis, and so on. Older women are more prone to arthritis, obesity, diabetes, osteoporosis, cataracts, heart disease, and urinary incontinence (a common and trou-

bling condition). If given before menopause, HRT may prevent osteoporosis but the claims that HRT is a valid form of therapy for all degenerative diseases of older women is of concern (Topo 1993). Osteoporosis is a major preventable cause of disability in more than 50 percent of women over 45 years and in 90 percent of women over 75 years. Alerting younger women to the importance of diet, the monitored supplementation of calcium and vitamin D, and weight bearing exercises is a simple means of prevention (Campaign for Women's Health 1993).

The WHO global program on tropical disease includes the investigation of the natural history and the stigma of disease on men and women. The new focus is to learn from the local women what they know and need instead of just telling them. There appears to be information that women have known for ages but which has been ignored by the health care providers. A case in fact is that of malaria. As far back as 1854 it was known by the Somali nomads that the mosquito bite brought deadly fever but the association was ignored. Forty years later an article published in the *Lancet* established the relationship between the mosquito and malaria (Washington Post 1993).

In the United States it has been recognized that women's health has been shortchanged. Research is needed for effective treatment; dosage, drug response, and natural history for diseases in women may be significantly different than in men. One example is how women respond to treatment for heart attacks. In the United States the involvement of women's groups at research institutions as policy makers and in government positions at all levels has resulted in more funds and more programs. There is now a shift toward a cost-conscious health care system that prevents illness, disease, and disability, with a strong emphasis on preventive care services for women's health.

CONCLUSION

There has been an increasing awareness that giving birth is both a natural and a family event and not a disease process, although it does have special risks (Rosenfield and Maine 1985). The importance of the emphasis on all aspects of this process (Table 11.4) is emphasized by WHO/UNICEF's recent "Safe Motherhood" programs. Its main elements are:

- Adequate primary health care and an adequate share of food for girls from infancy to adolescence.
- Universally available family planning to avoid unwanted or high-risk pregnancies.
- Good prenatal care, including nutrition, with efficient and early detection and referral of women at high risk.
- Assistance of a trained person for all women in childbirth, at home or in the hospital.
- Access to the essential elements of obstetric care at the first referral level for women at higher risk, especially those in emergencies of pregnancy, childbirth, and the puerperium. (Kwast 1991)

Table 11.4. Basic Services for Women

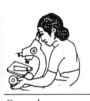 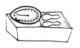 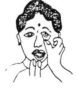 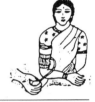

General	Pregnancy	Special birth services	Postpartum
Self health care	Preparation psychologically	Supervised assistance	Home visit to check lochia, diet, etc.
Sex education[a]		Minimal interference	
	Prenatal screening		Screen for anemia
Treatment of medical conditions (goiter, malaria, kidney infections, venereal disease, parasitic infestations, etc.)	Referral of high-risk women	Clear lines of referral	Maintain maternal health (including mental health)
		Select and supervise TBAs	
	Selective supplements		Advise on family planning[a]
Supervision of female circumcision (if it is an established practice)	Information on infant and child care, including breastfeeding[a]		Provide psychological support (especially postpartum depression and lactation problems)
Infertility services[a]			
Counseling (including family planning and genetic counseling)[a]	Abortions if desired or necessary		
Screening for cancer, diabetes	Recognize when to seek help (edema, decrease in fetal movements, etc.)		
Obesity programs			
Dental care			
Drug addiction programs	Hygienic measures		
Protection on the job			

[a]Men should be included.

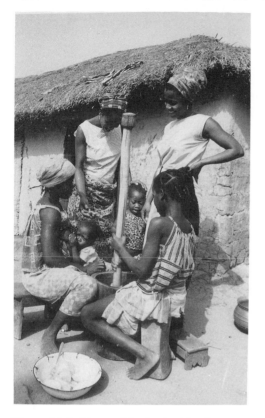

Figure 11.6. Home visits by health educators. When mothers and health educators home visit and exchange ideas, family health improves. The two educators in this photograph exchanged ideas and information while the village women pounded the daily supply of yams (UNICEF Photo, Berheim, Ivory Coast).

The ability of the medical system to treat women with obstetric complications will largely determine the success of safe motherhood programs (which should be called "safer" motherhood as motherhood is not "safe"). When difficulties occur, specialized obstetrical care is invaluable. A variety of methods to identify cases for referral to maternity clinics and hospitals for special care have been devised. In many countries, trained TBAs have this role. In industrialized countries, the degree of sophisticated testing (ultrasound and fetal monitoring, for example) has increased to the point where some obstetricians argue that the returns do not justify the extraordinary expense.

While in the West, doctors favor more tests, women are seeking alternatives to hospital deliveries and, often, an increased use of midwives. Birth centers are mushrooming everywhere, and home deliveries have increased as a reaction to the technical interference in what is usually a natural physiological process. Hospital deliveries in the United States are considerably more expensive than birth center deliveries, and the costs are even less than half for supervised home deliveries (Mehl et al. 1975–1976).

Each community should consider family preferences, available methods for rapid referral, action lines or outlined protocol, and resources. The situations differ greatly in a commercial medical system such as the United States, a free state-subsidized system such as Sweden, or a largely primary health care network as in many impoverished countries. The real need is for a balance between biological and traditional practices and for affordable modern technology when indicated.

While "services for women" are often interpreted to mean services for childbearing women, basic comprehensive services must be available to women at all stages of life. The care and education of women will lead to healthier and happier families (Fig. 11.6). Health services ultimately must aim to supply mature counseling for individuals before, after, and aside from the responsibilities of parenthood. This approach will not merely deal with physical disorders and disadvantages associated with childbearing but will help to raise the standards, improve the economics, and promote the progress of a community.

The empowerment of women through membership in women's groups in Bangladesh, for example, has resulted in a measurable increase in the status of their children and a dramatic increase in the survival of girls. Women were more able to influence decisions in their new role with their husbands as economic partners

(Sternin 1989). Development programs that have provided women with loans have increased their independence and income.

REFERENCES

Ampofo, D. A. (1969). Causes of maternal death and comments, Maternity Hospital, Accra, 1963–1967. *W. Afr. Med. J.* **18**, 75.

Baasher, T.; Bannerman, R. H. O.; Rushwan, H.; and Sharaf, I. (1982) *Traditional Practices Affecting the Health of Women and Children.* WHO/EMRO Technical Publication, no. 2, vol. 2. Alexandria, Egypt.

Baird, D. (1970). The obstetrician and society. *Am. J. Publ. Hlth.* **60**, 628.

Baumslag, N. (1989). *Infant feeding practices and trends.* U.S. Agency for International Development, Washington, D.C.

Baumslag, N.; Edelstein, T.; and Metz, J. (1970). Reduction of incidence of prematurity by folic acid supplementation in pregnancy. *Brit. Med. J.* **1**, 16.

BMJ (1970). Mothers of premature babies, editorial. *Brit. Med. J.* **2**, 556.

Brown, R. E., and Sandhu, T. S. (1969). Autopsy survey of perinatal deaths in Uganda. *Trop. Geogr. Med.* **18**, 292.

Campaign for Women's Health (1993). *Model Benefits Package for Women.* Older Women's League, Washington, D.C.

Chalmers, I.; Enkin, M.; and Keirse, M. (1990). *Effective Care in Pregnancy and Childbirth,* 2 vols. Oxford University Press, Oxford.

Chatterjee, M. (1991). Women taking control. *Multinational Monitor,* pp. 16–18.

Connor, B. H. (1970). Mothers and infants in Transkei. *Lancet* **i**, 768.

Dyhouse, C. (1981). Working class mothers and infant mortality, 1895–1915. In *Biology, Medicine and Society, 1840–1940,* pp. 73–89. Ed. C. Webster. Cambridge University Press, Cambridge.

Fleming, A. F.; Allan, N. C.; and Stewhouse, N. S. (1969). Haemolytic anaemia in pregnancy in Nigeria: Recognition by simple laboratory procedures. *W. Afr. Med. J.* **18**, 82.

Geber, M., and Dean, R. F. A. (1958). Psychomotor development of African children: The effects of social class and the need for improved tests. *Bull. Wld. Hlth. Org.* **18**, 421.

Ghosh, S., and Mohan, M. (1978). Screening for anaemia. *Lancet* **i**, 823.

Gibbons, G. (1981). Women at risk screening methods. *Mothers and Children* **1**, 4.

Gyorgy, P., and Burgess, A., eds. (1965). *Protecting the Pre-School Child, Programmes in Practice.* Tavistock, London.

Haroon, S. (1967). Problems of antenatal care in the tropics. *Brit. Med. J.* **1**, 617.

Harrison, K. A. (1979). Approaches to reducing maternal mortality and perinatal mortality. In *Maternity Services in the Developing World: What the Community needs.* Ed. R. H. Philpott. Proceedings of the Seventh Study Group of the Royal College of Obstetricians and Gynaecologists, London.

Heise, L. (1989). Violence against women. *The Hamilton Spectator,* April 26, p. A7 (Hamilton, Ontario, Canada).

Jelliffe, D. B. (1968). *Infant Nutrition in the Subtropics and Tropics.* Wld Hlth Org. Monogr. Ser., no. 28. Geneva.

Jelliffe, D. B., and Jelliffe, E. F. P. (1978). *Human Milk in the Modern World.* Oxford University Press, Oxford.

Jelliffe, D. B., and Jelliffe, E. F. P. (1989). *Community Nutritional Assessment.* Oxford University Press, Oxford.

Jelliffe, D. B., and Jelliffe, E. F. P. (1992). *Conjunctival Color Categorizer.*

Jelliffe, E. F. P. (1968). Low birth-weight and malarial infection of the placenta. *Bull. Wld. Hlth. Org.* **38**, 69.

Khan, E.; Wayburne, S.; and Fouche, M. (1954). The Baragwanath premature baby unit—an analysis of the case records of 1000 consecutive admissions. *S. Afr. Med. J.* **28**, 453.

King, M. H., ed. (1966). *Medical Care in Developing Countries.* Oxford University Press, Nairobi.

King, M. H. (1972). *A Medical Laboratory for Developing Regions.* Oxford University Press, Nairobi.

Kloosterman, G. J. (1978). De Nederlandse verloskunde op de tweesprong. *Nederlands Tijdschrift, voor Geneeskunde* **122**, 1161.

Kwast, B. (1991). The Safe Motherhood initiative. *Wld. Hlth. Forum* **12**, 1.

La Leche League International (1987). *The Womanly Art of Breast-Feeding.* 4th ed. Franklin Park, Ill.

La Leche League International (1991). *The Breastfeeding Answer Book.* Franklin Park, Ill.

Lawson, J. B., and Stewart, D. B., eds. (1967). *Obstetrics and Gynaecology in the Tropics and Developing Countries*. Edward Arnold, London.

Maitland, H. (1966). The Ngora maternity annex. *J. Trop. Pediat. Monogr.* **2**, 27.

Measham, D. M. (1992). *Toward the Development of Safe Motherhood Program Guidelines*. World Bank, Washington, D.C.

Mehl, L. E.; Peterson, G. H.; Shaw, N. S.; and Crecvy, D. C. (1975–1976). Complications of home birth. *Birth Fam. J.* **2**, 123.

Mootoo, C. L. (1967). Maternal mortality in Guyana. *W. Indian Med. J.* **16**, 139.

Neldam, S. (1980). Foetal movements as an indicator of foetal wellbeing. *Lancet* **i**, 1222.

PAHO (1969). *Iron Metabolism and Anaemia*. Pan American Health Organization, Washington D.C.

PAHO (1970). *Maternal Nutrition and Family Planning*. Scientific Publication no. 204. Pan American Health Organization, Washington, D.C.

Pearson, J. F. (1979). Foetal movement recording: A guide to foetal well-being, *Nursing Times* **75** 1639.

Philpott, R. H. (1972). Cervicographs in the management of labour in primigravidae. *J. Obstet. Gynec. Br. Common.* **79**, 592.

Philpott, R. H., ed. (1979). *Maternity Services in the Developing World: What the Community Needs*. Proceedings of the Seventh Study Group of the Royal College of Obstetricians and Gynaecologists, London.

Pop. Bull. (1969). A source-book on population. *Population Bulletin* **25**(5), special issue.

Rosa, F. W. (1970). International aspects of perinatal mortality. *Clin. Obstet. Gynec.* **13**, 57.

Rosenfield, A., and Maine, D. (1985). *Lancet* **ii**, 83.

Royston, E., and Armstrong, S. (1989). *Preventing Maternal Deaths*. WHO, Geneva.

Safe Motherhood News (1992). WHO, Geneva.

Shah, K. P. (1980). Appropriate technology in primary health care for better mid-wifery services. *J. Obstet. Gynaec.* **30**(1), 109.

Tibrewala, S., and Shah, K. P. (1978). The use of arm circumference as an indicator of body weight in adult women. *Baroda J. Nutr.* **5**, 43.

Topo, P. (1993). Climaterium. *WIPHN News* **13**, 3 (Bethesda, Md.).

Trussell, R. R. (1966). In *Medical Care in Developing Countries*. Ed. M. H. King. Oxford University Press, Nairobi.

Villar, J.; Belizan, J. M.; and Delgado, H. (1979). Monitoring foetal growth in rural areas: An alternative utilizing nonprofessional personnel. *Bull. Pan Am. Hlth. Org.* **13**, 117.

Washington Post (1993). Focus on Women, Useful Insights on Society and Illness, April 12, p. A3.

Williams, C. D. (1938). Child health in the Gold Coast. *Lancet* **i**, 97.

WHO (1965). *Nutrition in Pregnancy and Lactation*. World Health Organization Tech. Rep. Ser., no. 302.

WHO (1969). *The Organization and Administration of Maternal and Child Health Services*. World Health Organization Tech. Rep. Ser., no. 428.

WHO (1980). *Sixth Report on the World Health Situation 1973–1977*, part. One: *Global Analysis*. World Health Organization, Geneva.

WHO (1982). *World Health Statistics Annual*. World Health Organization, Geneva.

WHO (1988). *The Partograph: A Managerial Tool for the Prevention of Prolonged Labour*. Sec. 1: *The Principle and Strategy*. World Health Organization, Geneva.

WHO (1989). Preventing and controlling iron deficiency anemia through primary health care. World Health Organization, Geneva.

WHO (1992*a*). *Implementation of the Global Strategy for Health for All by the Year 2000*. World Health Organization, Geneva.

WHO (1992*b*) *Safe Motherhood*. World Health Organization, Geneva.

WHO (1992*c*) *Women's Health: Across Age and Frontier*. World Health Organization, Geneva.

Yao, A. C., and Lind, J. (1969). Effect of gravity on placental transfusion. *Lancet* **ii**, 505.

12

Health Services for Children

O Daman, O my mother, you who bore me upon your back,
you who gave me suck, you who watched over my first faltering
steps, you who were the first to open my eyes to the wonders of
the earth, I am thinking of you.
CAMARA LAYE, 1954

There is a tendency to emphasize the "young child health service" and the "under-5s clinic" or even "under-3s" clinic. These are the groups at highest risk; they need massive medical care and persistent supervision. Many health care workers, on the other hand, have found that contact with a population and continuity of care is maintained by general children's clinics or by family health services. It is, then, a matter for the health staff to focus attention and advice on the individuals and the age groups most at risk while trying not to exclude others who may need care. If the parents know that the child of 7 years who has worms will be treated, the child of 10 who is doing poorly at school will be examined, or the girl of 12 who is pregnant will be accepted for care, then the family concern becomes more realistic and effective.

Fragmentation of health care service can do harm and should be avoided as much as possible. Continuity, as expressed by the slogan, "comprehensive in aim and at risk in focus," seems paradoxical, but indicates the need to expand the range of activities as resources permit.

THE APPROACH TO CHILDREN

Parents, siblings, doctors, nurses, and other health workers vary enormously in their approach to children. In every setting, some are clumsy, frightened, resentful, sentimental, careless, ignorant, anxious, possessive, indifferent, scientific, analytical, fussy, observant, weary, bad, fair, good or excellent. Most people can learn how to approach a child, how to observe without looking too directly, how to talk and go on talking, or whistle or sing unashamedly, how to handle and examine, how to divert and interest, and how to attend to a child. To some, it comes more easily, but it needs experience and cannot be learned from a book. Health workers must learn how to approach a child and how to assess and improve the approach of individuals who are involved with children.

THE SERVICES

The health of the young child is intimately bound up with that of the mother. An imaginatively planned child health service therefore should cover a range of activities from family planning, through prenatal pediatrics, to the supervision of the health of schoolchildren and adolescents. In less developed areas of the world especially, much attention will have to be directed to young children, in the first five years of life. They make up about one-fifth of the total population in these countries and suffer a high rate of disease and death from preventable, infective, nutritional, and parasitic diseases, all acting together.

The organization of a health service for young children has to be based on the facts of life: large numbers of children sick with several diseases at one time, long distances and poor communications in predominantly rural areas, cross-cultural perceptions of health and disease, impoverished and ill-educated parents, inadequate staff of numerous types (and especially of the highly trained cadres), and limited equipment, facilities, and financial resources. For young children, especially toddlers, the situation is complicated by their relative immobility and the difficulties parents experience in carrying them to the hospital or clinic, especially if a younger baby has arrived.

Each section of a service for young children should cater to curative work, prevention of disease, and promotion of health. These must all be incorporated in training, teaching, and research concerned with practical fact-finding evaluation and improvement of services (Adeniyi-Jones 1958; Arnhold and Schneideman 1969; Backhouse 1966; Bell 1969; BMJ 1970; Inst. of Medicine 1982; Jelliffe 1957; Robinson et al. 1969).

In developing countries where young children are usually subjected to a progression of disorders, facilities for the treatment of disease are needed. At the same time, an exclusively curative approach has little effect on the fundamental picture. Paradoxically, a successful hospital treatment service creates its own problems, because an increasing flood of sick people makes it more and more difficult to divert some of the limited funds toward preventive aspects.

The MCH network will vary with local circumstances (Morley 1963, 1966; Welbourn 1956; Williams 1956) and in most places should be built on the existing infrastructure. In India the Integrated Child Development Service (ICDS) has done just this. Services are delivered at a community center, *anganwadi* (literally a "courtyard"), by community health workers. The program has been so successful in reducing mortality and the prevalence of malnutrition that it has been expanded (Lancet 1981, 1983). In rural areas, malnutrition was halved, and in urban blocks it decreased by 75 percent. The success of the program is attributed to the following factors:

1. Integration of nutrition, health, and educational services.
2. Inclusion of mothers and pregnant women in the program.
3. Provision of on-the-spot nutritional supplements for children up to 6 years old and for pregnant and lactating women (300 kilocalories, 15 grams protein, iron, folic acid).
4. Delivery of services through female residents trained for the work, who continue to receive on-the-job training.
5. Participation by the academic community in monitoring, evaluation, continued education, and supervision.

The program continues to improve by finding problems and developing solutions as part of its day-to-day activities and has identified the reasons for a proportion of children remaining unimmunized and malnourished. Some of the reasons were parental suspicion, lack of safe drinking water with frequent episodes of diarrhea, and interruption of feeding programs due to inadequate supplies because the roads are rudimentary and rain makes them impassable. These factors are now receiving attention. This program illustrates the importance of continuity of the services and intersectoral cooperation.

The aims, activities, and personnel of each unit should be integrated, so that they fit as far as possible into the overall plan for the service of the area. The practical system of liaison and referral devised should include care of the mother and family planning and should work with other groups and agencies concerned with improvement in schools and in village life. Frequently, particularly in larger tropical towns, there is a skeleton network of services for mothers and young children, but it is not coordinated, largely because the organizers of the component units are overwhelmed by their own immediate problems. A period spent in discovering the detailed activities of all MCH services in the area is invaluable, followed by continuing discussion on the best deployment of resources. This can sometimes be undertaken by an MCH committee to coordinate activities. In its new preventive-curative role, the hospital has an important part to play in an overall service for mothers and children, largely for referral of very sick children.

Experience in numerous countries has demonstrated clearly that a system of health centers is the only practical and economical way to carry a health service to scattered rural peoples and to crowded slum dwellers. The health center, whether of the bedded variety or not, is the basis of a realistic MCH service, especially if it is located in relation to the local population's needs and serves a defined area for home visiting (Robinson 1970; Rosa 1964; Stanfield 1966; Thomson 1962). Around it must be developed rural clinics, mobile or static, sufficiently near villages so that mothers can carry their young children from home to clinic and some form of home visiting activities is possible

(DeBeer 1966; Fendall 1969; Namboze 1966).

Outreach into the community may be undertaken by health personnel collaborating with various village schools, clubs, and organizations, such as those developed in some countries by a community development department, and wherever practical by home visits to mothers and young children at risk (Kark 1981; Stanfield 1967). To identify those most likely to be at risk, services must aim to reach 100 percent of the population.

"People's medicine" has always existed in communities but has often been ignored by the Western health care system. Recognition of the importance of reaching out into the community and providing basic health services to the vast majority rather than to the wealthy few can place hospital-oriented health care in the correct perspective—no longer the center but an essential component of a network serving villages and slums. Such a network of community-based health services integrated with nutrition, agriculture, and other sectors can make prevention of health disorders feasible. Community health workers are first-line health care providers (Fig. 12.1). They provide essential basic health services at the village level operating from a health post, a dispensary, or even their homes. Often each community health worker may be responsible for 100 to 200 families, depending on the terrain, population density, and number of workers available. In sparse areas with hilly terrain, deserts, and rain-drenched or roadless areas, fewer families can be covered. It is therefore important to assess the types of illness and transportation available before arriving at ratios.

Health workers cannot function in a vacuum; a network of dispensaries, health posts, subcenters, primary care centers, and maternities must be available and linked for continuity, referral, and supervision. Otherwise the hospital becomes inundated with patients suffering from

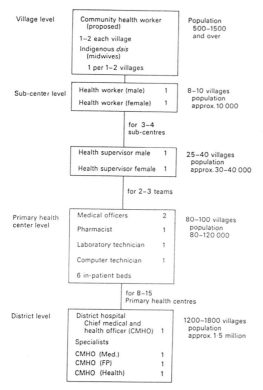

Village level	Community health worker (proposed) 1–2 each village Indigenous *dais* (midwives) 1 per 1–2 villages	Population 500–1500 and over
Sub-center level	Health worker (male) 1 Health worker (female) 1	8–10 villages population approx. 10 000
	for 3–4 sub-centres	
	Health supervisor male 1 Health supervisor female 1	25–40 villages population approx. 30–40 000
	for 2–3 teams	
Primary health center level	Medical officers 2 Pharmacist 1 Laboratory technician 1 Computer technician 1 6 in-patient beds	80–100 villages population 80–120 000
	for 8–15 Primary health centres	
District level	District hospital Chief medical and health officer (CMHO) 1 Specialists CMHO (Med.) 1 CMHO (FP) 1 CMHO (Health) 1	1200–1800 villages population approx. 1·5 million

Figure 12.1. Centers for primary health care. An example of a health delivery system in India. Patterns differ in each country and even in each region, depending on political system, financing, terrain, mobility, population density, and availability of trained health care personnel. In many countries making programs operational is the major problem. Source: Sharma and Chaturvedt (1978).

conditions that are preventable and most of which could receive better (or similar) care for less money and effort. As a rough guide, health posts serve 1,000 to 2,000 people; and eight to ten health posts should have at least one primary health care center for a population of 80,000 to 100,000. In each district of 1.5 million, eight to fifteen health centers are serviced by one district hospital (Sharma and Chaturvedt 1978). Although this is the goal, in many countries coverage of the population is still limited, including by terrain and population distribution. The urban elite still have the advantage (WHO 1980).

A difficult priority is the question of shifting funds for high-priced urban hospital facilities and technology to rural village care. Budgets have to be increased for staff, facilities, and supplies, such as drugs, vaccines, and food supplements to make health for all through community participation possible.

Care must be taken to ensure that false hopes are not raised. For example, in Swaziland the village health workers motivated the community to dig holes for slab latrines. The government was to deliver the concrete slabs. Pits were ready but the slabs were not delivered, and cattle fell into the pits and were injured.

HEALTH CENTERS AND OTHER SERVICES

Health centers cover a wide variety of establishments. They may be called dispensaries, clinics, maternities, health posts, or health stations. They may be mud huts, with insufficient protection from the weather, or well-equipped buildings with a water supply, electricity, X-ray equipment, and beds for cases in transit or for observation or delivery (maternities). Their effectiveness will depend more on the quality, organization, and training of the staff than on the physical amenities.

In the past, the dispensers, medical aides, or health officers may have had little or no training in mother and child care, and even less in nutrition and health education. This state of affairs is slowly improving, and the need for in-service training and refresher courses is recognized; health nurses and midwives too often need more practical training in child and maternal health and nutrition. If there is a little cooperation between hospital and medical school activities and the general staff, the staff from the health centers and the hospitals may be exchanged for short periods and so keep in touch with various aspects of health work.

Health centers exist to serve the whole population. Sometimes they are seriously overcrowded with adult patients. In this case, it is well to have certain times restricted to mothers and children only, and sometimes to children only. The main thing is to recognize the need for frequent, early medical care for young children and for continuing supervision of vulnerable groups.

Home visiting must be organized from and linked with the health centers. Supplies and equipment for health centers require constant attention too, and however modest the range of drugs and dressings may be, they must be kept in order, stocked in a quantity sufficient for needs, and dispensed economically to suit local conditions. Even in remote places, a patient can bring a clean bottle for medicine and a clean tin for pills or ointment.

The building and surroundings of the health center, as well as any living quarters associated with it, should be kept in good order, especially with respect to water supply and latrine maintenance. Every encouragement should be given to the staff to plant and maintain a garden, with some local medicinal herbs, and even rear poultry (preferably by the deep-litter method). This is the best form of visual aid for health education.

All health centers should be used not merely as convenient depots for obtaining medicines but for the preventive functions that they can perform. Enormous variations will be found in activities in different centers according to the amount of education, supervision, and genuine interest on the part of the health staff concerned. In one health center, the medical assistant spent his spare time helping to supervise the TBAs, collecting data on births and deaths, helping to improve a protected water supply, giving first aid and health classes to schoolchildren, and growing green vegetables, peas, beans,

and fruit trees in the garden around the health center. The range of potential activities is huge. Guidance and discussion with workers and the community can help in suggesting priorities.

YOUNG CHILD CLINICS

The basis of much practical work for young children—the under-5s—is health supervision, which permits preventive measures to be put into practice; for example, nutrition education and immunization permit infectious diseases to be recognized and treated early and malnutrition to be detected at an early stage by examination and regular weighing, so that appropriate measures may be taken (Vintinner 1968; Williams 1956; Yankauer 1961). Such supervision is based on the regular observation of young children at frequent intervals. Sometimes this may be carried out, at least in part, by home visiting, but usually, health supervision entails attendance of the mother and child at a young child clinic (YCC) (Morley 1963).

Depending on the distribution of population in the region, an appropriate network of children's clinics may have to be established by the fieldworker to serve the area (Kreysler 1970). Sometimes one clinic may be adequate, but if dwellings are widely scattered or if the area to be covered is large, YCCs may have to be held at several locations on different days of the week, in the form of mobile personnel serving nearby settlements. The network should aim to make the services available and accessible to as many people as possible. Peripheral clinics run by nurses or auxiliaries will permit frequent observations, advice, and treatment but must have supervision and a system of referral. These clinics also allow for home visiting, particularly to check on nonattenders and reasons for the lack of attendance. Many experiments are underway

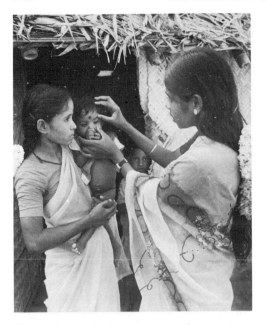

Figure 12.2. Bringing services to those most in need. A social worker on the outskirts of Madurai, India, makes home visits to examine the eyes of children for "white spots," a sign of serious vitamin A deficiency. UNICEF photograph by T. S. Nagarajan.

the preventive aspects of the clinic are the main priority, constantly before the eyes of the organizers of the clinic as their principal aim and concern.

YCCs should be organized to run in a certain sequence from one "station" to the next, often in the following order:

1. Registration.
2. Weighing and recording on growth chart.
3. Examination, diagnosis, counseling, and treatment.
4. Health education (especially concerning nutrition) by group and individual discussion/demonstration.
5. Immunization (if feasible).
6. Prescription issue of food supplements and/or medicine.

If facilities exist for simple laboratory tests, as may occasionally be the case, a separate station should be set up for this purpose. At a minimum, a microscope should be available and used to identify key problems, such as intestinal parasites.

Registration

Record systems should be simple and functional. A book at the clinic can list the names of those attending at each visit, together with a brief note of any procedure, advice, or decision on management (for example, home visiting required for a child at risk). A separate register for at-risk children is very useful.

Weighing and Recording

Experience suggests that a YCC card, often kept by the mother, is the best record of weight, nutrition, and health status. The mother should keep a card with the name and clinic number so that records can be found. It is rarely possible to keep an alphabetical or numerical roll. A large number of country-specific cards have been developed in recent years.

In general, two types of cards (growth charts) have been developed (Fig. 12.3).

in different parts of the world. The physical structure of these clinics is unimportant, provided they are near the people concerned, acceptable to them, and relatively weatherproof. They can be carried out in the open air, under a tree, in a school house, in a hut lent by the village, or anywhere else (Fig. 12.2).

Wherever the clinics may be, their function should be a combination of prevention and curative work, including examination, weighing, early management of malnutrition and infections, including respiratory infections and the management of dehydration, using ORT, prevention of important infectious diseases (immunizations, antimalarials if indicated), and, above all, health education, with special attention to nutrition. Inevitable in the early stages of expanding work, it is the sick children who will first come for treatment. In all cases, however, it is of the greatest importance to ensure that

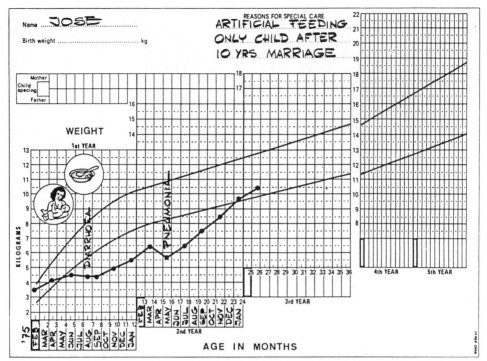

(a)

(b)

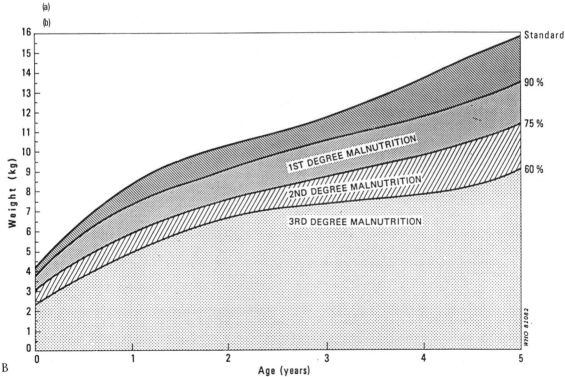

Figure 12.3. Two types of growth charts. (A) Morley-type Road to Health chart. (B) Gomez-type classification of malnutrition. Source: WHO (1981).

Modifications of the Morley Road to Health chart, as advised by WHO, are widely used. The aim is not so much to diagnose the child's illness but to see if the growth parallels the lines on the chart. Flattening out or a decline indicates the need for special attention. The other growth charts show several lines indicating a reference base and percentage levels below (for example 80 to 75 percent). On the front page of the growth chart used in Uganda, social identification data are recorded, with space available for recording information about immunizations and the issue of antimalarial drugs. The inner pages are divided into three columns for recording the date and the weight of the child, with a blank column for brief notes on feeding, results of examination, and advice given. When unfolded, the card contains a graph, on which the child's weight can be plotted. Three curves are marked on this: the standard (100 percent) and the 80 percent and 60 percent levels of this standard. Children's weights may be compared with these levels and appropriate action taken. Serial measurements may also be made to see if growth is progressing satisfactorily (Griffiths 1981; Morley and Woodland 1979; WHO 1981).

The growth chart can be an invaluable tool (Jelliffe and Jelliffe 1989); however, it must not be used just as a recording device but for counseling. The child is his or her own reference, and any growth change that is not upward on the chart needs observation and, if need be, investigation with the appropriate action taken, such as treating infection if present or improving the weanling's diet. The chart serves as the infant's first medical record. Social milestones, illnesses, immunizations, and antimalarials (if given) should be recorded, as well as other information pertinent to the infant's health. Attractive country-specific charts have been developed for recording appropriate additional information such as vitamin A supplements (Indonesia), chloroquine

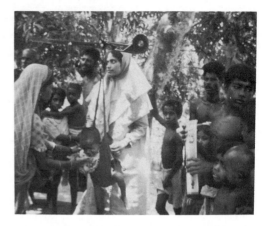

Figure 12.4. Women helping themselves and their families. With support and education, these women in a Bangladesh mothers' club have learned to monitor their infants' growth and development using an inexpensive, familiar, traditional beam balance scale.

prophylaxis (Malawi), and educational messages (breastfeeding, oral rehydration, and weaning foods).

In some countries, cards in a plastic cover have been issued to mothers. These cards act as permanent health records and are available if children attend a distant hospital or health center. Cards may well be lost, but if their importance in relation to the continuing care of their children is understood by mothers, they are often looked after conscientiously.

These cards also have considerable educational value regarding health and nutrition, especially the weight records, which unsophisticated mothers are able to appreciate. The importance of the cards can sometimes be increased if a very small, nominal charge is made for them.

In a mothers' club in Bangladesh, mothers in rural remote villages were taught to use a simplified beam balance scale, and a growth chart was issued at a small charge and proudly carried to and from the clinic (Fig. 12.4). Because many of the mothers are illiterate, 15-year-old schoolgirls act as recorders. It would be preferable, through functional literacy programs, to train mothers to

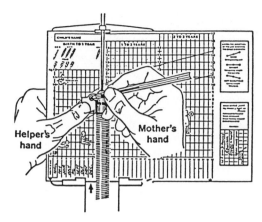

Figure 12.5. The Talc direct recording scale, designed to be used, even by illiterate mothers, in the home and the community. When the mother is involved in plotting her child's weight she is able to understand the meaning of the growth curve. Source: Morley et al. (1991).

record the weights themselves. Mothers in Ghana are using a new recording scale designed for the illiterate (Fig. 12.5) (Morley 1991).

In Bangladesh, the mothers' club members weigh infants by means of locally designed and manufactured beam balances. Local weights and beam balances are familiar to village people because they are used in the marketplace. Through this program, mothers monitor their infants; once they understand the linkages between diet, health, and growth, they are alert to problems. The club also has unexpected spin-offs, such as providing an opportunity for mothers to exchange ideas and experiences and to provide support for each other (Baumslag 1979).

Recording weight is not a simple task (Griffiths 1981; Jelliffe and Jelliffe 1990; Morley and Woodland 1979). Health workers must be taught to examine for edema, make sure that human errors are eliminated (such as the need to put the dot in the right place on the chart), ensure the scale is accurate and balanced, and, most important, pay attention to details such as whether the child is weighed with or without clothes (Table 12.1) (HHS 1980). The scale must be properly secured since the whole program can end in disaster if the child is dropped. Good training, supervision, and attention to detail are essential. If techniques are not standardized and precise, serial weighing may reflect measurement error rather than increased growth. The mother is not an appendage. She must be involved at all steps of the child's progress and not just encouraged to carry around a growth chart. The cooperation of the grandmother may also be invaluable.

The measure most commonly used is weight for age. Where this cannot be obtained, arm circumference can be used as a screening device (Griffiths 1981; Jelliffe and Jelliffe 1989). If height can be measured too, it is possible to differentiate between acute and chronic malnutrition. Height for weight is especially useful in infants whose age is not known (but whenever possible, "special events calendars" should be constructed to determine the approximate age). It is best to have the birthweight recorded, if available, because this is an important point of reference. A low-birthweight infant may be below the level of the standard reference population on the growth chart but progressing well in terms of individual weight gain, and a mother who is doing her best should not be discouraged (Morley 1979). In Jakarta, Indonesia, the referral of malnourished children or low birthweight infants is based on growth charts (Fig. 12.6) (Griffiths 1981).

Examination and Counseling

Children attending the YCC should be examined naked or with minimum clothes for signs of malnutrition and relevant infections. Whenever feasible, basic laboratory tests should be available for hemoglobin estimations, stool examination, and so on.

The history taken from the mother should inquire carefully into the child's

Table 12.1. Measurement Errors

Equipment	Improper and inadequate (for example, bathroom or spring scale, stretchable tapes, yardsticks not attached to table or wall)
	Failure to check the zero balance on the scale periodically
Technique	Failure to notice edema
	Weighing the child inconsistently (for example, sometimes with and sometimes without clothes)
	Improper positioning or extended head
	Measuring top of hair instead of top of head
	Putting the dot in the wrong place on the growth chart
	Not recording the measurements immediately and accurately
Training	Failure to understand the importance of precision and accuracy in terms of the individual's health progress in sequential visits
	Incorrect interpretation

Source: HHS (1980).

diet and tactfully discover the mother's attitude and beliefs.

Advice to individual mothers concerning their children's health, diet and need for supplementary food, immunization, or medicine is an important educational aspect, which may also benefit other waiting mothers who happen to be listening. If the interview mainly emphasizes illness, the preventive objective of the clinic may be lost.

Education

The clinic is an excellent site for education for individual parents and in well-

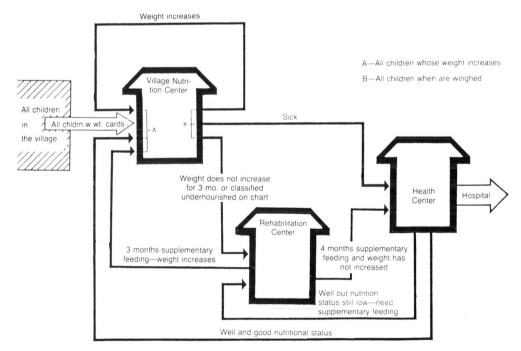

Figure 12.6. Nutrition referral. This is the system used by the Indonesian Family Nutrition Improvement Program (UPGK) of the Ministry of Health, Jakarta. Source: Griffiths (1981).

planned group discussion-demonstrations. A model garden and an improved, low-cost house adjacent to the clinic with plans available free to interested parents can be more valuable than any other form of visual aid, but is expensive and difficult to maintain.

Immunization

This will depend on the infectious diseases prevalent, the immunization activities of the particular program, and the methods used. Equipment should include appropriate syringes, disposable needles with special reference to the dangers of HIV infection, and cooling apparatus for the vaccines (Sabin and Stinson 1981).

Food Supplements

Supplies of food supplements should be available for children who require them. They may take the form of dried skimmed milk or other food supplements—for example, wheat-soy blend (WSB) or a source of some other nutrient, such as iron (as ferrous sulphate), thiamine, or vitamin A (from such sources as red palm oil or fish liver oil). Wherever possible, local foods should be used. The quantity given and the method of distribution must be planned beforehand and can often be made easier by prepackaging suitable quantities. Food supplements may be appreciated more if a nominal charge is made. The Salvation Army program in Kinshasa, Zaire, did just this; those who had no money were asked to provide some services, such as packaging the food supplements sold to parents with malnourished children.

Widespread distribution of food supplements is needed in emergencies, in acute refugee situations, or in severe food shortages (for example, famine or extreme poverty). In general, supplements should be issued selectively on defined indications with careful practical demonstration, nutrition education activities, and home visiting, when possible. Food supplements should be geared to local food habits, should encourage local food production, and, indeed, ideally should be produced locally. In some instances, the sale of small, cheap, subsidized saucepans and a teaspoon may be helpful in the preparation and feeding of sufficient quantities of semisolid foods designed especially for young children. Most important, food supplementation should not be the main activity of the health staff, as dependency results and overwhelming of the clinic's other functions. Moreover, the clinic may become identified only with handouts, and attendance will fall when none are given.

Treatment

The drugs available for treatment will depend on local health problems, funding, and distribution systems (Table 12.2) (WHO 1977). Paper should be used to wrap the tablets. Squares of newspaper can be prepared beforehand or small, inexpensive envelopes purchased. A packet of wooden tongue depressors should be available for dispensing ointment, together with a supply of small bottles and boxes.

Treatment should be as uncomplicated as possible—for example, a single large dose that lasts for a prolonged period, such as oral vitamin A (Christian Med. Comm. 1983; Cook 1970) or deworming in the clinic with piperazine. Careful instruction for the parents is essential. Treatment should not be directed solely at elimination of a problem but at prevention. Often the mother does not know what caused the illness and how to avoid reinfection. If certain conditions are common, there may be a need for special facilities, for instance, a rehydration room, an injection room, or on-the-spot first treatment for scabies. If any drugs are to be issued, the dosage schedule and method of administration will have to be taught to the mothers. This should be as uncom-

Table 12.2. Basic Drug List for Primary Care

Bacterial infections	Penicillin, ampicillin, tetracycline, chloramphenicol
Eye infections	Suphacetamide (10%), tetracycline eye ointment (1%), silver nitrate (1%), cortisone[a]
Skin disease	Gentian violet (1%), aqueous solution, benzyl benzoate emulsion, benzoic acid ointment, sulfur ointment, tetmosol soap, vaseline, kwell
Ear infections	Peroxide, sulfonamides, chloramphenicol
Diarrhea	Prepackaged ORS or bicarbonate, sugar and salt
Cough	Syrup with codeine
Fever or pain	Aspirin
Convulsions	Phenobarbital tablets and injections, paraldehyde
Worms, intestinal	Piperazine tablets, tetrachlorethylene
Hookworm[b]	Thiabendazole
Amebae, giardia[b]	Metronidazole
Malaria[b]	Chloroquine tablets, daraprim tablets
Tuberculosis	Streptomycin, isioniazid, ethambutol, rifampicin
Leprosy[b]	Dapsone, rifampicin, clofazimine
Schistosomiasis[b]	Niridazole
Vaginal infections	Vinegar
Insect bites or stings	Ephedrine[a], adrenalin[a]
First aid	Bandages, antiseptic lotion, specific antivenom[b] Where snake bite is a problem, vaseline
Vaccines	DPT, BCG, measles, polio
Supplements	Iron tablets preferably with vitamin C (for young infants, liquid form is preferable), iodized salt, thiamine, vitamin A, food supplements[b]
Bleeding	In childbirth: ergometrine Low-birthweight newborns: vitamin K injections

Note: The list should be specific for each region and regularly modified, according to local needs, including resistant organisms. Selection needs to be made based on the local disease priorities, the cost, and ease of administration.

[a] Small quantities needed for emergencies.

[b] Drugs needed only in specific areas or seasonally.

plicated as possible and in accordance with the local situation. For example, "four hours" is meaningless in clockless societies, whereas at "sunrise," "noon," and "sunset" is understandable.

HOME VISITING

In the early stages of setting up a health service, it is most important for a prospective home visitor or other health worker to wander around the slum, the village, or the rural area to see what is to be seen and to begin to make friends and contacts. Very soon, however, some organization will be necessary. It is useful to have a map of the area, even a hand-drawn one, and then to get districts, roads, and houses identified or numbered. The health worker must have priorities. The following order is a sound one: newborn babies, sick children, at-risk children (especially with abnormal growth curves), and all young children. The at-risk register must be carefully maintained (Morley 1966; Stanfield 1967).

Newborn babies should be visited as soon as possible after birth in the home or after return from the hospital. In the SINAPS project in Guatemala, the illiterate community health worker (*comadrona*) checked on the mother and newborn during a home visit and was able to record the infant's health status and refer mothers and infants if necessary (Fig. 12.7) (SINAPS 1982). Where a large proportion of births take place in non-

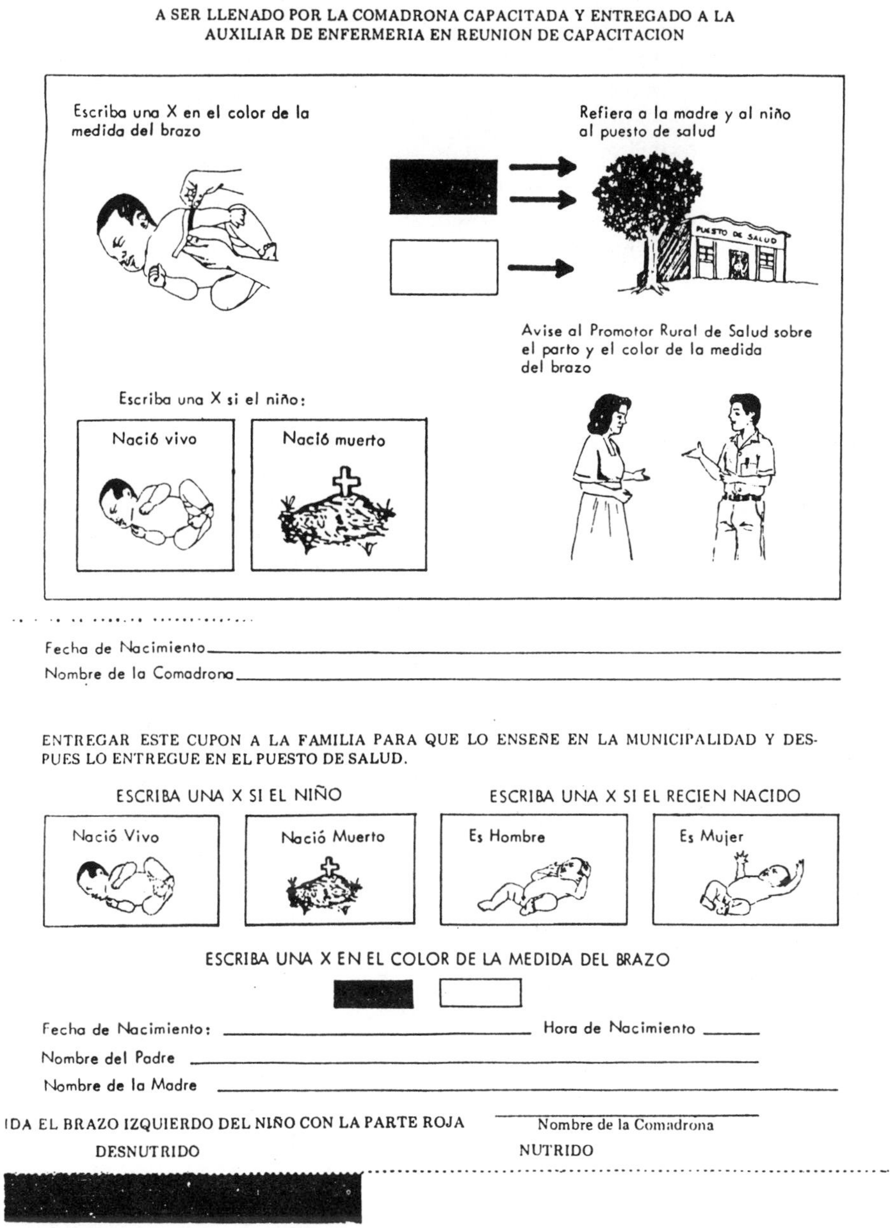

A SER LLENADO POR LA COMADRONA CAPACITADA Y ENTREGADO A LA AUXILIAR DE ENFERMERIA EN REUNION DE CAPACITACION

Escriba una X en el color de la medida del brazo

Refiera a la madre y al niño al puesto de salud

PUESTO DE SALUD

Avise al Promotor Rural de Salud sobre el parto y el color de la medida del brazo

Escriba una X si el niño:

Nació vivo

Nació muerto

Fecha de Nacimiento ________________

Nombre de la Comadrona ________________

ENTREGAR ESTE CUPON A LA FAMILIA PARA QUE LO ENSEÑE EN LA MUNICIPALIDAD Y DESPUES LO ENTREGUE EN EL PUESTO DE SALUD.

ESCRIBA UNA X SI EL NIÑO

Nació Vivo

Nació Muerto

ESCRIBA UNA X SI EL RECIEN NACIDO

Es Hombre

Es Mujer

ESCRIBA UNA X EN EL COLOR DE LA MEDIDA DEL BRAZO

Fecha de Nacimiento: ________________ Hora de Nacimiento ______

Nombre del Padre ________________

Nombre de la Madre ________________

IDA EL BRAZO IZQUIERDO DEL NIÑO CON LA PARTE ROJA

____
Nombre de la Comadrona

DESNUTRIDO

NUTRIDO

Figure 12.7. Recording form for home visiting newborn infants and their mothers. In SINAPS, an integrated health, nutrition, and family planning project in Guatemala, illiterate workers make home visits and monitor growth using arm circumference (measurements in the dark area indicate malnutrition). By this method, at-risk children can be identified. Source: SINAPS (1982).

institutional settings, measurement of chest circumference in accomplished with color-coded plasticized paper tapes with "above 2500g," "2000–2500g," and "under 2000g" categories. A nonstretch string with two knots 30 centimeters apart can also be used for screening. Another screening measure used by TBAs and community health workers is a respiratory timer. Infants with respiratory rates of fifty or more breaths per minute are diagnosed as having pneumonia (Morley and Brown 1992).

In Brazil, a home visit at seven to ten days has been found to be important to reassure mothers at that time, especially with regard to breastfeeding. Where the delivery has been undertaken by a trained midwife, the latter should make a home visit for postnatal care to mother and baby. The health worker must ensure that she is cooperating with whomever is in immediate charge of the delivery (doctor, nurse, midwife, or grandmother), especially if this attendant is of the traditional rather than medical variety.

The second priority is children ill at home. The health worker must make regular visits to the hospital and note the children and maternity cases from her area and their problems. Health center cards (or supervision or antenatal clinic cards) should always be sent to the hospital when the patient is admitted (for a record of evidence of loss of weight and previous instances of diarrhea). In fact, mothers should keep the cards themselves, although they need to have this use of the card explained to them. Dates of admission and diagnosis should be recorded on the card so that the information will be returned to the supervision center or clinic when the patient is discharged.

With a knowledge of her own district and its families, the health worker can concentrate on those most in need: the young mother with her first baby, the family where the father has absconded or

the grandmother has broken her leg, where there are personal, environmental, or economic problems. She can help the mother sponge down the child with fever, clean out a kitchen cupboard, or get a health inspector to deal with the rats in the yard. When she visits a family, she must look at all the members and make an assessment of the family resources and needs. It is easy to keep a box for the cards of special cases and ensure that nonattenders and others at risk receive needed care. In a small, thickly populated urban area, she may save time by going on foot. In a scattered rural area, transport is essential.

The home visit should be comprehensive enough to include the entire family and yet selective enough to concentrate on those most in need. Cooperation with other auxiliaries and community workers to reach individuals for health promotion and identification of cases at risk is also important. The sick should be treated before the disease becomes serious, and the baby identified before he or she is battered. However simple the system, the health worker must be able to count and analyze the case load, recording frequency of conditions and the effects of treatment and education.

Care of Sick Children in the Home

Home care services radiating from a hospital are all too rare. For years, health nurses, district nurses, and private nursing services have been providing home care in a number of communities—generally the more sophisticated and wealthy ones.

Some children's outpatient departments give meticulous instructions to parents about caring for the child at home. Some issue handbooks and pamphlets that may be of great help to the relatives, especially if they are literate. This is an aspect of child care that needs expansion, particularly in disadvantaged communities. Unless the health worker knows the home and its other inhabitants, it is very hard to give practical advice about care of the patient. Health workers who never visit in the homes are at a serious disadvantage.

In a teaching hospital, medical and nursing students should be required to make home visits to outpatients and previous inpatients and for routine supervision. They should begin by working with a health nurse in charge of a home care service. They must learn to make observations on the environment—mental, physical, economic, and geographical—and on the relatives' education, capability, and attitudes toward the patient and each other. Their observations will provide information on the causes of any existing disease and the history of the family and the patient. They should then be able to advise on the care of the patient. They may have to exercise some ingenuity in helping to construct a bed table, or provide suitable room temperature, and in devising an appropriate diet.

The possibilities for improving health care for mothers and children are infinite, and experience is positively the best teacher. Home visiting is certainly one of the most important aspects of the education of medical students, nurses, and all other health workers. A good health worker can transform a difficult household situation into one that is manageable and bearable through continuing supervision and support. Health workers must learn to understand what sort of help they should give in the various crises that arise. A family coping index can be invaluable (Choi et al. 1983) and should be developed for local conditions. Following is an example of such a checklist:

Do the family members recognize the need for and accept help?

Do they accurately perceive their life situation, including their health condition, and the current and potential results of the actions of themselves and others?

Do they have reciprocal support relationships?

Is their stress level low?

Did they use constructive methods in coping with previous life changes and stressful situations?

Do they fulfill family and societal roles?

Is the physical condition, including energy level, of each family member good?

Do they balance the need to be confident in their own and their family members' abilities with a realistic acceptance of their own and their family members' limitations?

Do they have mutuality in communication, interaction, and decision making within the family?

Some families may be stable, but they are never static. Where auxiliary workers are trained and employed on a neighborhood basis, they can be of great importance. In one area in Britain, it was recorded that the "home help" was the basis of health improvements. To provide this sort of care without being possessive, interfering, or despondent is indeed a valuable service.

It is useful to devise a booklet of standing instructions for health workers (especially students) about their responsibilities in home care, since they often have to work in some isolation. But no amount of standing orders or record keeping can replace experience in this field. Experience can do a great deal to develop maturity, common sense, and sensitivity.

Mobile Units

In the effort to "take health care to the people" mobile units have been experimented with (DeBeer 1966; Kimmance

1970; Namboze 1966; Vintinner 1968). In New York City, for example, mobile clinic vans are used to provide health care to homeless children (Gordon 1993, personal communication). Large, impressive vans, complete with modern conveniences, a laboratory, and even toilet facilities have been used occasionally. However, they cost a great deal of money to purchase, to run, and to repair and often have served only certain propaganda purposes. Moreover, they are unsuitable for the roads where they are most needed and are soon stationary, functioning as extra accommodation of the most costly variety. It is preferable to have mobile staff and static health centers. With a Landrover (or a less expensive motorcycle, canoe, or camel) and one or two boxes of equipment and drugs, a couple of health workers can count on going farther and faster.

A good plan is to develop a home base in every place to be visited. It may be located at the compound of the local chief, the teacher, the police station, or the traditional birth attendant's house. When the team arrives, they should find some place and some person who expects them, can assist, and can inform them of the local news and the local needs. Accommodation may consist of the most rudimentary type of shelter; they may set up their center under a convenient tree. The person who is to provide this focus of attention must be carefully chosen as a key part of a primary health care service. Regular visits on an appointed day will soon ensure good attendance. If the sick are treated, these mobile units will soon be able to collect useful information as well as provide immunizations, oral rehydration, some basic treatment, environmental improvement, and, slowly, health education. After a time they may be able to establish good medical care and continuing supervision when the people themselves offer to build some improved accommodation. Some communities have not only built a health post

but accommodation for the health worker, as well as provisions for her or his keep and training. Of critical importance too is the availability of transport for referral.

THE HOSPITAL

In developing countries hospitals of all sorts, large or small, rural or urban, attached to a main teaching center or otherwise, must be concerned with more than just the therapy of the great numbers of sick children who attend.

Even more than with health centers, the problem is how to integrate activities other than curative into the program when faced with large-scale floods of sick people (Kark 1981). This is always difficult, but prevention is of such ultimate importance to MCH in the community that it has to be introduced, preferably by a readjustment of hospital activities and, if need be, at the expense of some aspects of less obligatory clinical work.

Components of a Hospital Unit

A hospital unit for children often has an outpatient clinic, children's wards, and supplementary accommodation. Mothers should be admitted with young children not only for psychological reasons but also for their cooperation in patient care, to maintain communication, and for health education (Fig. 12.8). Outreach programs, home care, and follow-up home visiting arrangements may also be components.

Outpatient clinics. The first and foremost of the hospital units will frequently be a large-scale children's or family clinic, whose functions will include sorting and referral of cases, clinical and domiciliary treatment, and as much preventive work as practicable, such as health education and immunization.

Special outpatients departments will

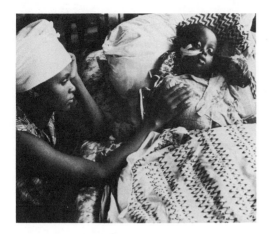

Figure 12.8. Admission of mother to children's ward can be invaluable. A mother's constant love and attention may be essential to the children's recovery, and her nursing assistance can be invaluable, especially where there is a staff shortage. WHO/UNICEF photograph by B. Wolff, Sierra Leone.

also be required in larger hospitals to which patients may be referred from the peripheral clinics. As well as a general referral clinic, other outpatient departments will usually be required for major problems. These vary from place to place but often include services to treat and prevent malnutrition and tuberculosis. In certain regions, particular conditions, such as sickle cell anemia in Africa, may require special services. It is important for these clinics to be related to priority public health problems for which economical and practical methods of prevention and management are available.

Service for newborns. The care of newborns lies in the frontier zone between obstetrics and pediatrics. With heavy pressure on both departments, it is usual for resuscitation at birth to be carried out by the obstetrician or midwife delivering the baby and for the routine care of newborns to be undertaken by the nursing staff of the midwifery wards. Rooming in, with the baby by the mother's side, should be the rule rather than separating

baby and mother, as often practiced in the Western world. Keeping the newborn with the mother is not only more natural but also encourages early and successful lactation and minimizes cross-infection.

In larger hospitals, the pediatrician may be called in to take over the care of neonates who are sick or born with abnormalities. Isolation facilities are needed for babies with infections, and in a larger hospital, a special care unit should be developed for low-birthweight infants, particularly those with special problems. The level of low-birthweight infants needing special care demands local definition and from a practical point of view depends on their ability to suckle. This level can vary from 4½ to 5½ pounds or generally under 2,500 grams. The scientific basis of the management of low-birthweight babies is the same as anywhere else: the control of environmental temperature and humidity, the prevention of infection, and progressive feeding methods to match the maturity of the babies' swallowing and sucking reflexes. Practical application has to be undertaken with simple apparatus and limited staff. One adaptation is a water mattress filled with heated water to warm preterm infants. It has been found to be just as effective as heated incubators and has the advantage of allowing mothers access to their babies (Sarman and Tunell 1989).

The most important aspect of management is to ensure that babies are breastfed on discharge if weeks of expensive, time-consuming care, followed by death from diarrhea and marasmus on return home, are to be avoided. This implies a need for sleeping accommodation for the mothers near the special care unit and their active participation in the feeding and care of their babies as soon as possible. Although there is a chance that infection may occur with mothers coming into the unit, the disadvantages are more than compensated for by the opportunities for health education, the advantages in feeding, and in using the mothers as nurses, especially because the mother will not only look after her baby but will supply built-in prevention of infection through breast milk. Infections can be minimized if the mothers are taught to take hygienic precautions.

Children's wards. The size, construction, and equipment of the children's ward depends on the age range and types of disease to be admitted. However, the disease pattern in developing regions is such that wards will usually be concerned principally with illness in young children.

Efficient hospitals can be built of cheap material at a fraction of the cost of the more traditional materials. The floors should be of some easily cleaned material. Buildings should be fly- and mosquito-proof and should be constructed with the local climate in mind, such as the need to catch the prevailing breeze and to avoid inundation during tropical storms. In very hot parts of the world, small units with air-conditioning, extra fans, or other cooling devices may be necessary. But it is not uncommon for hospitals in these countries to be erected with no consideration for the marked fall in temperature that can occur at night, particularly during the rainy season. In these circumstances, it is important to have glass windows that can be shut, and in some more upland areas, it is not uncommon for a children's ward to need a few warmed cubicles for children prone to hypothermia, particularly if they are malnourished.

The main ward should have sufficient space for cribs and beds with lockers for the patients' belongings and room for the mothers to sit during the day and to sleep at night. The space between beds should be about four feet. In view of the high incidence of infectious diseases admitted, barrier nursing is necessary, and some cubicles for such cases as typhoid fever provided. However, individual cubicles, or those for one baby with mother, are

difficult to supervise, and it is distressing for the mother to be isolated with her very sick child. When the type of infection makes it appropriate, it is preferable to have a few small wards each with four beds for the children and four for the mothers. The mothers can support, teach, and help each other, and these units can be supervised easily.

Other essential elements of the children's ward in a larger hospital are a treatment room (with facilities for instrument sterilization, apparatus for resuscitation, for blood taking, and other procedures, and good lighting); a teaching demonstration area (with space for benches or mats) for mothers, visitors, or students; a food preparation room (largely for mixing the milk-based mixtures used in the treatment of malnutrition); a small side laboratory (equipped to carry out the range of about ten tests that are needed rapidly); a centrally placed nurses' room with a view of as much of the ward as possible; and a play area, preferably out-of-doors, for convalescent children and their mothers.

Most of the ward should be equipped with simply designed, easily cleaned, sturdy cribs, with a small number of short beds for older children. Each crib or bed should have an adjacent locker. At night, subdued central lighting in the ward is essential, with either an individual light for each bed or a movable light that can be taken to a particular crib.

Equipment in some children's wards in developing countries is so inadequate that unnecessary inefficiency is the result. Frequently tested, simple beam balance scales are needed for weighing infants and toddlers. This is an extremely important, but often neglected, diagnostic measure in cases of malnutrition and for measuring improvement in many pediatric conditions, ranging from kwashiorkor, to the nephrotic syndrome, to tuberculosis. Diagnostic sets for looking at the eardrum, throat, and retina should be in working order with an effective battery and bulb, as well as easily available tongue depressors. Simple reflected light instruments should be available. There should always be a microscope handy for immediate inspection of blood, urine, sputum, and stools.

The use of various forms of disposable equipment is a matter of perennial debate. In many larger hospitals, it is cheaper, more efficient, and helpful in reducing cross-infection to use disposable plastic syringes, paper diapers (for diarrhea patients), wooden tongue depressors, and paper towels rather than the sodden, bacteria-laden pieces of cloth usually employed. However, it has been difficult, if not impossible, to convince administrators that extra immediate cost is more than covered by longer-term saving. The need for expensive disposable syringes has been made a priority by the increase of AIDS infection.

Children's wards should be well supplied with water, preferably with spaced sinks, in view of the fact that medical and nursing staffs frequently have to wash their hands since a high percentage of admissions have infected stools (including diarrheal diseases, typhoid, and poliomyelitis).

Organization and Management

The organization and management of children's wards in developing countries has to be undertaken in relation to six overlapping factors:

1. The limited finance available.
2. The pressure of admissions on inadequate accommodation.
3. The shortage of trained staff.
4. The likelihood of cross-cultural misunderstandings.
5. The need to introduce prevention into the hospital environment.
6. The need to develop the hospital as a training and research center.

Limited finance. It is imperative that priorities be developed for the establishment of the most essential health services for common problems that are remediable, and not for fashion, political visibility, or the personal research interests of the current pediatrician. Unfortunately, for political and prestige reasons, sometimes associated with misguided project-linked foreign aid, large, inappropriate hospitals have often been constructed for which neither staff nor finance for recurring expenditures are available. Although the basis of a health service should be a network of strategically located health centers, hospitals are needed at central points, preferably for selected children referred for special investigation or specialized services. However, the over-large chromium-plated glamour hospital distorts the outlook of both the population and administrators concerning future needs and possibilities, while swallowing disproportionately large amounts (often more than 20 percent) of a country's health budget. The erection of this type of building is an attempt to follow inappropriate foreign traditions. A hospital should be judged by its contents and activities rather than by the grandeur of its architecture. The danger is that the hospital outpatient departments will become swamped with cases that could be treated better in primary care centers, and this takes away from the delivery of specialized services.

The annual health budget of most developing countries is often limited to between $0.50 and $1.50 per capita. To be able to work within restricted finances, a hospital has to be constructed economically, deploy expensive personnel optimally, purchase only equipment that is truly necessary (with due regard to sturdiness), and have the equipment available where it will be required.

The drug bill in particular—always a major item in a hospital's recurrent expenses—must be supervised and scrutinized. In fact, the majority of treatment for most of the more usual complaints can be undertaken with no more than about twenty important drugs. Many countries make use of a standard list containing a limited number of drugs that can be used by all general-purpose health workers. This list varies and depends on the disease patterns and whether the drugs can be produced locally or must be imported. A pharmaceutical distribution project in Nigeria began with a list of twenty essential drugs. In Bangladesh, thirty drugs were chosen for local production, and Lesotho produces a hundred basic drugs (Christian Med. Comm. 1983).

The need for a drug list and the importance of the economics of therapy should be stressed continually in the training of all medical and health personnel. A difference of a fraction of a penny between one drug or another with a similar action may not be of significance in relation to the therapy of an individual but is of obvious financial relevance if it is to be used for hundreds of thousands of children. Economy in the use of supplies and drugs must be practiced and preached unceasingly. Staff trained in missions have experience working with limited funds and are often more economical than those trained in government establishments.

Admissions and inadequate accommodation. Admissions to children's wards, with certain minor regional variations and local seasonal fluctuations, have a characteristic pattern and usually pose similar problems. Typically, large numbers of seriously and acutely ill young children with repetitive and preventable diseases must be treated, such as those with diarrhea, respiratory infections, and malnutrition. However, the chief "illness" to be found is a composite of infection, malnutrition, and parasitism. Multiple diseases, each aggravating the other, are usual, and among children reaching the ward, there is a high mortality because of the multiplicity and severity of diseases, as well as the lateness of admission due to the initial use of village therapy and the long, ex-

pensive journey often required to reach the hospital.

The basic problem for the hospital staff is a heavy, remorseless pressure for beds. On rounds, the health professional is concerned more with who can be discharged than who is well enough to be discharged. An overcrowded children's ward (with two or more to a crib), with utterly overworked staff, can be counterproductive. In fact, the children's ward can become a "lethal factor" due to cross-infection and inadequate treatment (including feeding) (Jelliffe and Jelliffe 1970).

A rehabilitation unit or convalescent ward attached to the hospital can be most useful, in addition to organization of visiting nurses for home care. Obviously the solution to the overcrowded children's ward is to eradicate the preventable conditions by devising a primary chain of accessible health centers and rural clinics with home visiting, so that ill children can be dealt with earlier, while the illness is in a less advanced form (Cook 1970; Jelliffe and Jelliffe 1970).

As with all other aspects of medical treatment, selection plays a major role in the admission of children to the ward. Factors to take into consideration include the severity of the illness, the capability of the parents, the type of home, the distance of the hospital away from home, the probable length of the stay, and, most important, the treatability of the condition. Paradoxically, the first basis of ward treatment is to avoid it by devising methods of treating as many acutely ill children as possible in the children's clinic, health and day care centers, and homes. This can be done only by convincing parents that they should bring children for treatment early in the disease. In the ward itself, every effort should be made to make the best use of the limited beds by trying to wed efficient, economic, humane therapy, and investigations with the greatest possible turnover. Regular supervision is the key to improving health.

For many conditions, particularly dehydration and meningitis, treatment can be initiated fastest by developing a ward resuscitation area, often in a corner of the treatment room.

Routine management of all admissions may be general, with the temperature, weight, and hemoglobin recorded for each child, but it must also be standardized and clearly understood for all the diseases that are commonly admitted to the ward, such as pneumonia, anemia, and dehydration. Quite simple methods may cut days off hospitalization—for example, the use of an intragastric polyethylene tube to overcome the poor appetite in certain types of malnutrition, the collection of a stool sample for ova or blood by the insertion of a small glass tube or a drinking straw into the child's anus, with immediate examination of a slide prepared from the specimen. Simple technologies may improve prognosis—for example, radiant heat cradles for malnourished children with edema because coldness of the extremities is very common in these cases. The cradles can be improvised using a wire cage with a waterproof cover, warmed by a carbon filament lamp. All forms of therapy should be aimed at improved cost-effectiveness and speed of recovery.

Despite everything, however, it might be necessary to discharge children before they are ready. In that case, it is essential to review the possibilities of continuing care and supervision apart from inpatient treatment.

Supplementary accommodation. The need for continuing supervision, as well as the serious shortage of beds, can be met by having a convalescent unit (Burke 1969). Many centers have set up rehabilitation wards (nutritional rehabilitation units) for health education of mothers and the long-term care of malnutrition (Nat. Council Nutr. 1970). This type of approach is also extremely useful for patients with chronic ulcers or tuberculosis and for other children or their mothers, including ante- and postnatal cases. They do not need full-time nursing care, but they do need continuing supervision of diet, education, treatment, and activity. The patients may live at some distance; transport is expensive and journeys exhausting and hazardous; to leave the hospital prematurely without full treatment is to invite a relapse or a return to unsuitable conditions and influences.

The convalescent ward can be of a simple dormitory type, with more informality than is possible in a hospital ward where severely ill cases are being treated. Or it can be in the form of individual rooms and a veranda around a compound with sufficient washing and cooking facilities. This type of accommodation is often found at centers run by indigenous practitioners and is usually acceptable. Supervision must be regular. These wards can bring about great savings in staff, in time, and in hospital beds.

As an alternative, a child may be discharged from the hospital to stay in a nearby house and brought in daily for dressings, diet, or supervision. In some areas, a large proportion of patients will have relatives or friends in the town near the hospital and will welcome this type of arrangement. Wherever possible, the child should attend the nearest health center.

A third possibility is to establish a home care service. This has been practiced for many years at St. Mary's Hospital in London, where, as elsewhere, hospital care is costly. In Montreal, Canada, at the Children's Hospital, home care costs are a fifteenth of hospital care costs. Moreover, some children do better at home than in a hospital. The service is under the care of doctors and nurses based at the hospital, and at least one month's rotation is now required for all medical and nursing students in this program.

All such methods of supplementing expensive, and possibly unnecessary, hospital care provide valuable opportunities for health education for patients, parents, and personnel.

Records. In hospitals, records may of necessity be very simple (Cuthbertson and Morley 1962; Morley 1966). It is recommended that as much use as possible must be made of the observations of the mothers and the nurses. They will invariably respond if they find the doctor depends on others for collaboration. Special care must be taken to keep health nurses or clinics informed of the progress of patients referred by them. A family record can be most useful. Mothers should be well informed of the health of their children and the treatment given. This should be recorded on the Road to Health growth chart and explained to mothers when given the chart initially. The local health center must be informed as to what transpired in the hospital and what follow-up is necessary.

Staff shortage. All levels of staff in health services tend to be inadequate in number, especially those who are more highly trained, such as doctors and senior nurses. To deal with the situation realistically, it is necessary to employ trained personnel selectively, to make increased use of trained auxiliaries with practical experience, and to teach mothers home care of both the sick and the well.

Consideration of staffing studies in health services in developing countries clearly indicate that, whether traditionalists agree or not, the only hope of carrying the health services to the population is to employ practical trained personnel who do not fit into existing orthodox categories, to make better use of volunteers and part-time trained nurses, to train community health workers, and to enlist community participation. Community health workers can carry out an important, though limited, range of tasks under supervision. It could be economical and useful to recruit some of the discontented semi-educated young men and women who are found in increasing numbers in many developing countries. As King and associates (1978) say, "Delegate every task to the humblest member of the team capable of doing it satisfactorily."

Auxiliary-type workers might include trained ward personnel, children's attendants (ayahs, amahs), or clerks for children's clinics, who can be taught to keep a register, file records, weigh, and interpret. The use of auxiliary health workers actually has been the custom in most hospitals and health services in all parts of the world. These workers are essential and should be used widely.

Admission of mothers to hospitals. In many hospitals in developing countries the mother or other attendant is admitted with the sick child. This practice is often not appreciated by Western-trained senior nursing staff, who feel that a hospital is progressing if mothers can be kept out and the ward assumes an austere atmosphere of regimentation, although there are some indications of a changing attitude. Plainly, there are disadvantages and problems for both families and hospital when mothers are admitted with their children. It puts hardship on the rest of the family left at home, although extended families can often help out. In the hospital, mothers can be untidy, noisy, and disruptive of ward routine if facilities are not well organized. Moreover, they may occasionally interfere with the treatment by pulling out intragastric tubes or may continue surreptitiously to give harmful herbal medicines to their children. Moreover, when limited finance is a problem, the admission of mothers to the hospital implies an expenditure of capital to provide for accommodations, food, and use of facilities.

Nevertheless, the benefits of having mothers in the ward with their children far outweigh the disadvantages. Any child, especially one from a rural village, needs the mother's reassurance in the strange, disconcerting atmosphere of the hospital during what is often a frightening and painful episode. With the mother present, the child will rest, sleep, and feed better. Mothers are also able to undertake some important tasks, such as feeding, bathing, and changing their children, collecting samples of urine and stools, and drawing early attention to physical changes in their condition or to abnormalities in treatment. With instruction and supervision, mothers may learn to carry out these tasks well and to widen their range of activities. It may be possible to avoid intravenous rehydration by having the mother sit with the baby in her lap patiently giving teaspoons of oral rehydration fluid.

In the case of young children, particularly infants, the mother obviously needs to be admitted if the baby is being breastfed. The folly of undertaking prolonged, expensive treatment for neonatal tetanus or for prematurity is apparent if survivors are subsequently to die of diarrhea-marasmus because the mother's lactation has not been continued.

An important aspect of admitting mothers to the ward is that they are a target group for health education. If their children are recovering, the mothers may be open to new ideas gained by observation of ward routine, by individual discussion and counseling, and by group discussion and demonstration (Fig. 12.9). A further unappreciated advantage of having the mother in the ward with her young child is that she is immediately available when the patient is discharged. She should be able to receive advice on discharge with details of home treatment and diet and of the time and place for continuing supervision, at a health center or an outpatient department.

If mothers are to use children's wards, plans should be made to provide facilities for them. Mother-centered children's wards need arrangements for toilets, washrooms, baths, and sleeping accommodation. Feeding arrangements may take the form of a simple kitchen or the provision for hospital-cooked meals for mothers. Storage space will be needed for mothers' belongings and chairs or mats by the children's bedsides. A teaching area must be available, and this can double as a mothers' rest space. It can be inside the hospital or, in some climates, under a tree near the ward. Associated with the teaching area and close to the ward, it may be possible to have such visual aids as a demonstration kitchen, a low-cost model house, or even an improved garden (Fig. 12.10).

Play opportunities. Modern children's wards and outpatient departments emphasize the need for play areas, toys, and play supervisors. It may be hard for a poor country to give these a high priority, but even when no money is available for playthings or for personnel, it is more than ever the duty of the staff and the parents to ensure that the children get the attention and stimulation that they deserve.

In one poverty-stricken area, everyone collected old cotton reels to be strung on bits of colored string, old match boxes for building, mango seeds to be made into dolls' faces, rags for constructing crude dolls, cigarette tins with seeds for rattles, bits of wood sawed up for bricks, and calabashes and gourds for sand and for water play. Bamboo, cigarette boxes, and tins can be used for construction projects. A piece of wood with holes and seeds is all that is needed for the local game of warri (almost universal in Africa) or a board for checkers. Papers (even wrappers) can be used to make flowers for decoration.

In many hospitals in Africa, the health staff sing songs and tell stories and encourage mothers to join in. The nurses not only sing the local forms of nursery rhymes in their own language but make some up, like "listen to your heart beat tick, tick, tick," to help children understand some of the activities of doctors.

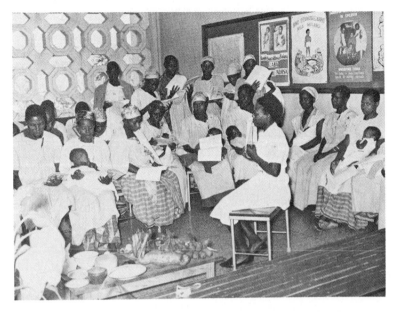

Figure 12.9. Listening and talking with mothers. In the children's ward, an MCH demonstrator discusses infant feeding with mothers. Experienced mothers with children recovering from malnutrition lead the discussion and demonstrate the preparation of weaning mixtures to mothers newly admitted to the Mulago Hospital, Kampala, Uganda.

The value of play cannot be overemphasized. There is no doubt that it has saved the lives of children who had lost interest in life. To have mothers and health workers cooperating in this valuable form of therapy is worthwhile, although mothers occasionally have to be taught to touch, talk, sing, and play with their infants. MCH centers, health centers, rehabilitation centers and MCH departments, day care centers, and convalescent centers can do much to encourage games, singing,

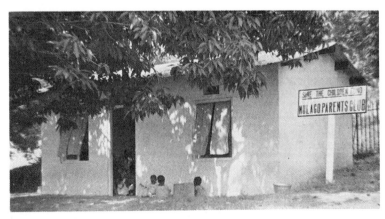

Figure 12.10. A model low-cost house, kitchen, and garden used for teaching purposes, adjacent to the children's ward at Mulago Hospital, Kampala, Uganda. A basic plan for the house was available at no cost for parents.

dancing, and individual play and even "play lessons," which stimulate growth and development in children, parents, and health workers alike.

Cross-cultural misunderstandings. Whenever a village child and mother are admitted to a modern hospital, a situation is created in which interaction occurs between two different cultural patterns, with considerable likelihood of misunderstandings. Health workers must learn about the cultures of the people they work with.

Pathology. Laboratory facilities are often minimal, but facilities for urine analysis and a microscope should be provided whenever possible. It is also necessary to have a postmortem room, for without the possibility of autopsies, many of the children who die will be inadequately diagnosed (Alderson et al. 1983). While this is something to aim for, it is not always possible for a variety of reasons, including cultural and religious beliefs.

Prevention, training, and occupational therapy in hospital. Historically, the hospital has been the main center of clinical, curative endeavor; however, prevention must be included as an equal partner. The preventive function of a children's ward is to avoid cross-infection, especially in malnourished children. They may have to be isolated and provided with hygienic measures, and immunizations may be a practical precaution, at least against some diseases, prior to the patient's discharge. For example, it may be possible to give BCG and a first dose of triple vaccine (DPT) to children as they leave the ward. At the same time, advice and directions can be given to mothers as to how they can take the child to a health center near their home to complete the remainder of the immunization.

Training. Hospitals in developing countries serve as training centers for medical students, auxiliaries, and the whole range of health personnel. Students and staff should also work in the community and with follow-up home visits.

REFERENCES

Adeniyi-Jones, O. (1958). The role of the hospital in the public health program. *W. Afr. Med. J.* **7**, 73.

Alderson, M. R.; Baylis, R. I. S.; Clarke, C. A.; and Whitfield, A. G. W. (1983). Death certification. *Brit. Med. J.* **287**, 444.

Arnhold, R. G., and Schneideman, I. (1969). The organization of a large urban dispensary in East Africa. *J. Trop. Pediat.* **15**, 18.

Backhouse, J. (1966). A follow-up clinic for children in a rural hospital in Tanzania. *J. Trop. Pediat. Monogr.* **2**, 74.

Baumslag, N. (1979). *Bangladesh Trip Report.* U.S. Department of Health, Education and Welfare, Office of Nutrition, International Division, USAID, Washington, D.C.

Bell, J. E. (1969). *The Family in the Hospital: Lessons from the Developing Countries.* U.S. Government Printing Office, Washington, D.C.

BMJ (1970). Children in hospital. *Brit. Med. J.* **2**, 302.

Brown, J. E., and Brown, R. C. (1979). *Finding the Causes of Malnutrition.* Task Force on World Hunger, Presbyterian Church, Atlanta.

Burke, F. G. (1969). The Pediatric Convalescence Hospital. (Pediatrics **45**, 879.

Choi, T.; Josten, L. V.; and Christensen, M. L. (1983). Health-specific family coping index for noninstitutional care. *Am. J. Pub. Hlth.* **73**, 1275.

Christian Med.Comm. (1983). Strengthening and regulating the supply, distribution and production of basic pharmaceutical products. *Contact* **73**, 2.

Cook, R. (1970). Is the hospital the place for the treatment of malnourished children? *J.Trop. Pediat.* **17**, 15.

Cuthbertson, W. F. J., and Morley, D. (1962). A health and weight chart for children from birth to five. *W. Afr. Med. J.* **11**, 237.

DeBeer, G. (1966). Mobile young child clinics in Buganda. *J. Trop. Pediat. Monogr.* **2**, 79.

Fendall, N. R. E. (1969). Health centres in Kenya. *E. Afr. Med. J.* **37**, 171.

Griffiths, M. (1981). *Growth Monitoring of Preschool Children: Practical Considerations for Primary Care.* Paper no. 3. American Public Health Association, Washington, D.C.

HHS (1980). *Weighing and Measuring Children: A Training Manual for Supervisory Personnel.* U.S. Department of Health and Human Services, Public Health Service, Center for Disease Control, Nutrition Division, Atlanta.

Inst. Med. (1982). *Community Oriented Primary Care.* Conference proceedings. Eds. E. Connor and F. Mullan. National Academy Press, Washington, D.C.

James, V. L., and Wheeler, W. E. (1969). The Careby-Parent unit. *Pediatrics* 43, 488.

Jelliffe, D. B. (1957). Notes on medical treatment in the child welfare clinic in India. *Indian J. Child Hlth.* 6, 752.

Jelliffe, D. B., and Jelliffe, E. F. P. (1970). The children's hospital as a lethal factor? *J. Pediat.* 77, 895.

Jelliffe, D. B., and Jelliffe, E. F. P. (1989). *Community Nutritional Assessment.* Oxford University Press, Oxford.

Jelliffe, D. B., and Jelliffe, E. F. P. (1990). *Growth Monitoring in Young Children.* Oxford University Press, Oxford.

Jelliffe, D. B., and Stanfield, J. P. (1968). Para-auxiliaries and medical manpower in tropical pediatrics. *J. Trop. Pediat.* 14, 199.

Kark, S. K. (1981). *The Practice of Community Oriented Primary Health Care.* Appleton-Century Crofts, New York.

King, M. et al. (1978). *Primary Child Care: A Manual for Health Workers.* Oxford University Press, Oxford.

Kimmance, K. J. (1970). Evaluation of the work of a mobile outpatient unit in Switzerland. *J. Trop. Pediat.* 16, 62.

Kreysler, J. (1970). Rational development of an "under fives clinic" network. *J. Trop. Pediat.* 16, 48.

Lancet (1981). Editorial: Child health. A coordinated approach to children's health in India. *Lancet* i, 650.

Lancet (1983). Editorial: Child health. A coordinated approach to children's health in India: A progress report after 5 years (1975–1980). *Lancet* i, 109.

Morley, D. (1963). A medical service for children under five years of age in West Africa. *Trans. Roy. Soc. Trop. Med. Hyg.* 57, 79.

Morley, D. (1966). The under-fives clinic. In *Medical Care in Developing Countries.* Ed. M. H. King. Oxford University Press, Oxford.

Morley, D., and Brown, R. (1992). Breathing rate and pneumonia. *Brit. Med. J.* 304, 637.

Morley, D., and Woodland, M. (1979). *See How They Grow.* Oxford University Press, Oxford.

Morley, D., et al. (1991). Talc direct recording scales. *Lancet* 338, 600.

Namboze, J. M. (1966). Mobile young children's clinics in Kasangati Health Centre defined area. *J. Trop. Pediat. Monogr.* 2, 75.

Nat. Council Nutr. (1970). *Nutritional Rehabilitation Through Maternal Education.* Report of a Working Conference, National Council of Nutrition, Bogotá.

PATH (1989). Leprosy. *Health Technology Directions* 9, (3), 1.

Robinson, P. (1970). Children's hospitals. In *Diseases of Children in the Subtropics and Tropics,* 2d ed. Ed. D. B. Jelliffe. Edward Arnold, London.

Robinson, G. C.; Shah, C. P.; Argue, C.; Kinnis, C.; and Israel, S. (1969). A study of the need for alternative types of health care for children in hospitals. *Pediatrics* 43, 866.

Rosa, F. W. (1964). Some practical approaches in the child health clinics of Gondar, Ethiopia. *J. Trop. Pediat.* 9, 113.

Sabin, E. and Stinson, W. (1981). *Primary Health Care Issues: Immunizations, International Health Programs.* American Public Health. Association, Washington, D.C.

Sarman, I., and Tunell, R. (1989). Providing warmth for preterm babies by a heated water filled mattress. *Arch. Dis. Childhood* 64, 29–33.

Sharma, R., and Chaturvedt, S. K. (1978). India. In *Basic Health Care in Developing Countries.* Ed. B. S. Hetzel. Oxford University Press, Oxford.

SINAPS (1982). *Integrated System of Nutrition and Primary Health Care.* Final Report. Institute of Nutrition of Central America and Panama, and Ministry of Public Health, Guatemala.

Stanfield, J. P. (1966). Initial experience with a multi-purpose children's clinic in a rural area in Buganda. *J. Trop. Pediat. Monogr.* 2, 73.

Stanfield, J. P. (1967). Organization of MCH services in developing regions. *J. Trop. Pediat.* 13, 59, 102.

Thomson, F. A. (1962). The reasons mothers take their children to a health centre (appraisal of work done at a health centre in Mengo District, Uganda). *J. Trop. Pediat.* **7**, 107.

UNICEF (1990). *Children and AIDS: An Impending Calamity.* UNICEF, New York.

Vintinner, F. J. (1968). A mobile rural health service program in Central America and Panama. *Am. J. Publ. Hlth.* **58**, 907.

Welbourn, H. F. (1956). Child welfare in Mengo District, Uganda. *J. Trop. Pediat.* **2**, 24.

Williams, C. D. (1956). Maternal and child health in Kumasi in 1935. *J. Trop. Pediat.* **2**, 141.

WHO (1977). *The Selection of Essential Drugs.* World Health Organization Tech. Rep. Ser., no. 615.

WHO (1980). *Sixth Report on the World Health Situation, 1973–1977,* Pt. One: *Global Analysis.* World Health Organization, Geneva.

WHO (1981). *Guidelines for Training Community Health Workers in Nutrition.* WHO Publication no. 59. World Health Organization, Geneva.

WHO (1991). *Child Health and Development: Health of the Newborn.* World Health Organization, Geneva.

Yankauer, A. (1961). Prospectus for a child health service built around paediatric clinics. *J. Trop. Pediat.* **6**, 122.

13

Health Services for School-Aged Children

To free oneself is nothing. The arduous thing is to know what to do with one's freedom.
ANDRE GIDE, 1930

Millions of children do not have the opportunity to attend school (Fig. 13.1) and many have to work in the labor force (ILO 1979). Increasingly, governments are giving education a higher priority.

While not in the precarious state of health of the infant and pre-school child, school-aged children are frequently poorly nourished and suffer from a variety of parasitic and infectious diseases. They often have tiring household duties and a long walk to school on an empty stomach. Older children are undergoing the physical and emotional stresses of adolescence, and the girls often are preparing for childbearing and child rearing.

Schoolchildren still are (or should be) growing rapidly, and this deserves consideration, for mental capacity and initiative depend on health and nutrition, and national development depends in the final analysis, on education. Schools are important for introducing new ideas and attitudes that can have an impact on the health and well-being of the entire community. By definition, schools should be places of change where young pupils expect to acquire new knowledge and additional skills. Their course of study should

include not only practical subjects but philosophy, history, economics, ethics, human behavior, and human relations.

Children in developing countries mostly attend day schools. This impressionable group is exposed to a new "ecology" for half their waking hours. Economically, logically, and administratively, this is the time and place for health education, which can lead to long-term results in the children themselves, in their homes, and, most important, in the next generation. Schools should emphasize children's attainment of health knowledge, as well as acquisition of certificates. In this important process, the teacher is the key figure. The primary sites for the development of new ideas concerning education in health and nutrition are the teacher-training colleges, in both their basic program and in refresher courses.

Schoolchildren are subject to special stresses. They are exposed to types of information and to exertions that may be quite different from their previous, traditional concepts of life and living. Even to sit on chairs and benches is exhausting for someone used to sitting on the floor. Whereas in the traditional village life every

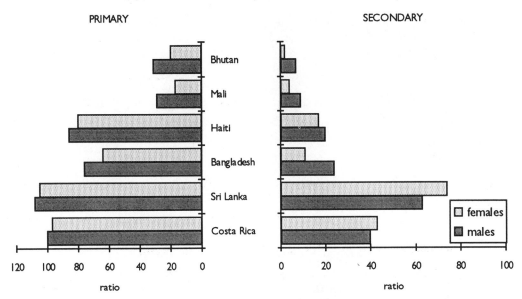

Figure 13.1. Children enrolled in schools in selected countries, 1986–1989. In countries such as Mali and Bhutan, a high proportion of children are in the work force. Outreach programs are needed for them. Source: UNICEF (1992).

single interest, idea, and activity is shared with the family, the children now acquire ideas and concepts that they cannot easily share. They may be exposed to new standards of behavior and choices.

In some countries, as many as nine out of ten children grow up unable to read or write. Although the proportion of children in primary schools has been increasing in less developed countries, only 62 percent of children were enrolled in primary schools compared with 94 percent in more developed areas (ILO 1979). More males than females are enrolled, and the difference is increasing substantially as the educational level rises (Fig. 13.1). The low enrollment of girls in less developed countries reinforces their educational deprivation (Figure 13.2).

A large number of children aged 5 to 15 years are outside the school system. They are engaged in the labor force from an early age in both the informal and formal work force, mainly in agriculture but also in cottage industries, textile mills,

and other activities such as carpet making. The number varies regionally. Children working in hazardous occupations should receive health education and screening organized through the health center whenever possible.

CHILD LABOR

In developing countries, one of the motives for having many children is economic necessity. The welfare of the family often depends on how much each member can contribute to the family income. Thus, children enter the work force early in life (Fig. 13.3). According to estimates by the International Labour Organization, there may be more than 100 million children betweeen the ages of 8 and 16 in the labor force in the developing countries (Fig. 13.4).

Working conditions depend on whether the work is agricultural, industrial, within the family, or for an unrelated employer.

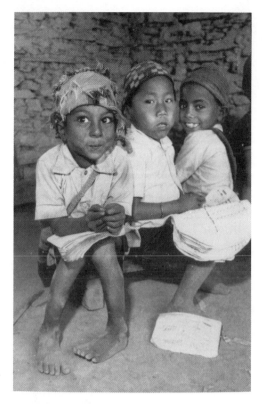

Figure 13.2. More girls need to be educated. More than 100 million children of school age (60 million of them girls) never step into a classroom. UNICEF photograph Wright.

It is not unusual to find children working ten or more hours per day, six or seven days a week. With expanding industrialization, children are employed in dangerous environments where they come into contact with toxic substances and carry heavy loads.

In addition to unfortunate social and emotional consequences and missed educational opportunities, children who are overworked or work under poor conditions face serious health risks. Because of their lower endurance and muscular strength, children tire more easily and become more vulnerable to accidents, toxic substances (such as pesticides, lead, solvents, mercury, glue in leather factors) or dust diseases (skin or eye irritation, bronchitis) and tuberculosis. Growth disorders can result from heavy loads and prolonged awkward body positions. A study in Japan showed growth stunting among children who began work before age 14, as compared with workers who did not work until age 18 (ILO 1979). When children are overtired and undernourished, their resistance to infections is lowered.

Laws and labor regulations have been promulgated to protect children from exploitation and harmful working conditions; however, there are numerous loopholes and exemptions regarding certain branches of the work force (especially in agriculture), light work, cottage industries such as textiles and glass, and family businesses (ILO 1979).

Along with the need for strengthened protective legislation, educational systems should be based on the reality that many children must combine work with school. If this is not recognized, efforts to establish compulsory education will be futile. Unfortunately, the exploitation of cheap child labor helps to maintain low wages throughout the economy. The elimination of this system would threaten many vested interests, and this is a major obstacle to change (Standing 1981), but not a reason for ignoring the problems or failing to suggest measures of prevention. Health services personnel should recognize these problems and be aware of social services and other agencies that could assist these children.

PLANNING THE SCHOOL HEALTH SERVICE

Organization

The development of a school health program poses problems, some of them common to all projects and others are peculiar to this alone (Bennett and Lutwama 1966). Administratively, the health of schoolchildren often falls between two ministries—those of health and education. It may not fit neatly into the budget,

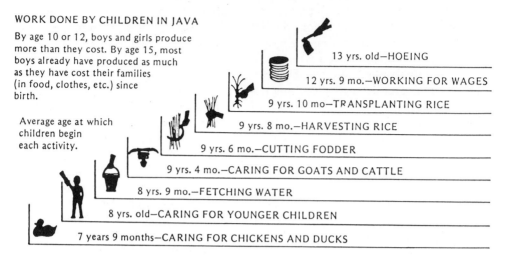

WORK DONE BY CHILDREN IN JAVA

By age 10 or 12, boys and girls produce more than they cost. By age 15, most boys already have produced as much as they have cost their families (in food, clothes, etc.) since birth.

Average age at which children begin each activity.

13 yrs. old—HOEING

12 yrs. 9 mo.—WORKING FOR WAGES

9 yrs. 10 mo—TRANSPLANTING RICE

9 yrs. 8 mo.—HARVESTING RICE

9 yrs. 6 mo.—CUTTING FODDER

9 yrs. 4 mo.—CARING FOR GOATS AND CATTLE

8 yrs. 9 mo.—FETCHING WATER

8 yrs. old—CARING FOR YOUNGER CHILDREN

7 years 9 months—CARING FOR CHICKENS AND DUCKS

Figure 13.3. Children in the work force, Java. Many children enter the work force early in life. Source: Werner, D. (1982).

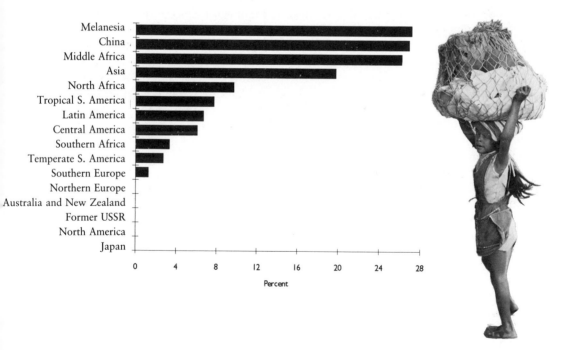

Figure 13.4. Percentage of children aged 10 to 14 in the labor force, selected countries, 1975. A large number of children in poor countries enter the work force at an early age. There may be as many as 100 million children in the labor force in the Third World, often working in hazardous conditions. Source: ILO (1977).

administration, or policy of these two government departments. Both see the need and would like the direction (though not the expense) to be within their own ministry. Often this dichotomy results in a chronic impasse and few beneficial results. The success of such programs depends on interdepartmental liaison and collaboration. Various divisions of responsibility are possible, sometimes with a joint advisory committee guided by an MCH adviser.

Liaison with other MCH activities should also be developed. This collaboration may lead to opportunities for establishing more day nurseries and creches for the children of both school and health service staff. In addition, these nurseries would provide opportunities for older children to gain experience in child care, baby-sitting, first aid, nutrition, and care of the sick, the young, and the old.

A school health service should also maintain cooperation with administrators, agriculturalists, industrialists, and judicial and religious authorities.

Finance and Staff

Most developing countries have only token school health services that reach a limited area—often only in the major cities. In the context of a restricted national budget, the launching of a new or expanded school health service may be difficult, particularly in view of the many other development programs. However, the need for the maximum benefit from schooling for national, social, and economic development and the opportunity presented to acquire new ideas are forceful arguments that are quite likely to appeal to administrators and politicians.

The service suggested has to be so devised to use, as far as possible, existing organization and staff, and with only minimal increase in expenditure. Teachers themselves, part-time workers (particularly married nurses), and various types of medical auxiliaries are likely to be the main source of staff, with the limited involvement of doctors for referral and for assistance with planning and organization.

Priorities

The practical aims of a school health program have to be established for the circumstances found in a particular country. All too often, a school service is initiated in a less well-to-do country as the mirror image of an old-style service in a European or North American country. This service will frequently emphasize routine medical examinations, which, with limited staff and inadequate facilities at referral centers, usually degenerate into an endless, almost pointless, routine of inspection of some children once during their schooling, with no possibility of correcting the large numbers of abnormalities or deformities discovered. Classically, this consists of a solemn search for advanced caries in schoolchildren when only one dental surgeon exists in the country or for eye defects when no remedial care is available. Before screening, it is necessary to make sure curative services are in place.

Assessment of Priorities

Before planning a school health program, an assessment of priorities must be made by investigation of the available literature and reports and, if possible, by a survey of a statistical sample of schools in representative areas. The number of children requiring special services, such as children in the labor force or exceptional children, should be determined.

Health problems. A rapid assessment of health problems can be made by observing the condition of the children, their teachers, and the premises. Among the children, the younger age groups will show more general malnutrition, skin infections, enlarged spleens, oral sepsis, anemia and possible lethargy, and poorer clothing than the older children. The quality of the teachers can usually be assessed on general appearance and behavior toward the pupils. Defects in the premises are even more obvious. A comparison should always be made between numbers on the roll and numbers actually in school and the causes of absenteeism.

A more detailed survey of schoolchildren to assess their main medical problems may be practical, based on clinical examination for stigma associated with malnutrition and for those of obvious treatable diseases (for example, skin infection, or ear discharge); chronic, potentially remediable defects (for example, deformities following poliomyelitis, talipes, poor vision, dental disease, hernia); and past medical history (for example, vaccination scar, indigenous medical incision, enlarged spleen) (Brown and Wilks 1967; Kamel 1961; Lowenstein 1963). Nutritional anthropometry can include weight and height, sometimes with other measurements; of these, the arm circumference and the triceps skinfold seem particularly useful (Jelliffe and Jelliffe 1989). Basic laboratory tests should include hemoglobin estimation, a tuberculin test, and stool examination for intestinal parasites, together with a thick blood film for malaria in endemic regions.

After preliminary surveys, the main medical priorities can be identified. These often include skin infections, undernutrition, intestinal helminth infection, malaria, tuberculosis, and, in some places, leprosy. Schistosomiasis is usually more common in schoolchildren than in younger age groups.

It may be feasible to try to obtain information on some aspects of the past history and on certain social details, such as the distance traveled to school, the method of transport, and the meal pattern at home in relation to school hours.

Finally, an assessment should be made of the presence, extent, and usefulness of existing health services for children at school. This can begin with inquiry at medical and educational headquarters but can be judged more realistically by observing and questioning teachers at schools.

Environmental problems. Assessment of the environmental problems at schools should be made in preliminary survey work, including investigation of the water supply, excreta disposal, cleanliness, accident hazards, and space and shade for recreation.

A variety of factors can affect school health, including epidemics of communicable diseases, natural or man-made disasters, teachers' strikes, suddenly increased absenteeism, and water shortage; all of these may entail special measures devised by the health authorities. Health workers who know the schools and the types of personnel involved will be in a good position to decide on the priorities.

Educational problems. Some educational problems can be assessed theoretically by prior study of the curricula of both teachers and children, but practical aspects can be gauged only by visits to schools.

The knowledge and interest of schoolchildren may be tested by questionnaire or by asking students to pose their own questions. The results reveal the range of the children's knowledge and things that worry them or are especially lacking.

FUNCTIONS OF THE HEALTH SERVICE

Health Services for Schoolchildren

These have three major components: environmental protection, health promotion, and health education (Table 13.1). Routine examinations should be reduced to a minimum, possibly on admission and prior to leaving school. They should be limited to important signs of remediable conditions, and records should be simple

Table 13.1. School Health Programs

Environmental protection ⟷	Health protection and promotion ⟷	Health education

Maintenance of safe, sanitary buildings and grounds	Periodic medical examinations
	  Screening
	  Growth monitoring
	  Referrals
		Health education in school curriculum

Adequate refuse disposal		Integration of health education with other subjects and programs
Protection from flies, mosquitos	Emergency care	Special programs
Safety patrols, accident prevention	Mass immunization	First aid

Hygienic cooking facilities, hand washing	Care of exceptional children	Child health
		  Family planning and sex education
		  Responsible parenting
		  AIDS, tuberculosis

	Health services for teachers	
	Physical fitness program	In-service health education for teachers, training teachers to recognize common problems
	School garden	

	Extension of services to the community
	  Outreach to children not in school
	  Child-to-child program
		Participation of community health personnel in school programs

		Parent education
		Cooperation and coordination with community health education programs

Source: Modified from Hanlon (1974).

and uncluttered. Parents should be invited to attend when these examinations take place.

Schools can represent a valuable, easily accessible focal point for immunization, particularly the "one-dose" type of vaccination against measles, hepatitis, and TB.

Simple first-aid facilities, appropriate to local needs, should be made available. Both teacher and pupils should learn how to use them.

Teachers should be taught how to recognize the main causes of illness and how to refer students to the nearest health center. Children with physical or mental impairment should have special consideration, even if only by such minor adjustments as by arranging for the child with poor vision or hearing to sit in the front row. The severely disabled require special schools, but these are rarely available, and, in any case, it may be unwise to alienate a child from his or her family. It is generally preferable to provide special services in the regular school setting.

MCH staff, including health nurses, will be responsible for the school health program, including clinic work, examinations, and, when feasible, home visits to deal with absenteeism. Lines of communication must be established so the health nurse is supervised and can obtain consultative services. Volunteers can also be utilized. Special attention should be given to the younger children.

Time permitting, health staff may be available to advise on vocational training, further education, and job opportunities and may assist with the work of voluntary organizations, such as the scouts and guides, YMCA or YWCA, and the Red Cross, and promote recreational and leisure activities.

Health Services for Teachers

Schoolteachers should have a physical examination commencing duty and then periodically, with reference to certain infectious diseases, particularly tuberculosis. Arrangement for the expeditious treatment and supervision of teachers and their families is important in itself, but also because teachers have a major role as scouts for ill health among their charges. The teacher's housing, toilet facilities, and water supply need supervision. The way in which teachers behave and their home surroundings are more likely to influence children than classroom lectures.

Finally, the curricula for teacher training colleges, refresher courses, and special seminars should be prepared in concert with the health authorities. Textbooks used in colleges and schools that have a bearing on health should be realistically geared to local conditions and should be repeatedly surveyed.

Environmental Control

The health staff should be able to advise on the construction and position of school buildings and their water supply, toilets, and classroom accommodation, including lighting and equipment. Attention must be given to playing fields, gardens (for food production and biology classes), cooking facilities (for school meals and for practical home economics), and sometimes an infirmary.

Accident prevention must be incorporated in environmental considerations, including the dangers of falls, cuts, traffic accidents, drowning, burns, and snake bite.

Environmental control is one of the most important aspects of a school health program. The routine use of simple but effective toilets and water for hand washing and cleaning of teeth is practical health education at its best. With good relations between teachers, parents, and health staff, it is sometimes possible to obtain the cooperation of pupils and parents in improving the school premises and surroundings.

Health Education

A great deal of better health education (WHO 1980) could be achieved by teaching first aid, home nursing, child health,

and sex education in schools as part of the curriculum.

Advice and assistance may be given in the teaching of such subjects as hygiene, first aid, home economics, nutrition (including breastfeeding), biology, sex (including AIDS), mental health, civics, home nursing, responsible parenthood, horticulture, and local priority health problems (e.g., schistosomiasis in some areas) to children, parents, and teachers, school nurses, and voluntary workers. Health professionals may also help in such teaching and in discussions on a number of social issues, such as further education, population problems, the mass media, war crimes, drug addiction, smoking, delinquency, typhoid, hospitals, patent medicines, and advertising.

Cooperation with the parent-teacher association, school committees, and local councils may help these organizations to appreciate the needs of schoolchildren. Sports and games, arts and crafts, singing, dancing, and acting, both traditional and contemporary have a part to play in growth and development.

Planned health education should be incorporated into the children's teaching program by both teachers and available health staff (see Appendix 4). Informal health education should be a part of daily school life, with clean surroundings, simple but adequate toilets (that are used), and, in some places, a school meal to set the example, although this often poses practical difficulties.

Nutrition

The nutrition of schoolchildren can be assessed by health staff during medical examinations, from clinical history and signs, from weight or other measurements, or by the teachers themselves if they keep simple serial weight records or merely spot and refer to the health staff very thin, underweight pupils. Undernourished children must be referred for investigation, treatment, or home supervision—whichever is most feasible (Jelliffe 1967; Jelliffe and Jelliffe 1989).

Nutrition education should be incorporated into all aspects of classroom work, with such subjects as science and home economics and with practical activities, such as preparation of school meals and the upkeep of gardens. School lunches are sometimes widely organized, but are expensive and pose problems of food storage and lack of staff and facilities for cooking and serving. However, sometimes they can be organized, at least on a short-term basis, with the help of simply cooked and inexpensive local foods or donated supplies.

Through individual advice or through the parent-teacher association, it may be possible to advise parents to supply a packed lunch or snack for their children. This could consist of a cooked root vegetable with beans and vegetable sauce; puffed or boiled rice with sprouted gram; soybean cakes with bread or rice; a hard-boiled egg or a handful of roasted peanuts with a couple of bananas—the possibilities are infinite. Too often the child is given some money to take to school and spends it unwisely on fizzy bottled drink and a sweet cake. Sometimes it is possible to control the hawkers or contractors supplying the schoolchildren and to insist on the supervision of what they sell, as well as its preparation. It may be possible to suggest items that are both appealing to children and nutritionally sound.

Milk is a valuable supplement to the diet, but some children may not be used to drinking it. Moreover, its distribution and consumption will have to be supervised and its flavor modified.

School gardens and experimental agricultural plots, fish ponds, and rabbit or hen keeping can be made the basis for nutrition education (Fig. 13.5). Problems may, however, arise with pilfering, care during holidays, and disgruntled students who consider the work to be forced labor. It is difficult to make sure the best of the produce raised is for the children, not the staff. In areas where water is scarce and the ground is hard, this project is not feasible.

CONCLUSIONS

Each school health program has to be devised within the limits of available resources, realistically aligned to major remediable problems, and viewed in relation to the probabilities of return on the investments of restricted staff and funds. The competing claims of more vulnerable groups, especially very young children, have to be weighed against each other constantly setting priorities (Jelliffe 1967).

Selection within the activities suggested will vary with circumstances, but three main approaches may often be valid: health education, health screening, and immunization. Much depends on the teachers and on the relevance of the training they give to health and nutrition education, through the curriculum, through school activities (such as meals, gardens, and environment), and, perhaps most important of all, through personal example. Much, too, depends on the health staff's recognizing and referring pupils in need. The doctor interested in MCH must make every effort to influence the curricula in teacher training colleges.

Certainly one of the greatest priorities in improving the health of schoolchildren is less developed areas is more appropriate training for teachers, still constrained by restrictive curicula and examinations from overseas and by irrelevant textbooks designed for Europe or North America decades ago. MCH staff can help at the ministry level with guidance for more appropriate books and curricula and in the field with advice and participation in school activities.

Innovative school health programs are being carried out in many parts of the world. In Tanzania, a pilot project extended benefits to the schools' villages

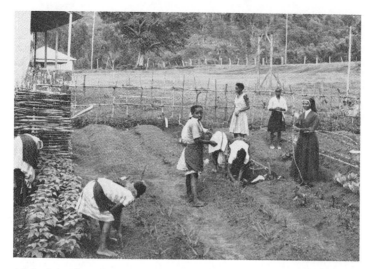

Figure 13.5. School garden for food and nutrition education, Ethiopia. Photograph by Dr. H. A. P. Oomen.

through community participation, child-to-child extension, and public education. The project emphasized coordination with village health committees to improve water supplies, sanitation, public health educations, and school garden production (Berger and Ngaliwa 1983).

When school attendance is low and the social environment poor, the health needs of children who do not attend school are likely to be more acute than those of children at school. Because the number of children with no formal schooling is increasing, this is a growing problem that must not be ignored (WHO 1980). In an agricultural area of Nepal, 7 out of 100 primary school pupils were girls. By secondary school, there were only 2 out of 100. Girls who attended primary school did so for only one or two years because they were needed for work in their homes and were married off at young ages. An innovative program by UNESCO held classes for young girls after late fall and harvest for 160 days to improve the educational and social status of women (Fig. 13.6). It taught them how to improve their health and hygiene and that of their families. Initially, attendance at the classes

was low and irregular, and there was a lack of qualified teachers. Now thousands of girls have passed through the program, and the classes have become important to the community (WIPHN News 1991).

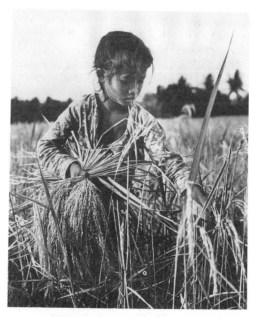

Figure 13.6. Adaptive education programs for young girls working in the fields. Source: ILO CO2.2 Indonesia.

School health programs can play a key role in maximizing community health resources and protecting children from health hazards in the workplace and in the community. Child-to-child programs can be organized to train children in simple techniques of nutritional surveillance, early oral rehydration therapy, and basic preventive care, first aid, and sanitation. Their knowledge may then be passed to siblings and neighbors who do not attend school (Aarons and Hawes 1979).

REFERENCES

Aarons, A., and Hawes,H. (1979). *Child-to-Child*. Macmillan Press, London.

Bennett, F. J., and Lutwama, J. S. (1966). Organization of MCH services in developing regions, I: Health services for school children. *J. Trop. Pediat.* **12**, 16.

Berger, I. B., and Ngaliwa, S. (1983). "Mradi Wa Afya Mashuleni": The Tanzania school health program. *J. School Hlth.* **53**, 95.

Brown, R. E., and Wilks, N. R. (1967). *A Survey of Primary School Children in Uganda*. Kampala, Uganda.

Gurney, J. M. (1969). Anthropometry in action, III. Simple tool for assessing the growth of school age children. *J. Trop. Pediat.* **15**, 9.

Hanlon, J. (1974). *School Health in Public Health*. 6th ed. C. V. Mosby, St. Louis.

ILO (1977). *Labor Force Estimates and Projections 1950–2000*. International Labour Organization, Geneva.

ILO (1979). *Children at Work*. International Labour Organization, Geneva.

Jelliffe, D. B. (1967). Principles in intiating a school health service. *J. Trop. Pediat.* **13**, 1.

Jelliffe, D. B., and Jelliffe, E. F. P. (1989). *Community Nutritional Assessment*. Oxford University Press, Oxford.

Kamel, W. H. (1961). A school health survey in Alexandria, Egypt. U.A.R. Part IV. Health questionnaire. *Alexandria Med. J.* **7**. 133.

Lowenstein, F. W. (1963). Nutrition and health of school children in a Brazilian Amazon town (use of certain indicators for rough evaluation). *J. Trop. Pediat.* **8**, 88.

Pop Ref. Bur. (1980). *World's Women Data Sheet*. Population Reference Bureau, Washington, D.C.

Standing, G. (1981). Child labor revisited. In *ILO Information*. International Labour Organization, Geneva.

UNICEF (1990). *Meeting Basic Learning Needs: A Vision for the Nineties*. Background document for World Conference on Education for All, Thailand, UNICEF Interagency Commission (UNDP, UNESCO, UNICEF and World Bank). UNICEF, New York.

UNICEF (1992). *State of the World's Children*. Oxford University Press, Oxford.

Werner, D., and Bower, B. (1982). *Helping Health Workers Learn: A Book of Methods, Aids, and Ideas for Instructors at the Village Level*. Hesperian Foundation, Palo Alto, Calif.

Werner, D., and Bower, B. (1992). *Helping Health Workers Learn: A Book of Methods, Aids, and Ideas for Instructors at the Village Level*. 2d ed. Hesperian Foundation, Palo Alto, Calif.

Williams, C. D. Experiments in health work in Trengganu, Malaya. In *Primary Health Care Pioneer: The Selected Works of Dr. Cicely D. Williams*. 1986 Ed. N. Baumslag. World Federation of Public Health Associations and UNICEF. Washington.

WIPHN News (1989). Nepal: Empowering girls. *WIPHN News* **6**.

WHO (1980). *Sixth Report on the World Health Situation, 1973–1977*, Pt. One: *Global Analysis*. World Health Organization, Geneva.

14

Special Programs

Special programs are of two main types: those that deal with an emergency situation that is likely to be temporary and those that attempt to meet certain needs over and beyond the established services that should be routinely available for mothers and children.

Emergency programs are organized in cases of natural disasters such as flood, drought, earthquake, and high winds and of human-made disasters, such as war, civil disorder, and refugee situations. In cases of epidemics too, such as poliomyelitis, measles, cholera, and sleeping sickness, particular measures are necessary.

A different type of special program is indicated for disabled children and their mothers, for orphans or abandoned children, and for such conditions as leprosy, tuberculosis, or AIDS, which are of particular danger to children. These are, for the most part, chronic problems, and their treatment and prevention must eventually be incorporated into ongoing and expanding health programs. Special programs are needed for special problems (Bell 1969; WHO 1980a) to meet individual and community needs.

Assessment centers, established in a number of countries, are useful in helping primary health workers to utilize specialists and analyze the needs of patients. They are also valuable to health planners in defining the areas of greatest need for expansion of services and appropriate training.

REFUGEES

Pregnant and lactating women and small children often are the most dependent members of any population and the least able to defend themselves against war and natural disasters. In Africa alone in 1991, there were at least 5 million people needing refugee assistance out of 15 million refugees in the world. More than half were children (Simmonds 1983; USCR 1991). Moreover, the number of refugees and displaced persons is increasing. In Eastern Europe, there were already 3 million refugees in the former Yugoslavia in 1992. Kurdish and Somalian refugees require much assistance. Refugees are at great risk for diseases. They face problems of alienation, depression, overcrowding, change of life-style, fear, anxiety, and lack of educational and health services. Not only have they lost their life assets, their familiar milieu, and loved ones, but they have suffered severe deprivation and hardship and now face total dependency, at least temporarily. Women refugees are often sexually abused and may even be expected to provide sex for food or medicine.

Generally refugee camps start during wars or droughts and famines as stopgap measures, but many of them become permanent settlements; examples are the Palestinian refugee camps and those on the Thai-Cambodian border. They provide basic shelter, health care, food, safe water, sanitary disposal of waste and refuse, social services, and education as well as general social and religious activities. A major problem is coordination, especially of the donors, who each want to run their own show. Clear lines of communication and action and definition of roles (especially of volunteers) must be established, preferably with a national governmental control agency or committee. It is essential to make attempts to repatriate, absorb, or resettle the population as soon as possible and to recognize that the camps are only a temporary solution (Fig. 14.1).

Great care and attention must be paid to the selection and training of personnel. Expatriate health workers need to concentrate on training of refugees as practical workers. When Western physicians and nurses without experience of the health care problems of developing countries enter the refugee scene, they often attempt to provide inappropriate high-technology services and may promote detrimental practices, such as bottle feeding for newborns. At one camp in Thailand, infant formula was provided for babies up to 6 months old, after which they were forced on to weaning foods exclusively, and malnutrition resulted (Olness 1981). Fortunately, these practices are changing as an international

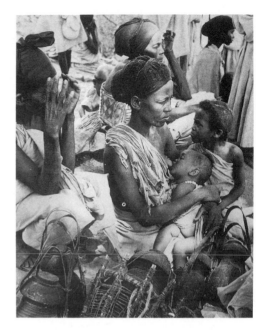

Figure 14.1. Refugees need support, health services, and education as well as food. Malnutrition, diarrhea, and disease are common problems in refugee camps. UNICEF Ethiopia photograph, Campbell.

protocol is becoming established for health care in refugee camps. In Somalia, apparatus for artificial infant feeding was banned from refugee camps. In some camps, mothers who have lost their infants have been encouraged to breastfeed orphans, with benefits for both the infants and mothers. Breastfeeding has helped these women with their depression and given them a purpose in life. The camp itself may disturb family relationships, as happened in Ethiopia, where mothers and daughters were left in the camps during the Sahelian drought while fathers and sons looked after the livestock and searched for water and food (Baumslag 1981).

The use of donated foods that are inappropriate, not well tolerated, or are habituating (e.g., preferring Norwegian sardines in oil to local fish) has to be recognized. Refugees have been provided with food imports even when they have not needed food, as was the case with the Guatemalan earthquake when food aid replaced the local foods and laborers waited in line instead of working in the fields. These hand-outs served as a disincentive to local food production, and the people's request for shelter and not food was ignored (Baumslag 1981). It is imperative to analyze the situation in each refugee group before prescribing for it.

Where food is needed, careful analysis must be made of local resources. Donated food should be screened to avoid outdated items or inappropriate food such as chicken tetrazzini (provided for Rwanda refugees), tinned sardines in oil, or noodles and tomato sauce. In one program, dog food was made available. In Somalia, corn raised for pig food was donated and could not be eaten until hand mills were obtained to grind it. For food distribution, cultural acceptance must also be considered; pork rind for Muslims would be intolerable, and when pregnant Cambodian women were provided with milk as a supplement, they would not drink it for cultural reasons.

Water often constitutes a major problem in refugee camps and may have to be rationed or its source protected. Careful attention must be given to sewage disposal and waste, as well as to the nutrition status of the refugees, as priorities. There is a danger of development of diseases such as meningitis, dysentery, typhoid, and diarrhea where overcrowding and poor living conditions prevail. Most of the children will have to be vaccinated against communicable diseases. Another major problem is to find work for the adult refugees and to provide educational programs for the children. Activities have to be organized to maintain mental and physical health and develop self-esteem, hope, and self-reliance.

The possibilities for providing health education in refugee camps are great, and refugees are typically ready to learn to provide their own health care. The Cambodian or Khmer refugees are a case in point. Many of the Khmers expected to be repatriated to Kampuchea, where during the time of Pol Pot most Western-trained physicians were killed. Camp residents were recruited as health assistants, and training courses for health professionals were implemented, as well as retraining of midwives (Levy 1981). The opportunity to assist the community to learn to deal better with problems of mothers and children should be a primary goal of MCH programs, whether in stable communities or in the setting of refugee camps.

For the growing number of refugees, food aid is not enough; household food security and peace are essential.

SUPPLEMENTARY FEEDING PROGRAMS

These programs do not attack the root cause of malnutrition, poverty, which in the long term can be alleviated only by food security (ICN 1992). The term *supplementary feeding* has been used to cover a variety of activities—short term or of prolonged duration—aimed at various age groups, ranging from vital emergency relief in disaster situations to the frantic disposal of unwanted and embarrassing surpluses in overworked clinics (Bengoa 1967; King 1966). Ideally, they should not replace the local diet but should be given short term and selectively (Fig. 14.2).

There is no doubt that in times of acute food shortage, supplementary feeding can be invaluable, but as a rule, it has to be extremely carefully and selectively administered, or it will do more harm than good (Rush 1982). Historically programs were developed by UNICEF to feed war-ravaged countries and, later, children in developing countries. The food originally distributed was surplus unfortified milk powder. From 1954 to 1970, bilateral and voluntary agencies took over the programs, distributing

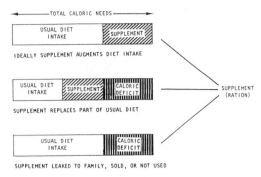

Figure 14.2. Supplementation programs.

cereals, oil, and foodstuffs such as tinned sardines. In the 1970s the World Food Program entered the arena with new programs (Bailey and Raba 1976). In less developed countries, over $750,000 million was spent to provide 125 million children with food (Berg 1973). The United States is the biggest contributor, and since 1954 has provided $26 billion of food assistance to foreign nations.

Food assistance has been growing, and so have loans. Some countries are deeply in debt, and their dependence on U.S. food imports, especially wheat, is enormous, while production of local staples is depressed. Inequitable food distribution is at the root of the problem; wasting scarce resources on importing, storing, and transporting costly, often inappropriate food will not solve the problem (Lappe and Collins 1977).

Recent disenchantment with the use of ill-defined, widespread supplementary feeding programs has stemmed from their lack of effectiveness, their high hidden costs to governments (for transport, storage, and staff time), their diversion of health staff from major activities, the resulting dependence psychology, the depression of local food production, and, in the case of dried skimmed milk, the decrease in breastfeeding (Mora et al. 1990). The overenthusiastic distribution of unfortified skimmed milk, in spite of the availability of breastmilk, has resulted in widespread xerophthalmia and blindness.

New initiatives have been implemented that make the use of food aid in MCH more rational. In countries such as Zaire, MCH programs try to use only local foods. Food is prescribed as a medicine for selected cases, not dished out as a universal panacea. Programs in Sudan have been integrated into the general MCH clinics. Food supplements are given to children under 2 years of age and to severely malnourished children under 5 years. Studies have shown that in mildly malnourished children, more harm than good is done by giving food supplements to the families because the families give the infant the food as a replacement rather than as a supplement. Furthermore, studies have shown that school feeding programs do not reach those most in need and do not significantly affect the nutrition status of the participants (Beaton and Ghassemi 1978).

It would seem axiomatic, but is not always so, that a supplementary feeding program should be based on knowledge of the local forms of malnutrition and the factors responsible. Supplementary feeding is essential for treating severely malnourished children and for malnourished mothers in the last trimester of pregnancy, to improve birthweight and lactation. A clear knowledge of the causes of the malnutrition affects the decision whether to undertake a supplementary feeding program and affects the program's form and content. Blanket distribution is to be condemned.

Feeding programs often have political goals and at best can be considered only an emergency measure for short-term use. Basically there are two main types of feeding programs: take home and on site.

Take-home programs can reach a wide population. The food, however, is often shared by the family and cannot easily be targeted to one individual. Administration costs may be less, but larger rations have to be given. The danger of such programs is that clinics serve as food distribution sites, and mothers come for food, not for health care and education. The effects on a well-established, carefully organized MCH clinic may be disastrous as a struggling mass of women try to get hand-outs; when there are none, clinic attendance may drop markedly. To top it all, the food may be used for other purposes and not to improve the nutrition status of the individuals for whom it was originally intended. It may be sold or diverted to the rest of the family or even to the military.

On-site programs may provide handouts or prepared meals. This type of program is often very demanding of staff time and facilities. Storage is a major problem and expense, and few children or pregnant women can be reached. However, one can ensure that the supplement is ingested. Nutrition rehabilitation centers, "mothercraft centers," or village nutrition centers are directed at the malnourished child, and programs involve nutrition education of mothers in low-cost buildings (Bengoa 1967). There are two types of on-site program: residential and, more usually, day care. Essentially, mothers can see the recovery of their own children and others with a diet of locally available food mixtures they have prepared themselves. The recovery is obvious visually on growth charts and, funds permitting, by before and after photographs.

There are problems with this type of facility, including stigmatization of the family and the limitations on the number of children who can be admitted. Irrespective of how these units are organized, they are relatively costly. The idea of using facilities separate from the health center for nutrition rehabilitation was to show that malnutrition is due to poor food intake, as mothers do not see inadequate feeding as the cause. Follow-up is necessary to see if lessons learned are applied.

Primary prevention is the best solution, or failing that, rehabilitation in the home setting wherever possible. Well-trained community workers at the village level can assess the household situation and individually tailor practical programs to village needs and potential. In such areas, some type of nutrition rehabilitation unit or child-feeding center may or may not be feasible or possible. Such activities can occur at or adjacent to a health center or hospital.

A study of nutrition programs in developing countries found that 50 percent used imported foods (Karlin 1976), such as cereal-legume mixes blended from high protein foods (wheat-soy blend or corn-soy milk). Interestingly, these blends are not always used in the country of origin. They are costly and not always culturally acceptable. For example, in Bangladesh a fish-soy-protein mix was not accepted because it smelled so bad. The fish-soy concentrate separated on standing, and the fish portion was sold to farmers as fertilizer (Baumslag 1981). New foods have to be tested for acceptability in the setting where the product is used. Furthermore, the ingredients must be locally available if needless expense, waste, and harm are to be avoided.

A variety of weaning foods processed from local ingredients are now produced at the village level in many countries. These can be very simple mixtures (for example, corn–red bean flour in Haiti) or as individual foods in plastic packs for mothers to cook together (for example, rice, mung bean, dried fish, and oil in the Philippines). Some weaning foods have been produced commercially and distributed at relatively low cost (Jelliffe 1984). However, they have not had the success anticipated because they have always been too costly for the main target group—the very poor.

Local resources vary. In some areas, communities may benefit more from new or improved roads for market accessibility than from feeding programs. In the Jamkhed project in India (Arole 1977), people were motivated to identify and help solve their problems by using their own resources for feeding. Villages donated land for food production. In Madagascar, community cooperatives were developed with the money obtained from selling donated food.

It is critical that habituation and dependency on foreign foods be avoided at all cost. Efforts should be aimed at locally increasing the availability and geographical and financial accessibility of basic foods—usually the staples and major legumes, vegetable oil, and breast milk—especially through improved storage, gardens, better utilization at the household level, and increased equity.

IMMUNIZATION PROGRAMS

The pattern of ill health in early childhood in developing regions is dominated by the cumulative burden of interacting malnutrition, parasitism, and infectious diseases.

Long-term preventive programs must be based on parental education, improved health supervision, and medical care. At the same time, immunization against locally important childhood infections should form an essential part of MCH services. The priority of immunization campaigns needs careful thought and scrutiny. For example, the threat of an epidemic of yellow fever calls for an immediate campaign. The control of other endemic diseases may be initiated by a campaign but must be followed by ongoing programs within the regular health service.

An immunization campaign can be attractive; it appears to be clear-cut, achievable without major change in behavior, fairly simple, and comparatively cheap. A campaign may be directed against several important infections at one time, including whooping cough, measles, tuberculosis (for women and children), tetanus, and poliomyelitis (Schofield et al. 1961). All are serious causes of mortality and require large-scale, continuing national expenditure.

Immunization programs, particularly against poliomyelitis, are often willingly given financial support by politicians, who consider them to be clearly and dramatically visible activities directed toward the control of identifiable conditions, which are often understood and feared by the electorate in general. Indeed, there is still some hope of worldwide eradication of poliomyelitis. This understandable emphasis can be used to focus attention on the need for continuing MCH services.

Such programs not only reduce morbidity and mortality from specific infections but at the same time help to decrease the overwhelming case load on the limited curative resources of the health services. Moreover, they may also be considered in part to be "nutritional immunization campaigns" because they minimize the burden of several nutritionally important conditioning infections on young children during a period of cumulative stress, often in the second year of life (Karzon and Henderson 1966; Morley et al. 1961). However, they pose considerable problems and disadvantages that are often unappreciated. In particular, short-term mass campaigns may lack the means for continuity of effort when the often financially well-endowed, enthusiastic initial project is over; the necessary follow-up program to cover dropouts and children born subsequently may be lacking, with the result that mass immunity may decline over succeeding years, leaving a highly susceptible child population in a more dangerous state than before. Even more important, ill-considered immunization campaigns channel too much money and staff time toward one activity, to the exclusion of effort in the fields of education and health supervision.

Plans must be made early on to ensure continuity through both existing and newly developed MCH services (Gonzales 1965). In fact, one of the most important by-products of mass campaigns should be the stimulus to the development of long-term, ongoing MCH services. Notable in this regard has been the Preschool Protection Program in Ankole, Uganda, which was slowly transformed from a mobile immunization campaign into a network of MCH clinics (Cook 1968; Moffat 1969).

A concerted global effort is being made toward universal child immunization (UCI) through the Expanded Program of Immunization (EPI) and as part of the child survival initiative. Resources and training are being directed particularly toward improving the quality and stability of the vaccines, distribution, outreach, and education of health workers (PAHO 1981; WHO 1980*a*). In many countries, the EPI and Child Survival programs integrated into primary health care have significantly reduced the incidence of communicable disease. Estimates are that 3.2 million child deaths are averted each year from measles, pertussis, and neonatal tetanus. Coverage levels have also been increased in India through the Integrated Child Development Services (ICDS) (Lancet 1983).

In other areas while there have been substantial gains, UCI efforts have not been as successful as desired. For example, in developing countries only 30 percent of the pregnant women immunized against tetanus have received the two doses of tetanus toxoid as recommended by WHO/UNICEF.

A WHO/UNICEF goal to immunize 90 percent of children by the year 2000 seems unattainable at this point for a number of countries, including Haiti (Fig. 14.3). A common problem is the high drop-out rate (ranging from 5 to 60 percent) from the first to the third dose of DPT and polio vaccines (WHO 1992). An advantage of EPI-type programs is that they are satisfying and quantifiable to funding agencies.

Adapted Schedules

Immunization schedules employed successfully in Europe and North America are neither appropriate nor practicable in less developed areas. It is difficult for mothers to attend often enough due to long distances, cross-cultural misconceptions about time intervals, and a heavy work burden in the village, together with shortage of staff in health centers, making this type of schedule impractical (Table 14.1) (Cook 1966; Morley et al. 1961; Stanfield 1967, 1970).

Much work has been undertaken to develop and assess the compression of immunization schedules for the youngest age groups possible, by the simplest, most economical methods (Table 14.2). Selection of the most appropriate schedule depends on many considerations, including whether the clinic services are mobile or stationary (WHO 1992; Sabin 1981).

Additional questions of priorities have arisen with the development of expensive vaccines against hepatitis B and rota viruses. Similar questions will be posed when (and if) a vaccine against malaria becomes available.

Major Immunizations

Vaccines against measles, polio, and tuberculosis must be kept refrigerated from the point of manufacture to the point of injection. A super-vaccine that may be given as one shot will, hopefully, be developed in the future.

A hepatitis B vaccine is being used in Southeast Asia and the Middle East.

Immunization against tuberculosis is controversial (Ebrahim 1982; WHO 1980*b*). BCG is probably useless or nearly useless for protection against pulmonary tuberculosis (TB prevention trials 1979). The problem is that the effectiveness of BCG is not as clear-cut as that of measles or polio vaccination. There are a variety of vaccines in use, none of which is standardized. Moreover, special syringes are required at extra expense, and adverse reactions such as nasty scars at the injection site with axillary lymphadenitis alarm mothers. Anaphylactoid reactions too have been described (Tshabalala 1983). In view

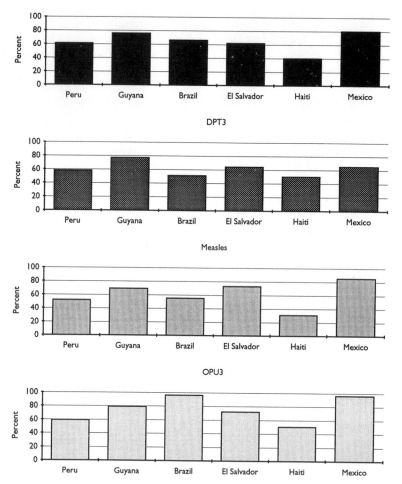

Figure 14.3. Percentage of Latin American children under 1 year of age receiving BCG, DPT, Measles, and OPV3 (oral polio vaccine, three shots), 1989. Source: PAHO (1990).

of these side effects, it is not surprising that many mothers do not bring their children to clinic after BCG vaccination. Inclusion of BCG warrants careful consideration because its effectiveness is clearly at a different level of proof from other vaccines commonly in use. There is, however, a constituency in many countries who are devout believers in BCG. Research is underway to improve the effectiveness of the BCG vaccine.

As whooping cough occurs in such a severe and lethal form in infancy, immunization should be given as early as possible, commencing from 6 weeks to 3 months—preferably early, since peak mortality is in the first six months. Triple vaccine (DPT), containing tetanus and diphtheria toxoid as well as pertussis vaccine, is customarily used; it is cheap and widely available and gives increased coverage of two other infections.

Although most authorities advocate the use of DPT, it has been associated with severe neurological damage attributed to impurities in the pertussis vaccine (Cody 1981). In infants, whooping cough is a difficult diagnosis to make, and hence the risk-benefit ratio is difficult to measure.

Table 14.1. Incomplete Immunizations: Reasons and Solutions

	Reasons	Solutions
Education of the public	Health staff failed to explain need for four visits in first year; one dose thought to be enough	Make immunization part of integrated primary health care
	Mother alarmed by unexpected side effects, not forewarned	Make education part of individual immunization routine
	BCG ulcer serves as deterrent	Involve community leaders in educational campaigns
	Rumors, illness, or death blamed on immunization	
Training of health staff	Records not properly filled in	Improve health staff understanding of need for accurate records
	Infectious hepatitis and abcesses develop due to infected needles	Improve training in injection techniques
	Health staff not trained to educate the public adequately	Train staff in methods of education
Logistics and support	Records lost	Improve record-keeping system
	Vaccine available sporadically	Coordinate field activities with ministry of health
	Unstable vaccine used—health service is no longer trusted	Monitor and supervise storage
	Family has no access to health care	Improve rural primary health care delivery system
	Vaccine improperly stored with ineffective refrigeration	

An improved form of the vaccine is expected to reduce the adverse reactions.

Poliomyelitis in developing countries still retains the picture of infantile paralysis' seen in nineteenth-century Europe, with most cases occurring between 6 months and 3 years of age. Although it does not have the direct or nutritional

Table 14.2. Sample Immunization Schedule for Clinics

Age	Immunization[c]
3 months	1st DPT,[a] 1st polio
4 months	2d DPT[a] 2d polio
5 months	3d DPT, 3d polio
9 months	Measles
13 years and over (females)[b]	Antitetanus toxoid—two doses,

Note: The routine schedule for vaccination listed above should be modified according to zero conversion rates, when known, and age-specific attack rates. Children with moderate undernutrition should be included.

[a] At the EPI Asian meeting in Manila 1983, it was decided that DPT can be given at 6 weeks. Limited data suggest that three doses have been found to induce fourfold greater antitoxin levels than two doses.

[b] For primary vaccination of pregnant women, second dose at least six weeks after the first and at least four weeks prior to the expected delivery.

[c] The use of BCG is being questioned.

killing potential of measles or whooping cough, it is a costly, disabling disease in relation to the individual family, the community, and the national health budget if rehabilitation services are planned. This is particularly so if contrasted with the relatively low cost and simplicity of immunization with modified live vaccine given by mouth from about 6 weeks to 3 months of age on three occasions, at four- to six-week intervals. Vaccination against poliomyelitis also is usually very acceptable to communities because parents generally recognize and fear the condition.

Measles has a high importance because it has a direct mortality and because it is potentially a nutritional conditioner in the etiology of kwashiorkor (Morley et al. 1961). Live measles vaccine—for example, the "further attenuated" and heat-stable strains administered in a single dose—are effective, safe, and relatively inexpensive ($0.10 per dose). Dogma has it that infants under the age of 6 to 8 months seldom contract measles, presumably because of the persistence of maternal antibody by tran-

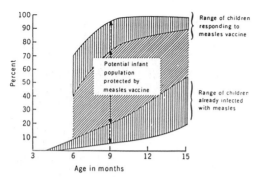

Figure 14.4. Effectiveness of measles vaccine administered to children 6 to 15 months of age in developing countries. Seroconversion rates following measles vaccination at 6 to 12 months are variable. Therefore, it is impossible to recommend a single age for the administration that would be optimal for all countries. The available data support giving the vaccine at 9 months in most developing countries but should not prevent health workers from administering measles vaccine to 6- to 8-month-old malnourished children who are at high risk of complications from natural measles and may not return for immunization at 9 months of age. Age-specific data, coupled with seroconversion rates, should be used to modify the recommended age for routine vaccination. Source: Halsey and Quadros (1983).

splacental transmission. This may not be so in developing countries.

Data collected from urban, peri-urban, and rural locations in Natal/Kwa Zulu in South Africa showed a positive correlation between population density and the percentage of measles cases at 8 months or less (Loening and Coovadia 1983). Therefore, it may be important to immunize urban infants against measles earlier; early vaccination may, however, result in primary vaccine failures and the children will have to be reimmunized later (Fig. 14.4).

In areas where tetanus is an important public health problem, women of childbearing age should be immunized with two doses of antitetanus toxoid at four-week intervals. For pregnant women, the second dose should be administered at least four weeks before delivery. Tetanus toxoid given during pregnancy has been shown to raise protective antibody levels in newborns (Sabin and Stinson 1981).

Schoolchildren are an easily accessible group and should be given primary immunization with DPT, polio, and measles vaccines if they have not previously received them. The decision to carry out a school immunization program, and its scope, must weigh the relative accessibility of this age group against the expense and the priority needs of other age groups. Usually limited resources need to be channeled to less accessible, more vulnerable young children. While schooling is available to most of the population, compulsory vaccine prior to registration has proved useful. Special programs are needed to reach vulnerable groups such as migrant and street children.

Immunization has dramatically reduced many of the communicable diseases; however, adverse reactions are often ignored or go unrecorded. In order to minimize these problems and to achieve maximum coverage of the population, immunization programs must be integrated into the health care system and monitored.

An accurate record-keeping system is essential, with individual records at the health center for cross-reference with the vaccination card kept by the mother. Mothers must be informed as to the purpose of immunization, the schedule, and what to expect. For example, a rash and fever, easily controlled with aspirin, can occur eight to twelve days after the measles vaccination. A local reaction with fever and crying eight hours after the DPT shot is common. Reactions to oral polio vaccine are rare. One in every million experiences paralysis similar to polio. To obtain cooperation and complete treatment, parents must be well informed and understand that return visits are necessary. Otherwise, incomplete coverage or incomplete vaccination results (Sabin and Stinson 1981).

DISABLED CHILDREN

The most severely disabled children include the poorest of the poor and the most neglected of the neglected (Burress and Perlman 1980). Due to war and civil disturbances, more and more children and their mothers have been disabled. Until recently in some cultures, children with disabilities were hidden from sight. Sometimes mothers believed that they had been given the evil eye, that they had been cursed, or that they had seen a monkey when pregnant.

Working with the Disabled

Physicians and health professionals were, and to a large extent still are, ignorant of what can be done to improve the quality of life of the disabled child and the family. Attitudinal negativism on the part of health professionals can be not only detrimental but also soul destroying.

Where only half of the children without disabilities survive to maturity, prevailing attitudes often lead to their neglect. In harsh circumstances, such as the Kalahari desert, !Kung women buried physically deformed infants at birth even if the child was alive. In so-called enlightened countries, disabled children are often abandoned, neglected, or abused. However, these children should be considered special or exceptional children. Attitude and community support can go a long way to developing them to their fullest potential if resources are made available.

It has been argued that money is better spent on prevention of blindness than on a school for the blind; however, both are needed and complement each other. In an unusually disadvantaged part of Africa, blind children in the community rarely survived. A school was started with about twenty small children who were fed, taught to read and write using braille, sing, make baskets, look after themselves,

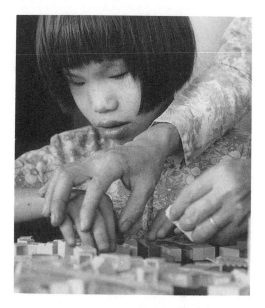

Figure 14.5. Helping children to realize their full potential. A blind Vietnamese girl receives a manual dexterity lesson as part of rehabilitation. Prevention of and early screening for vitamin A deficiency will reduce the incidence of blindness in developing countries. UNICEF photograph by J. Danios, Vietnam.

and carry out domestic chores. They were cheerful and active and often went back to their own families for days at a time. The families were enormously impressed that these children could read when they themselves could not, and their once fatalistic and hopeless attitude changed. They became interested in the possibilities of good medical care and eager to find out how blindness could be prevented or how their children could live happier, more productive lives.

One in ten children may be blind, deaf, or mentally retarded, or they may have other difficulties in learning, moving, seeing, hearing, or developing social relationships as a result of some physical or sensory impairment (One in Ten 1992). The challenge to health workers is to find ways to address the special problems of these children through community primary health care systems (Fig. 14.5). Of the 150 million disabled children, 120 million are in developing countries, where 93 percent of all disabled persons (adults and children) lack access to rehabilitation of any kind (One in Ten 1992). In Zambia a house-to-house survey showed large numbers of children are affected. Forty percent of the disabled children were physically disabled, 20 percent had vision problems, and 20 percent had hearing problems. In addition, 10 percent had learning disabilities and 10 percent multiple disabilities.

Simple screening techniques can be used in the community to identify problems and their causes so the necessary services and support can be implemented (Werner and Bower 1992). Most of the physical and mental impairment of children in developing countries can be prevented (Table 14.3). The disabilities are mainly due to inadequate nutrition, faulty child-bearing practices, preventable infectious diseases, including micronutrient defi-ciencies (iodide and iron), toxic chemicals (lead, mercury), and accidents. Measures such as improved support for MCH services, health education, disease control, and improved nutrition and environmental control of pesticides and chemicals can make a difference. Specific primary health care measures include the prevention of xerophthalmia, endemic goiter, and accidents, the control of trachoma, and immunization against poliomyelitis and measles.

Concurrently secondary prevention must be pursued. Early case finding means that the severity of contractures, birth defects, accidents, and other problems can be averted, arrested, or minimized. New information and techniques can be modified locally, and the child can thus be helped to reach a fuller potential (Ober and Thangavelu 1981).

Much can be achieved by ingenuity and adaptation. In China, bicycles have been adapted through simple modifica-

Table 14.3. Measures for Effectively Reducing Disabling Conditions: Selected Pointers

Primary preventions
  Supervise antenatal and birth practices
  Provide good nutrition (iodine in the maternal diet, vitamin A, folate, and zinc)
  Immunize against severe infections that cause disability (measles, polio, tetanus, whooping cough, diphtheria)
  Treat infections early (meningococcal meningitis, gonococcal ophthalmitis, tuberculosis, yaws, Hansen's disease, trachoma)
  Prevent accidents in home, workplace, and community (prevent drug and alcohol abuse, use fireguards, ensure occupational safety)
  Discourage consanguineous marriages
  Monitor community for chemicals (pesticides) and drugs
  Avoid chemical and drug exposure to fetus (smoking, lead, mercury, pesticides, alcohol, thalidomide)

Secondary prevention
  Educate the public to avoid stigmatization
  Detect early (through surveys and surveillance, screen older mothers)
  Train health workers for positive attitude, recognition, and action
  Develop appropriate technology for rehabilitation (effective for 80 percent at local level)
  Develop methods and materials to treat and train community in rehabilitation
  Train the child in home environs, preferably in local school when school aged
  Find ways to help child contribute to and belong in community (sheltered employment, independent living units)
  Employ fair practices
  Provide rights of access
  Provide relief care

Note: For these measures to be effective, efforts must involve all concerned ministries, including health, education, and labor; as always, selection of the most effective measures is needed when resources are limited.

tions so paraplegics can be mobile, by hand pedaling instead of foot pedaling. A wheelchair model designed for use in developing countries and has helped to increase the mobility of physically impaired children considerably. The chair is made of bicycle parts, bamboo, canvas, and wood (Int. Rehabil. Rev. 1983).

There is growing recognition that disabled children can develop skills and abilities to a far greater extent than previously thought possible (Mittler 1983). Ideally a team approach is needed, with health professionals, specialists, parents, and community volunteers working together. Even in the absence of specialists, just knowing what has been done elsewhere and how it was done has resulted in adaptations. Fashioning prostheses from used tires has provided incredible mobility—even climbing a tree. Such improvisations may not be as aesthetic as costly commercial limbs, but they function as well. Constant stimulation is important, as well as trying for small gains through a breakdown of tasks and giving strong praise to the child for a lot of effort and maybe little progress.

Early recognition and treatment of disabilities through local programs have begun in some countries involving relevant sectors such as physical therapy, health, and nutrition within the primary care setting. The Portage guide to home teaching is a successful example of such a program. It was originally developed in a remote rural area of the United States, but is being adapted to meet the needs of countries that lack specialized services (such as the Caribbean Islands and India). The program involves a home visiting service in which selected community workers with only one week's intensive training visit families to help them teach the disabled child to set and reach short-term goals within the space of one or two weeks. Simple developmental checklists are used to help the community worker and parents pinpoint what the child can do in key areas of development, such as self-care skills, communication, play, and social development (Weber et al. 1975).

It is important to determine prevalence of disabilities through surveys in order to estimate the type of program and resources needed. The prevalence measures the tip of the iceberg of the diseased, chronically disabled children. Thus, the presence of one cretinous child may indicate that about 2 to 4 percent of children may be iodine deficient and a larger proportion of children may be impaired neurologically. In the case of cretinism (associated with mental retardation, deafness, and stunted growth), iodine administration prenatally can reduce the prevalence of these conditions. In many countries, including Myanmar and Vietnam, endemic cretinism is still a serious problem (One in Ten 1983; Stein 1981). Programs may make the problems worse, leave them unchanged, or improve them; hence, it is important to monitor the effects constantly.

Much can be done, but first awareness of the problems and change of attitudes are essential. In parts of Nepal, a community worker walked through a village hand in hand with a disabled child to demonstrate that disabled children are loved and cherished and that their condition is neither medically nor socially contagious (Mittler 1983).

Prevention

Causes of disabling conditions must be identified wherever possible. Toxic metals such as lead, mercury, or pesticides can cause mental retardation and neurological damage. Minamata's disease (WHO 1972) would have been prevented had more attention been paid initially to the clustering of cases in Japan. They were passed off as cerebral palsy and attributed to poor birth practices. Fortunately, in Japan, the umbilical cord is customarily stored in a special box. Thus, scientists were able to go back and analyze the chemical content of the dried umbilical cord. They found a high mercury level, proving that the so-called cerebral palsy was intrauterine mercury poisoning.

Health workers should be aware of marriage patterns or reproductive trends in a particular community that may influence the prevalence of certain disabilities, especially mental retardation. In parts of India, it has been estimated that 30 percent of cases of mental retardation are attributable to consanguineous marriages. Down's syndrome, a common form of mental retardation, is more common in children of older mothers. Although it may not be possible to change marriage and childbearing customs, children in these high-risk groups should be screened early so that families can understand and assist the child in reaching his or her developmental potential (Mittler 1981).

Health professionals, parents, and teachers must be educated to prevent stigmatization of disabled children and to improve their physical and psychological treatment. For example, many people are afraid of epilepsy. They should be taught how to handle a seizure so as to protect the child from injury. Old practices such as using tongue depressors cause more harm (damaged teeth) than good, since a large amount of pressure is necessary to open a jaw in the clonic phase of a grand mal seizure.

For children with severe disabilities, it may be necessary to provide residential care, particularly as the community becomes more urbanized. For these children, it is essential to monitor the quality of care constantly and to ensure that they are not neglected or abused.

Programs for early detection and therapy are of little use if the child grows up only to be neglected as an adult. Whenever possible, the disabled should be gainfully employed, however limited the job—often by using his or her unaffected faculties. Supervised, sheltered employment should be developed and disabled persons trained to be as self-supporting

as possible in their society. In a southern African community, a plant nursery was organized where mentally retarded epileptics could be productive and self-supporting while working and living under supervision.

Programs are needed at all levels, from early detection in villages to support and coordination by ministries. Activities and resources of voluntary, private, and government agencies should be incorporated into community MCH services.

Not only do the disabled have limitations imposed on them by their condition, but by society and often by health professionals. This situation is improving with prevention and new attitudes toward rehabilitation, so individuals can enter the mainstream and be as independent as possible (Baumslag and Yodaiken 1972; Joint Comm. on Intl. Aspects of Mental Retardation 1980; Wolfensberger 1975).

MENTAL HEALTH

Every culture has definitions of normal and abnormal behavior. In developing countries, there is usually an indigenous system for diagnosing and dealing with aberrant behavior and mental disease within the local cultural context. Different communities have differently defined forms of mental and psychological abnormal behavior.

Integration of mental health services with general health services has been the key to providing mental health care to a widely dispersed population with limited resources. Initiatives involving nonmedical community members, such as traditional healers, teachers, and religious leaders, have been undertaken in many countries, including Colombia, India, the Philippines, Senegal, and Sudan (Asuni 1975; WHO 1975). Treatment within the community by primary health workers, even for more severe mental disorders, is now a realistic alternative to institutionalization, which was often inhumane. In some countries "psychiatric villages" have been created, where brief periods of intensive treatment can be given in a setting that is familiar to patients from rural areas. Other countries are stressing the creation of small psychiatric units, staffed by nonspecialists, in general hospitals.

In Western culture mental health programs traditionally have been very fragmented and usually deal with a specialized problem in isolation from the family unit or the community. Problems of alcohol and drug abuse, suicidal crises, depression or stress, and childhood behavioral disorders are often dealt with by vertical programs, and are recognized too late to be effectively treated.

An integrated family-oriented health care service can address psychological problems at the primary care level, focusing on early recognition of emotional and psychological disturbances. A young child may not develop full mental capacity if early mental stress or lack of stimulation goes unrecognized. Mental illness of family members may affect marital relationships, parenting, and physical health.

The trend toward urbanization has been described as a major stress factor contributing to psychiatric disorders as families become isolated from their traditionally extended family support. Studies in London have shown that working-class women are particularly vulnerable to depression, and as many as one in five need psychotropic drugs (Ebrahim 1982). Contrary to popular belief, rural women may be under at least as much stress as their urban counterparts. A study in a mountainous region of El Salvador revealed that 67 percent of women of childbearing age had at some point been prescribed tranquilizers. Most of these women exhibited signs of anxiety neuroses stemming from a cycle of early and frequent childbearing and tragic losses, poverty, poor health, and circumstances of life that were stressful beyond reason. The

men in this region suffered an extremely high rate of alcoholism (Harrison 1982).

Prevalence and types of psychological stress and mental illness vary from one community to the next. Problems should be diagnosed in each area and family-oriented mental health programs designed to meet local needs. Community support groups play an important role in any mental health program; they offer a means of communication and acceptance that is critical to coping with or recovering from the illness. The most well-known group is Alcoholics Anonymous. Support groups have also been helpful for such problems as drug abuse, family violence, chronic depression, and phobias.

In certain situations, family stress may have a negative impact on child rearing:

1. Frequent pregnancies (several preschool children at home).
2. A premature or low-birthweight infant or a physically or mentally disabled child.
3. A single-parent household or the equivalent (parent away physically due to job, service, or abandonment; parent away psychologically).
4. Financial strain.
5. Emotionally disturbed (depression, anxiety, schizophrenia) or mentally retarded parent.
6. History of alcohol or drug abuse.
7. Marital discord.
8. Social immaturity of parent (adolescent).
9. Warfare, community, and political unrest and violence.

Many of the risk factors are similar to those leading to child abuse. In addition to family violence, these stressful conditions can lead to neglect, emotional deprivation, lack of stimulation, failure to thrive, malnutrition, learning disabilities, low expectations, difficult social relationships, and socially unacceptable or delinquent behavior.

When a family or individual is

undergoing a crisis, either short term (divorce, birth, death, acute illness) or long term (chronic illness, mental or physical disability), a healthy pattern is evident if the crisis is being dealt with satisfactorily:

1. An initial period of stunned denial. The family cannot hear what is being said to them.
2. A period of confusion, anxiety, and frequently resentment of the sick family member.
3. A period of recovery and reorganization.

Supporting help from health professionals depends on the stage of stress and can alleviate unnecessary strain and facilitate readjustment (Baumslag 1973).

The sensitivity and training of health workers is critical to their effectiveness in dealing with mental illness. More than in the physical realm, the health worker's degree of success depends on attitudes toward the patient, the family, and the type of illness. Subconsciously, most people impose their own cultural values and attitudes on those with different life-styles. A word association test can be used to uncover negative attitudes and is the first step toward changing them. This is also a useful technique for assessing a patient's own concepts, attitudes, and priorities or for helping a family to deal with stressful situations such as death (Baumslag 1973).

Because mental health is somewhat ill defined, the tendency for many health programs has been to neglect it. However, a health care program is not complete unless it addresses mental health issues. By improving knowledge of health and natural processes and by creating habits of observation and consideration for the needs of others, especially the young and the helpless, we can change behavior. Mental life is what makes life valuable (Gruenberg 1980), and a health worker must be concerned with the whole person.

ORPHANS

Of the 2 billion children in the world today, 70 million live without families (UN 1982). In countries such as New Guinea in the past, if the biological parent died, there was no difficulty in finding substitute parents (Mead 1930). The same was true in Ghana in the 1930s, where abandonment was rare. Currently in Latin America, at least one in five children are abandoned (40 million), in Asia 20 million, and 10 million in Africa. With increasing urbanization, these numbers are expected to rise. Many children in urban areas have become street children.

The problems of the street children have been created by poverty with erosion of traditional values, a breakdown of family structure, rapid urbanization, high birthrates and no adequate method of child spacing, and unwanted children. Family responsibility, especially among teenagers, shows marked variability in different cultures.

Children without families, street children, abandoned or abused children, refugees, and those working under intolerable conditions constitute a hidden or infrequently recognized source of mortality and morbidity. These children are frequently exploited. Newer approaches to neglected children stress the importance of integrating the child into the family and community through foster homes, when feasible.

PROGRAMS FOR UNMARRIED AND ADOLESCENT WOMEN

There are areas where women who have become disabled by disease or by incompetent midwifery (perineal tears, fistulas) are rejected by their families, especially their husbands, and live, or usually die, under terrible conditions. Improved obstetrical and medical services should reduce the number of such tragedies, but as long as they exist, the department of maternal and child health should provide rehabilitation or shelter for them and persuade the families that these unfortunate women need health care as well as consideration.

One of the most serious problems women suffer is vesico-vaginal-fistulas (VVF). A special center in Nigeria has been developed for women with VVF through the Nigerian National Women's Federation. The center provides surgical services for the women and has attempted to support itself through the work of the patients. The women make detergents, soaps, and body creams for their own use and for sale to support the center (WIPHN News 1991).

In some parts of the world, a girl or woman who has in the slightest degree infringed the cultural code of behavior—even if she was raped—may be killed, brutally punished, or expelled from her tribe or family. Every country and culture has its own methods of dealing with these problems, but unless provisions are adequate, the girl often has a choice only between suicide and prostitution. In Italy there is the *brefotrophio,* generally attached to a convent, where a mother can stay before her illegitimate baby is born and for some time after. In India, Latin America, and many other areas, there are homes where these girls can live and learn some type of craft. In Europe and North America, there are numbers of homes where they receive medical care and continue their education and training so they can support themselves. However, in the United States and other countries, there is often no follow-up, and after giving birth, these women find themselves alone with their infant and no means of support (Baumslag 1981).

Whatever may be accepted in a permissive society, it is still the woman who pays the price and who needs special protection because of her reproductive faculties, actual or potential. Some of the eternal truths are contained in the tritest of songs: "Plaisir d'amour ne dure qu'un instant, Chagrin d'amour dure toute la vie" ("Even when there has been no pleasure to start with—only fright and shame").

Problems relating to the permissive society and the generation gap have created a special need for adolescent pregnancy prevention programs. Early and out-of-wedlock childbearing is a problem in many parts of the world, with negative consequences for both the young mother and her family (Field 1981). Studies of infants born to teenage mothers indicate that these infants are a high-risk group due to such factors as low socioeconomic status, poor nutrition, no support from the father, lack of prenatal care, and a higher rate of pregnancy and delivery complications. There is a higher incidence of low-birthweight infants among adolescent mothers (Monkus and Bancalari 1981), as well as evidence of more long-term developmental problems (Broman 1981).

The existence of special programs indicates that the preventive need is not being met. Education on family planning and responsible parenting should be incorporated into the school curriculum of adolescents. For those who work, educational campaigns can be channeled through women's groups, religious and educational societies, political organizations, and labor unions. Information about their own bodies and nonjudgmental family planning counseling and assistance must be available (Sarrel 1980).

Another aspect of primary prevention is vocational training. With the rapid social changes occurring worldwide, it is most often adolescents, especially girls, who have no job prospects and have recourse only to childbearing or the sex trade as a means of enriching their lives.

DAY CARE CENTERS

Where mothers work, child care programs should be developed to meet specific needs identified by parents and the community, such as day care, seasonal care (in rural areas), industry-based child care facilities, nursery schools, temporary care of children whose mothers are in skills training programs, and other modalities such as neighborhood home-based care, housing complex care, and drop-in care for occasional need (Fig. 14.6). These programs need medical supervision, health care linkages, provision for immunization, screening, and referral, and guidelines to ensure a sanitary and nutritious environment, as well as on-site training of staff.

While alternative care is recognized as important, a study in six developing countries on the child care needs of low-income mothers revealed that less than 1 percent of children have access to day care centers, and those who are cared for are, typically, not from low-income families (Overseas Education Fund 1979). Among the constraints listed were cost of services, lack of transportation, and additional clothes and supplies that made creches out of reach of most low-income families. Hours of operation and the inability to take sick children further limited their usefulness. In general families preferred sending children more than 3 years old if given an option. Many were concerned that the factory was not a safe environment for their children and preferred community-based centers. Whether their fears are justifiable is difficult to determine in the absence of data, but it is clear that children who live near toxic or harmful chemicals can be at risk for poisoning. In a study of a Texas community exposed to a lead smelting plant, a group of children living near the plant

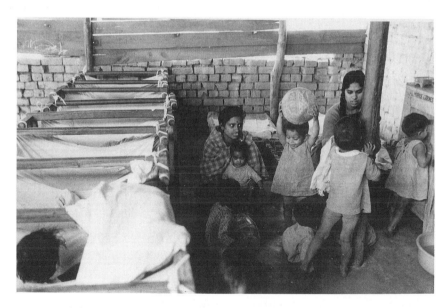

Figure 14.6. Mobile day care. Mobile health care in New Delhi provides custodial, medical, and nutritional education services to children of nomadic laborers and health services and education to the parents. Unless these centers have adequate facilities (space, toilets), use trained staff, provide potable water, maintain sanitary standards, and are well supervised, they become traps for infection, especially lethal to bottle-fed infants. Furthermore, child abuse and sexual assault have been reported to occur in some day care centers. As a safeguard, mothers should have ready access to children, lactation breaks for breastfeeding should be provided, and family involvement should be ensured. Israeli kibbutzim ensure care and safety of their children while parents work. UNICEF photograph by A. Heymann, India.

had high levels of lead in their blood, lower IQs, and early evidence of neurological impairments as elicited by a finger-wrist tapping test (Landrigan et al. 1975).

Day care centers should be the focus of health and nutrition education and can play a direct role in improving intellectual development and physical well-being of children under age 5. In addition, they can be a source of employment and education for the mothers and the community (WHO 1983).

Creches are a fundamental aspect of large-scale industry in countries such as Russia and Cuba (where many are excellent) and among the jute mills of Bombay and silk factories in China. Moreover, they can be important in facilitating continued breastfeeding as well as family planning and should be available to health center and hospital staff too. While in socialist countries government attention is given to child care for working mothers, in capitalistic countries it is usually the mother's sole responsibility (WHO 1980a). Child care services should at least be extended to low-income mothers, especially to those in domestic employment.

CHILD-TO-CHILD PROGRAMS

The fact that 350 million children in developing countries were beyond the reach of even a minimum of essential services led to the development of an outreach program for school-aged children. The children helped with the health of other children, especially siblings, and learned basic preventive measures appropriate for their community (Aarons and Hawes 1979). They learned the causes of death, accidents, and disease and how to prevent them through simple measures.

Use was also made of "health scouts," taught how to collect data such as the number of children immunized or nutritionally at risk or to identify malnourished children (through the use of arm circumference measurements). Scouts have also helped to screen children for visual and hearing impairments through simple charts and games (Werner and Bower 1992).

Children are an enthusiastic and fertile source of health education and promotion and can work with health workers and teachers in changing attitudes and practices in the community. Examples of child-to-child activities include accident prevention, understanding children with special problems, and care of children with diarrhea. Children constitute an important form of outreach hitherto untapped.

BABY SHOWS

Old-style "baby shows" or competitive pageants are revolting and incompatible with human dignity. To most mothers, their babies are the best in the world. The mothers who genuinely need encouragement are those who manage to cherish difficult and unresponsive children. They should be considered and supported in every way. Among poorer communities, it is remarkable how an occasional trivial mark of recognition, according to the situation, can be appreciated as true encouragement. A Christmas party or other culturally appropriate occasion, rather than a baby show, to which all diligent parents (and a good many others) are invited with their children appears to be a popular method of expressing goodwill and mutual interest.

AIDS PROGRAMS

There is no cure for AIDS, and the only prevention available is behavioral change. As well as health education, there is a growing need for compassionate care. TASCO, an AIDS support organization in Kampala, Uganda, provides hope, compassion, and practical support to families affected by AIDS. Many of its volunteers are themselves HIV positive or have lost relatives to AIDS. These volunteers are supplied with kits that include rehydration salts to prevent diarrhea dehydration and home care kits containing soup, antiseptic cream, and protective rubber gloves. Counseling sessions and home visits, particularly to families who cannot read government posters and leaflets, are carried out by trained volunteers. The program trains health workers, religious leaders, and volunteers basic counseling skills.

TASCO volunteers visit families daily. They have found that when time is spent with family members, explaining how the virus is contracted and talking through the family's fears, the family is better able to cope with caring for the sick. The tradition of families taking care of ill family members is being threatened by fear of AIDS.

TASCO provides some employment for AIDS victims. It sponsors a project, with funds and schooling, directed at grandparents who support orphaned children. TASCO is also developing a project to enable women who have lost their husbands to become economically independent.

In addition to material support, volunteers provide eggs and milk to patients for protein and selected low-cost medicines that include herbal remedies. This extraordinary program was started by a woman who nursed her AIDS-infected husband.

CONCLUSION

MCH services should assist women and children of all ages to make the best use of amenities and opportunities, actual and potential, and to show consideration for the rights and feelings of others. Special programs need to be considered or special aspects emphasized and integrated into primary health care in order to ac-

complish this, as soon as and as much as is possible. The danger is that each field, from services for the disabled to malaria control to AIDS prevention, wants its own program. Unless funding mechanisms encourage integration of special programs into primary care, much effort and resources will be wasted.

REFERENCES

Aarons, A., and Hawes, H. (1979). *Child to Child*. Macmillan Press, London.

Arole, R. S. (1977). India: The comprehensive rural health project, Jamkhed. In *Community Action: Family Nutrition Programmes*. Ed. D. B. Jelliffe and E. G. B. Jelliffe. Proceedings of a Joint IUNS/UNICEF/ICMR Working Conference, Hyderabad, India.

Asuni, T. (1975). Existing concepts of mental illness in different cultures and traditional forms of treatment. In *Mental Health Services in Developing Countries*. Ed. T. A. Baasher et al. World Health Organization, Geneva.

Bailey, K. V., and Raba, A. (1976). Supplementary feeding programmes. In *Nutrition in Preventive Medicine*. Ed. J. M. Bengoa. World Health Organization, Geneva.

Baumslag, N. (1973). *Family Care*. Williams & Wilkins, Baltimore.

Baumslag, N. (1975). *Report of the State Task Force on Maternal and Infant Nutrition*. Report of the Chairperson, Department of Human Resources, Atlanta, Georgia.

Baumslag, N. (1981). *Supplementary Feeding*. Lesotho National Workshop on Breast-Feeding. Trip Report Contract no. PDC-0262-1-00-1011-00. Office of Nutrition, U.S. Agency for International Development, Washington, D.C.

Baumslag, N. (1982). Food distribution. In *Famine in Africa*. Ed. J. P. Carter. Pergamon Press, New York.

Baumslag, N., and Yodaiken, R. E. (1972). Social aspects of care of special people. *New Engl. J. Med.* 286(a), 220.

Beaton, G. H., and Ghassemi, H. (1978). Supplementary feeding programmes for young children in developing countries. *Am. J. Clin. Nutr.* (Suppl.) 35, 864.

Bell, J. E. (1969). *The Family in Hospital: Les-*

sons from Developing Countries. U.S. Government Printing Office, Washington, D.C.

Bengoa, J. M. (1967). Nutrition rehabilitation centres. *J. Trop. Pediat.* **13**, 169.

Berg, A. (1973). *The Nutrition Factor.* Brookings Institution, Washington, D.C.

Broman, S. H. (1981). Long-term development of children born to teenagers. In *Teenage Parents and Their Offspring.* Ed. K. G. Scott, T. Field, and E. Robertson. Grune & Stratton, New York.

Burress, J. A., and Perlman, L. G. (1980). *Developments in Services for Handicapped People in Africa.* People to People Committee for the Handicapped, Washington, D.C.

Cody, C. L. (1981). Nature and rates of adverse reactions to DPT and DT immunizations in infants and children. *Pediatrics* **68**, 650.

Cook, R. (1966). Comprehensive immunization in rural areas. *J. Trop. Pediat. Monogr.* **2**, 13.

Cook, R. (1968). The Ankole Pre-School Protection Programme, 1964–67. Mimeographed. Kampala, Uganda.

de Ville de Goyet, C.; Seaman, J.; and Geijer, U. (1978). *The Management of Nutritional Emergencies in Large Populations.* World Health Organization, Geneva.

Ebrahim, G. J. (1982). *Child Health in a Changing Environment.* Macmillan, London.

Field, B. C. (1981). Socio-economic analysis of out-of-wedlock births among teenagers. In *Teenage Parents and Their Offspring.* Ed. K. G. Scott, T. Field, and E. Robertson. Grune & Stratton, New York.

Fitzgerald, S., and Gowers, P. (1983). Blueprint for success: The Gambian immunization programme. *Wld. Hlth. Forum* **4**, 79.

Gonzales, C. L. (1965). *Mass Campaigns and General Health Services.* Wld. Hlth. Org. Publ. Hlth. Pap., no. 29.

Grant, J. (1992). *The State of the World's Children 1992.* UNICEF, New York.

Gruenberg, E. M. (1980). Mental disorders. In *Public Health and Preventive Medicine.* 11th ed. Ed. J. M. Last. Appleton-Century-Crofts, New York.

Halsey, N. A., and Quadros, C. A. (1983). *Recent Advances in Immunization: A Bibliographic Review.* Scientific Publication no. 451. PAHO, Washington, D.C.

Harrison, P. (1982). Mothers in distress. *Co-Evolution Quarterly* **26.**

Haxton, D. P. (1982). Introductory remarks.

Rehabilitation International/UNICEF Seminar on Childhood Disabilities: Policies and Programmes. *One in Ten* **2**, 2.

Hull, H. F.; Williams, P. J.; and Oldfield, F. (1983). Measles mortality and vaccine efficacy in rural West Africa. *Lancet* **i**, 27.

ICN (1992). *Major Issues in Nutrition Strategies.* Theme paper no. 1, Improving household food security. FAO/WHO, Rome.

Int. Rehabil. Rev. (1983). National news wheelchair for developing countries. *International Rehabilitation Review* **2**, 6.

Jelliffe, D. B., and Jelliffe, E. F. P. (1981). Refugee medicine. *Sciences* **4**, 14.

Jelliffe, D. B., and Jelliffe, E. F. P. (1984). The principle of multimixes. In *Advances in International Maternal and Child Health,* vol. 4. Ed. D. B. Jelliffe and E. F. P. Jelliffe. Oxford University Press, Oxford.

Joint Commission on International Aspects of Mental Retardation (1980). *Mental Retardation: Prevention, Amelioration and Service Delivery.* Ed. A. D. B. Clarke and P. J. Mittler. International League of Societies for the Mentally Handicapped (for World Health Organization), Brussels.

Karlin, B. (1976). *APHA Summary on the State of Art of Delivering Low Cost Health Services in Less Developed Countries.* American Public Health Association, Washington, D.C.

Karzon, D. T., and Henderson, D. A. (1966). Current status of live attenuated virus vaccines. *Adv. Pediat.* **14**, 121.

Kimura, M. and Kuno-Sakai, H. (1991). Pertussis vaccine in Japan. *J. Trop. Pediat.* **37**, 45.

King, M. H., ed. (1966). *Medical Care in Developing Countries.* Oxford University Press, Nairobi.

Lancet (1983). Child health: A co-ordinated approach to children's health in India, Progress report after five years (1975–1980). *Lancet* **i**, 109.

Landrigan, P. J.; Whitworth, A. F.; Baloh, R. W.; Stathehling, N. W.; Barthe, W. F.; and Rosenblum, B. F. (1975). Neuro psychological dysfunction in children with chronic low level lead absorption. *Lancet* **i**, 708.

Lappe, F. M. and Collins, J. (1977). *Food First, Beyond the Myth of Scarcity.* Houghton Mifflin, Boston.

Lechtig, A.; Habicht, J. P.; Urrutia, J. J.; Klein, R. E.; Yarbrough, C.; and Martorell, R. (1975). Effect of food supplementation during pregnancy on birth weight. *Pediatrics* **56**, 508.

Levy, B. S. (1981). Working in a camp for Cambodian refugees. *New Engl. J. Med.* **304**, 1440.

Loening, W. E. K. and Coovadia, H. M. (1983). Age-specific occurrence rates of measles in urban peri urban and rural environments implications for time of vaccination. *Lancet* **2**, 324.

Mead, M. (1930). *Growing Up in New Guinea*, Peter Smith, Magnolia, Mass.

Mittler, P. (1981). Finding and helping severely mentally handicapped children in developing countries: Summary of discussions. *Int. J. Men. Hlth.* **10**, 107.

Mittler, P. (1983). Meeting the global challenge of mental handicap. *Int. Rehabil. Rev.* **2**, 4.

Moffat, D. (1969). The Ankole Pre-School Protection Programme, 1964–67. mimeographed, Kampala, Uganda.

Monkus, E. and Bancalari, E. (1981). Neonatal outcome. In *Teenage Parents and Their Offspring*. Ed. K. G. Scott, T. Field, and E. Robertson. Grune & Stratton, New York.

Mora, J. O.; King, J. M.; and Teller, C. H. (1990). *The Effectiveness of Maternal and Child Health Supplementary Feeding Programs: An Analysis of Performance in the 1980s and Potential Role in the 1990s.* Logical Technical Services, Bethesda, Md.

Morley, D.; Woodland, M.; and Martin, W. J. (1961). Measles in Nigerian children. *J. Hyg.* (Lond.) **61**, 115.

Ober, J. K. and Thangavelu, M. (1981). The need for the appropriate technology approach in lower extremity orthontics in India. *Appropriate Tech. for Health* **9**, 4.

Olness, K. (1981). A health outreach to a refugee camp: Perspectives for would-be volunteers. *Pediatrics* **67**, 523.

One in Ten (1983). Overview programming for childhood disability. *One in Ten* **2**, 6.

One in Ten (1992). A few alarming facts about childhood disability. *One in Ten* **2**, 52.

Overseas Education Fund (1979). *Child Care Needs of Low Income Mothers.* Final report: *A synthesis of Recommendations from an International Conference.* USAID grant TAG-1413. Washington, D.C.

PAHO (1981). *Immunization and Primary Health Care: Problems and Solutions.* Report on regional meetings of the Expanded Programme on Immunization, Scientific Publication no. 417. Pan American Health Organization, Washington, D.C.

PAHO (1982). *Health Conditions in the Americas, 1977–1980.* Pan American Health Organization, Washington D.C.

PAHO (1990). *Health Conditions in the Americas.* Pan American Health Organization, Washington, D.C.

Rush, D. (1982). Effects of changes in protein and calorie intake during pregnancy on the growth of the human foetus. In *Effectiveness and Satisfaction in Antenatal Care.* Ed. M. Enkin and I. Chalmers. Clinics in Developmental Medicine nos. 81/82. Spastics International Medical Publications, London.

Sabin, E. and Stinson, W. (1981). *Primary Health Care Issues: Immunizations.* American Public Health Association, Washington, D.C.

Sarrel, P. M. (1980). Who speaks for prevention? In *Maternity Care in Ferment: Conflicting Issues, the Edith C. Blum Memorial Seminar.* Ed. M. Kelly. Maternity Center Association, New York.

Schofield, F. D.; Tucker, V. M.; and Westbrook, G. R. (1961). Neonatal tetanus in New Guinea: Effect of active immunization in pregnancy. *Brit. Med. J.* **2**, 785.

Simmonds, S.; Vaughan, P.; and Gunn, S. W. (1983). *Refugee Community Health Care.* Oxford University Press, Oxford.

Stanfield, J. P. (1967). Organization of MCH services in developing regions, VI. Special programmes—immunization. *J. Trop, Pediat.* **13**, 102.

Stanfield, J. P. (1970). History taking and clinical examination. In *Diseases of Children in the Subtropics and Tropics.* 2d ed. Ed. D. B. Jelliffe. Edward Arnold, London.

Stein, Z. (1981). Why is it useful to measure incidence and prevalence? *Int. J. Men. Hlth.* **10**, 14.

Swedish Nutr. Fdtn. (1970). *Proceedings of a Symposium on Emergency Feeding.* Swedish Nutrition Foundation, Stockholm.

TB prevention trials (1979). Madras trial of BCG vaccines in South India for tuberculosis prevention. *Indian J. Med. Res.* **70**, 349.

Tshabalala, R. T. (1983). Anaphylactic reactions to BCG in Swaziland. *Lancet* **i**, 653.

UN (1982). *Urban Basic Services: Reaching Children and Women of the Urban Poor.* Report by the Executive Director of UNICEF. E/ICEF/L.1440. United Nations Economic and Social Council, 1982 session, New York.

UNICEF (1990). *Children and Development in the 1990s.* UNICEF sourcebook. United Nations, New York.

UNICEF (1991). *1991 UNICEF Annual Report.* UNICEF, New York.

USCR (1991). *World Refugee Survey 1991.* U.S. Committee for Refugees, Washington, D.C.

Weber, S. J.; Jesien, G. S.; Shearer, D. E.; Bluma, S. M.; Hilliard, J. M.; Shearer, M. S.; Schoringhios, N. E.; and Boyd, R. D. (1975). *The Portage Guide to Home Teaching.* Cooperative Educational Service Agency, Portage, Wisc.

Werner, D. (1988). *Disabled Village Children: A Guide for Community Health Workers, Rehabilitation Workers and Families.* Hesperian Foundation, Palo Alto, Calif.

Werner, D., and Bower, B. (1992). Children as health workers. In *Helping Health Workers Learn,* 2d ed. Hesperian Foundation, Palo Alto, Calif.

WIPHN News (1991). Women's International Public Health Network. *WIPHN News* 10, 7.

Wolfensberger, W. (1975). *The Principle of Normalization in Human Services.* National Institute on Mental Retardation, Toronto.

WHO (1972). *Health Hazards of the Human Environment.* World Health Organization, Geneva.

WHO (1975). *Organization of Mental Health Services in Developing Countries.* Wld. Hlth. Org. Tech. Rep. Ser., 564.

WHO (1980a). *Sixth Report on the World Health Situation, 1973–77,* Pt. One: *Global Analysis.* World Health Organization, Geneva.

WHO (1980b). *BCG Vaccination Policies: Report of a WHO Study Group.* Wld. Hlth. Org. Tech. Rep. Ser., no. 652.

WHO (1983). *Global Medium-Term Programme for Family Health.* Sixth general programme of work covering the specific period 1978–1983. FHE/79.4. World Health Organization, Geneva.

WHO (1992). *Implementation of the Global Strategy for Health for All by the Year 2000.* 2d ed. 8th Report on the World Health Situation. World Health Organization, Geneva.

World Summit for Children (1990). *The World Summit for Children.* UNICEF, New York.

15

Organization

*I say to you today . . . that in spite of the difficulties and
frustrations of the moment I still have a dream.*
MARTIN LUTHER KING, JR., 1963

There is a general recognition that basic health is a part of overall development and no longer a privilege but a right. The danger, however, is that people's expectations will be raised beyond societies' capabilities to respond. The pressing challenge lies in our ability to organize available knowledge and technology, adapting them to local needs and finding practical ways to solve global problems of health care coverage (Smith 1978). Services must be decentralized, rationalized, given priorities, adapted, and supervised through better management with more equitable distribution of services. Health guidelines have to be developed, a policy decided on, and legislation passed. There should be a long-term plan.

Currently in many developing countries, less than 20 percent of mothers and children have access to health care, and millions of children are not fully immunized (USAID 1992). Hence, the objectives should be: (1) to extend existing services; (2) to make them inexpensive so that adequate and easily accessible coverage is possible; (3) to organize in such a way as to attract the majority; and (4), most important, to reach those most at risk. Services should be comprehensive geographically and functionally family oriented. They must be economically feasible and geared to felt needs.

This is a formidable task. Priorities should be aimed at the groups at risk, building on existing advantages with phased, enlightened expansion. No countries would claim that they have as yet achieved all their goals. Failures have occurred mainly because so few of the authorities, national or international, have given much time or attention, understanding, or priority to this subject or because of rising costs and other social issues. National planners have to be persuaded that children are a good investment and that a healthy population is a necessary component of economic development.

Fragmentation of MCH services and lack of communication have obstructed good work, comprehensive care, and continuity. Feedback and interaction must exist among hospitals, health centers, and home care services; among doctors, nurses, community health workers, social workers, agricultural extensionists, nutritionists, and health educators; among government, municipal and local authorities; and among private practitioners. Any obstacles can be surmounted by improved organization (Breslow 1969; Roemer 1991). In each country, public health should be considered and clearly defined. In one country, it is accepted as the health of the public as a whole, while in another, it is stated to be any procedure in which the patient does not pay the doctor directly.

Even in Scandinavia, where mother and child mortality rates are low, overlapping of services occurs, and many problems remain to be solved, among them, delinquency, suicide, drug abuse, violence, and child abuse. It has been said that developed countries have a high standard of living and a low standard of everything else. To aim merely at reducing mortality and morbidity is not enough.

MCH cannot be organized as an independent service. These services form a part of the hospital and health center activities. In addition to providing MCH services, a medical officer may have to serve a whole district and supervise all the hospitals and dispensaries, as well as any local environmental sanitation or disease control programs. Medical and health staff will require general training and supervision, as well as adequate mobility.

Care of women and children may be available as a community- or state-organized service. Private doctors and voluntary workers have been the pioneers, but all over the world results have shown that it is the government-organized structure that can produce spectacular improvements through a wide range of services.

Public health officers trained under inappropriate European or North American systems tend to believe that MCH is exclusively preventive and not curative. Therefore, they are not always interested in individual services, instead stressing mass services, such as the maintenance of water supply and pest control. Certainly these services are important, but

the individual has sometimes been neglected. Moreover, public health officers are often under a different chain of authority from the curative services staff, and this may cause difficulties in coordinating activities.

The best solution for overall organization is to have a planning unit in the ministry of health, which can examine the extent and content of the MCH services and the needs for the care of women and children in hospitals, health centers, and home care, in training programs, and in distribution and supervision of staff. Of primary concern is to guarantee equitable allocation between the relevant regions and districts, as well as economic groups.

There is a desperate need for suitable courses to be available at medical institutions for postgraduate education in the area of health service management and support. Some universities have reoriented their undergraduates toward family medicine and community medicine.

Often women and small children receive no special attention (even where those under age 5 account for 50 percent of the total mortality) unless particular interest exists in MCH at the policymaking level. If there is a children's ward in a hospital, it may be the area with a leaky roof. Forceful characters sent by international organizations will introduce projects well funded in electron microscopy, even in incubators for the premature, and divert limited resources from pressing common health problems. Programs for training health professionals and community health workers are often deplorable in child care and nutrition.

The MCH planning unit should examine all aspects of the health services that affect women and children. Close scrutiny will lead to more rational planning, save money and personnel, and extend the benefits of MCH services (WHO 1969, 1980). This would entail close collaboration with medical and nursing schools and with voluntary agencies and would incorporate work in the spheres of nutrition, health education, mental health, pediatrics, obstetrics, preventive or social medicine, statistics, and hospital administration. Services should be organized and coordinated by the MCH planner. In short, MCH planners should:

Plan a long-term MCH program, based on available background information and guided by the continuing collection of health data and statistics.

Direct, guide, and evaluate all activities that have a bearing on the health of children and families.

Advise the government on MCH problems and ensure that political and administrative leaders are aware of them.

Locally adapt guidelines for use in the health services.

Advise on, and support, appropriate legislation relative to mothers and children.

Diplomatically coordinate the activities of various governmental, volunteer, and university groups with activities in the health care of mothers and children, and in related training programs, without interfering with their prescribed duties.

Establish suitable training and refresher courses and seminars for all types of staff and voluntary workers.

Develop logistics for MCH services, especially supervision, communication, and supply distribution.

Maximize community participation.

Defined standards of care, however simple and tentative, are needed for guidance in local circumstances, and such guidelines are valuable in training programs. In many cases, however, the only "standard" is that of trying to do the best one can with what one has to improve the content and the extent of services. Vital and social statistics may prove to be the best and the only valid standards—and collecting such information may take time.

Until such time, developments need to be guided by the imperfect information attainable.

COMPREHENSIVE CARE

It is easy to talk about combining preventive and curative medicine but not always simple to implement (Morley et al. 1983). Generally, the first goal is to ensure that the sick are accommodated, diagnosed, and treated. But continuing supervision is essential. By sending nurses or community health workers out to hold weekly clinics in temporary accommodation (someone's garage, the veranda of a school, an unused shop, or house) or in rural areas, mothers whose infants are most in need of care can be persuaded to bring their babies at least once every month and nurses encouraged to provide home visits. In these small, local centers, supervision can become a social occasion while mutual education is fostered (Fig. 15.1).

For mothers who can bring their babies to the clinic only occasionally and see the health worker for just a few minutes, there is much to recommend the small, local, informal clinics. Minor treatments can be given on the spot; the health professional can visit the neighborhood and learn to know the families, their births and deaths, and their hazards. They will know the mothers and children recently discharged from hospital, and those referred to the outpatient department, and will be aware of any special care that is needed.

Babies change so rapidly in the first year of life that they should be seen frequently and regularly. Some mothers may be willing and even anxious to come every week, especially with the first baby. Furthermore, if use is made of neighborhood auxiliaries and voluntary workers, the demands on health staff need not be excessive. Health workers learn which families are most in need of supervision and

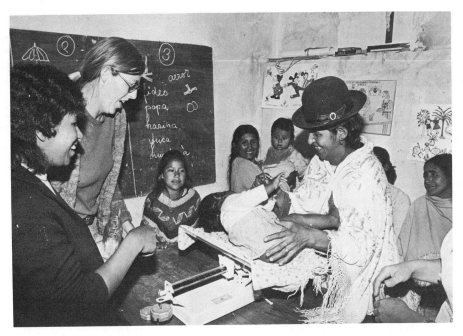

Figure 15.1. Comprehensive care and supervision—a social occasion. This weekly well-baby clinic is one of the activities of the mother's club in Irupana, Bolivia. UNICEF photograph by Cerni, Bolivia.

advice and can emphasize frequent attendance accordingly. Flexibility and good observation will ensure that those most in need receive the care that is necessary throughout episodes of health and ill health (Klarman 1967; Stewart 1959).

By establishing small clinics in neighborhoods, it is often possible to find an experienced mother who, in addition to the auxiliaries, will give neighborly help to the less experienced. Minimally trained aides and auxiliaries, with the encouragement of informal guidance and assistance, can help spread interest and knowledge in child care in gradually wider circles. Education is a process of growth; it cannot be expected to produce instant results.

Comprehensive care will foster good health in rural societies (Klarman 1967), as well as urban and industrial communities. People who are separated from their traditional modes of life, with all their protection and sanctions, need some form of organization that will help them make better use of available sophisticated technological developments.

Doctors, nurses, midwives, and students can work in wards and outpatient departments and follow up with their patients in health centers or homes (or with private doctors). This coordination gives the health staff an opportunity to correlate the diseases with the conditions that produce them. It varies the work load and makes the work more interesting and stimulating. Above all, it makes for better medical care and supervision. Care becomes more comprehensive, as well as more comprehending.

FACT FINDING

MCH planners must collect and make use of relevant information from local vital statistics on existing health services, types of staff and their training, the needs

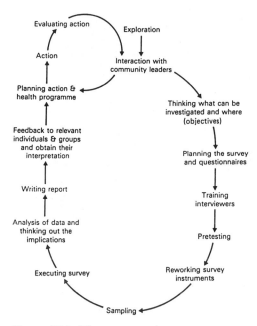

Figure 15.2. The process of community diagnosis and health action. Source: Bennett (1970).

of mothers and children, local economics, nutritional patterns, local attitudes, education, and traditions. More information than appreciated may be available or may await investigation, at least in approximate form, in the records of hospitals, in young child and prenatal clinics, and in health centers. Moreover, it is usually possible by minor modifications in record keeping and in the supervision of data collection to start a system for the collection of information (Brolly 1982). Information thus obtained from the health services or from existing demographic studies may be biased and incomplete but will give a broad idea of the overall picture, indicating those geographical areas not adequately covered and suggesting the need for more detailed investigation (Fig. 15.2).

As well as statistics showing the dimensions and forms of illness and deaths in women and children, information is required on the distribution and function of different components in the health service, on staff, training, and efficiency, and

on the effect of government policies on MCH services.

The MCH planner must weigh the imponderables and immeasurables. Educational, agricultural, and social workers as well as religious leaders, anthropologists, and indigenous practitioners should be consulted, so that appropriate activities based on their specialized insights can be undertaken in concert rather than in competition.

NATIONAL HEALTH PLAN

The MCH planner will have a major task in convincing the authorities of the need for developing MCH and the potential results (Arnold 1969; Bryant 1969; Cashman 1969; Klarman 1967; Mills 1983; Navarro 1969; Reinke 1972; Williams 1955). Health administrators have recognized the language and quantitative reasoning of economists and can state the case in terms that will convince economic planners and politicians that MCH services are not only "consumer" social services but play a key role in any national development plan (Abel-Smith 1968). Goals and objectives need to be laid down and the effect and the cost of the activities evaluated (Gish 1975; Reinke 1972).

Some countries have shown remarkable results with relatively small budgets. The former Soviet Union trained 30 percent of medical officers specifically for child care. Recent evidence suggests that services were less than satisfactory in many of the Eastern European countries. Czechoslovakia had an IMR of 133 immediately after World War II; by 1967 it was 17, and in 1990 it was reported as 11. In Poland, in 1935, life expectancy was 41 years, in spite of the devastation of World War II, including the deaths of many of the doctors; it rose to 68 by 1968 (Pop. Ref. Bur. 1983). These results have been achieved largely by an improved standard of living with emphasis on mother and child care and the importance of continuity of care. This is also allegedly true for China's health care system, which deserves close study and unbiased observation (Churchman 1968; Horn 1969).

The communist countries enforced a type of regimentation of staff and patients that would not be tolerated elsewhere and is breaking down now. It is also true that the attention to child health was accompanied by indoctrination—largely political but also fostering civic responsibility.

Gradual improvements in education, economics, and productivity will raise the standard of living. This is a slow process, and if it is not speeded up by vigorous MCH programs, then many disadvantaged families will remain disadvantaged. On the other hand, with good and realistic organization at a national level, the gross inequalities and inadequacies could be fairly rapidly and fairly inexpensively overcome.

The need everywhere is for an appropriate form of a interlocking, regionalized, satellite system that embraces home care and visiting, health centers and hospitals, and administration from the central, national, ministerial level, to the intermediate, regional level, and to the peripheral, local, or district level. The system should be based on clearly defined responsibilities, workable techniques of referral and supervision, and continuity of education.

Priorities and Rationale

The first priority is to have the idea of comprehensive care accepted at the highest political and administrative levels as an important component of any plan for national development (Bryant 1969; Churchman 1968; Dunlop and Caldwell 1977; UNICEF 1967). The second is to identify the areas and the age groups chiefly at risk and to categorize available resources of personnel, money, and materials (Djunkanovic and Mach 1975).

After that, methods of organizing the services and training the appropriate personnel may be instituted and gradually expanded and improved.

It is essential to seek cooperation with those working in other related fields. Voluntary societies can provide much help. International organizations, such as WHO, the Food and Agriculture Organization (FAO), the United Nations Educational, Scientific, and Cultural Organization (UNESCO), and the United Nations International Children's Education Fund (UNICEF) (Abel-Smith 1968; Robinson 1957; Stewart 1959; UN 1970; UNICEF 1963; UNICEF 1967; WHO 1969a, 1969b) may be consulted and will provide sources of help; so will voluntary international organizations such as the Save the Children Fund, CARE, International Planned Parenthood, Wellstart, and many others.

Pilot projects, demonstration centers, and feasibility studies are necessary and should always allow for expansion. Too often demonstration centers become show centers, demonstrating only that they are too elaborate, isolated, expensive, or atypical to be reproduced anywhere else.

Hospitals should be improved not only with the idea in mind that they should provide better and more appropriate treatment for women and children, but that they should act as the centers from which the organization of family care and supervision may radiate. This organization will avoid fragmentation of services and will provide centers for the continuing education and training of various grades of personnel, as well as practical, relevant research, investigation, assessment, and placement.

Adaptation

This is necessary at every turn. Needs must be studied, staff trained, and services organized to meet all needs (Finau 1983; Newell 1975; Williams 1955; WHO 1976).

There has been a tendency to develop a number of specialties and subspecialties and for intricate analytical work and laboratory research to be given the highest prestige, with accompanying salaries and career advancement. Hospitals have been the training institutions for doctors and nurses and tend to produce large numbers of specialists, subspecialists, and research workers. But in all areas there is a need for more health professionals who are generalists and can appreciate the local priorities and need for adaptation (Huntington et al. 1992).

Priority activities in a MCH program have to be adapted culturally, financially, logistically, and technically to the local epidemiology, to the ecology of the area, and to the staff and resources likely to be available (Bryant 1969; Churchman 1968; UNICEF 1967). Adapted programs can vary greatly for the same disease in different ecologies, depending, for example, on cultural factors, road communications and population distribution, available numbers and levels of staff, and funds.

A preventive program against tetanus of newborns in a country with adequate communications and deliveries performed by indigenous midwives could be based on education and supervision of these birth attendants; however, in the New Guinea Highlands, where the infection is common, there are few roads, close domestic contact with animals, and self-delivery in the homes, immunization of women, especially in pregnancy, requires the highest consideration (Schofield et al. 1961). Kuru is a slow viral disease with neurological symptoms that occurs in a New Guinea tribe when family members eat the infected brain of a dead kinsman as part of the death ceremony. The prevention of kuru depends on discouraging cannibalism.

Health education activities must be appropriately adapted (Stewart 1959). The nutrients young children require are probably similar all over the world, but adaptation is required in trying to achieve the correct intake in areas with different cultural, economic, and culinary backgrounds and with varying patterns of food production and availability. The services developed must be adapted to the demographic characteristics of the area and to the distribution and mobility of the population, their involvement with daily, intermittent, or seasonal activities, and distances and available transport.

In general, services must be stripped of nonessentials because universal limitations of funds, staff, time, and large numbers have to be dealt with by insufficient numbers of junior staff. Simplicity, economy, and effectiveness are the aims.

Let us look at a population of 1 million in a Caribbean country as an example. Only 30 percent of the mothers and children receive any supervision through MCH clinics, the IMR is 80, and only 30 percent of dying children are seen by a doctor. Is it better to start an open-heart surgery unit, or to expand the MCH services so that they can include 70 percent of the population at risk and to raise the numbers of hospital beds for mothers and children by 20 percent? Should there be extensive services to deal with major problems or costly intensive care for a few? The question is being debated in Oregon in the United States, where it is argued that antenatal care for many women is more important than a liver transplant for one person.

It is not likely that 100 percent of all mothers and children will need or demand treatment, supervision, or advice. Vital and health statistics, or, in the absence of these, surveys and crude observation will indicate the areas and types of need. MCH services should be available to all those in the vulnerable groups who require them, and they should be sufficiently widespread and responsible to seek out those at risk, to ensure that the helpless and neglected are not exploited but receive care and support.

Relation to Other Groups

MCH services can form a spearhead for fostering physical, mental, and social advancement, and they should be extended to all families. But physical, mental, and social well-being depends not only on MCH workers. Somatic medicine, as elaborated by the employment of an increasing number of specialists and subspecialists, also remains a function of the health department.

The development of mental and social care must be shared with colleagues in the fields of education, agriculture, housing, public works, transport, and practically all other enterprises. Social workers, for instance, have a valuable reinforcing role in recruiting the aid of the community, in cases with and without physical problems. If social assistance, financial relief, special equipment or transport, employment, or mental assessment is necessary, the health worker can apply to the appropriate worker in cases of need, if such services exist in the particular area.

In some areas, moreover, there may be very little in the way of state funds or pensions, charitable societies, orphanages, convalescent homes, or special schools available for those in need. The health authorities should then work with the social assistance or welfare workers to assess the priorities and thus ensure that the available resources are used in the best possible way and with the minimum danger of creating dependence. The private sector should not be forgotten as a possible resource.

Evaluation

Evaluation should be an ongoing process (Reinke 1972). It is used to measure the effectiveness of a program, based on available data. At all stages, those involved must help in deciding which data to collect and how to collect them. The method should ensure that the information is as comprehensive as possible and readily retrievable. Data may be obtained from many sources using a variety of techniques: surveys, observational studies, questionnaires, spot checking, utilization studies, staff ratios, and cost-effectiveness.

The litmus test of a good plan is whether resources allocated, buildings built, people trained, and new activities introduced meet goals and lead to an improvement in the health of the population, so it is important to have baseline data to asses whether goals are met. This has been done very simply in the PVO Child Survival Program. Evaluation may involve assessing the size of the problem, determining the causes, analyzing the workers' load to improve efficiency, assessing attitudes and knowledge of the community or health staff, or measuring the utilization of health services. A number of verifiable indicators can be used for evaluation (Table 15.1). When evaluation is comparative, baseline data must be collected before programs are changed or introduced, and definite measurable goals must be set. Throughout the planning process, everyone should be involved in evaluating the efforts: whether they are in the right direction or whether a change of course is necessary (Mills 1983).

Where utilization patterns are measured, correlations may be erroneous. For example, measuring the number of condoms distributed in a family planning program does not reflect utilization but only distribution, and at that only the number handed out. In immunization programs, counts of doses distributed instead of the number of fully immunized children will create erroneous impressions, which could be disastrous. In the case of food rations, programs often measure the number of rations or portions handed out, not the number of recipients, which can also be misleading. Sometimes evaluation focuses on a variable that may not be directly correlated with the mea-

Table 15.1. Examples of Verifiable Indicators

Cost accounting	Close watch of expenditures on various items, e.g., personnel, facilities, equipment, and supplies
Community participation	The extent of participation, particularly of the underprivileged, and involvement in the community and the activity should be included. Furthermore, the acceptance and perception of the program activities by the community and their real enthusiasms are important.
Coverage	The percentage of the target population to whom the activity has become available
Utilization rate	The number of the target population who actually participated in the activity
Health status	Infant mortality; 1- to 2-year-old mortality. Maternal mortality. Prevalence and case fatality, rates of major identifiable diseases, e.g., diarrhea, measles, pneumonia. Immunization rates
Nutritional status	Clinically obvious cases of malnutrition, night blindness, anemia, goiter, anthropometry, e.g., review of serial weight records on charts or arm circumference measurements
Reproductive patterns	Birthrate, abortions, perinatal mortality, acceptance of contraceptive methods, number of traditional birth attendants retrained, number of midwives
Environmental health	Availability of safe drinking water, proportion of households with latrines, number of standpipes, rates of intestinal parasites in young children
Staff	Number, type, and distribution of personnel; availability, training (initial and in-service), performance, productivity, motivation, job satisfaction task analysis, workload
Logistics	Transportation, communication, administration, supervision

Source: Modified from Jelliffe and Jelliffe (1985).

sure used, such as food rations and improved nutrition status. The measure may not take into account other changes, such as the building of a new road, protection of the water supply, or different seasons; thus, the conclusions may be wrong. Whatever is measured must be clearly defined, with stated objectives and measurable clear-cut goals put into a realistic time frame.

Evaluation of health activities generally should measure:

Efficacy: Can it work? Does the service do more good than harm to the people who comply with the recommendations or treatments?

Effectiveness: Does it work? Is it acceptable and useful to those who are offered the service?

Availability: Is it reaching those at risk or in need?

Efficiency: Is it worth doing? Is it the best buy for the money spent, compared with other things that could be done with the same resources? Usually it is best to use more than one indicator as a cross-check (Bomgaars 1978).

Much progress has been made in evaluation techniques. Formerly one looked only at the number of doctors per population or the number of people immunized, and mortality was a prime focus. Now morbidity and behavioral and attitudinal indicators are proving valuable in assessing health services and upgrading them.

Health plans require evaluation. In Latin America ten-year goals were set in the early 1970s to provide a safe water supply in urban areas to 80 percent of the population (measured by connected water supply) and to 50 percent of the rural population (measured by either water connections or standpipes). Review of the data revealed that services had successfully been provided to 170 million persons in urban areas but to only 37 million rural inhabitants. Urban progress is close to the goal; the rural goal is far from being achieved. When the data are disaggregated (Fig. 15.3), it can be seen that ten of twenty-five countries achieved the 80 percent goal in urban areas but only seven of twenty-five reached the 50 percent goal in rural areas. The differences are more dramatic when one considers the wide discrepancy in standards between rural and urban areas. In rural area easy access to water was defined by having wither standpipes or water connections available. However, when the urban areas were evaluated, only water connections were counted (PAHO 1982). Although there has been an increase in the availability of access to clean water, the least developed countries continue to lag behind (Fig. 15.4). Through approaches like these, health care can be evaluated and causes of deficiencies determined.

Where water is available, it may be helpful to assess the incidence of diarrheal disease episodes in communities and to determine causality by looking at the way water is stored, how long it is stored, in what storage facilities, and how the water is used. Feachem and associates (1978) in Lesotho found that providing access to water was insufficient. Hygiene education was also needed.

Progress in the provision of sewage services has been limited, especially in rural areas (PAHO 1982). Flush toilets have been built where there is no water to operate them. It is helpful, therefore, before plunging in and wasting millions of dollars, to establish acceptability and

perceived needs. Behavior modification may be required or cultural practices considered. In Pakistan in the Afghan refugee camps, it was found that the cost of latrines would be much higher than in some other countries since men and women would require separate facilities (personal communication, M. A. Javed 1984). Even the presence of latrines may not prevent some of the parasitic infestations if dirt or leaves are used in lieu of toilet paper.

Management Supervision

There is a wide range of activities aimed at maximizing the effectiveness of health system at all levels. Areas of primary importance are continuous supplies, adequate staffing and supervision, and efficient communication. The availability of drugs, for example, can be a major problem in rural and developing areas, but improved management and supervision can ensure a more continuous supply, better distribution, and quality control.

One of the reasons cited for poor attendance at rural health centers is the chronic shortage of drugs and supplies, which undermine the morale of the medical staff and destroy the confidence of the people (Cassels 1983). In many rural clinics, even simple supplies like iron tablets are frequently unavailable, while in the ministry, supplies may be plentiful. Local drug supplies often deteriorate under poor storage conditions (Table 15.2). For example, ergometrine, used to stop uterine bleeding after birth, absorbs moisture and then deteriorates. Another problem is the tendency to overprescribe available drugs in a shotgun approach of multiple drug therapy when only one drug is necessary or to treat diarrhea with expensive and unnecessary antibiotics when oral rehydration would be more appropriate and effective (Christian Med. Comm. 1983).

Research in rural Cameroon showed

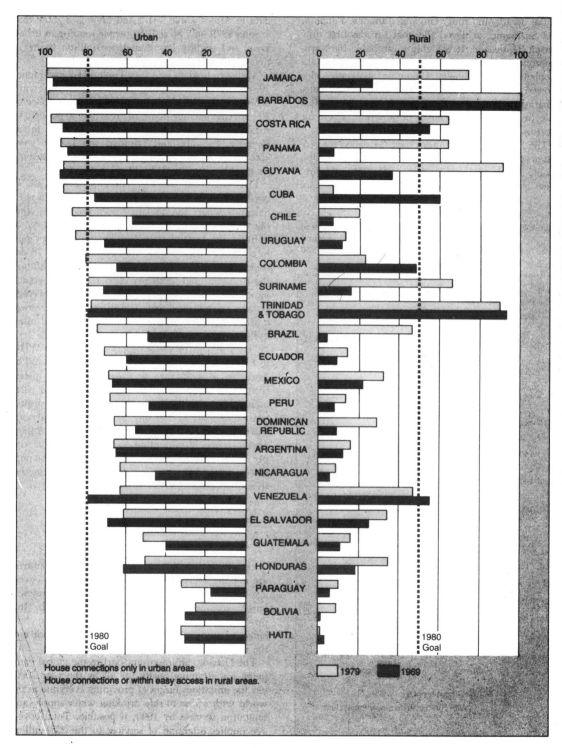

Figure 15.3. Evaluation of goals set. Population served by water supply in Latin America with goals established for 1980 under the ten-year plan. Source: PAHO (1982).

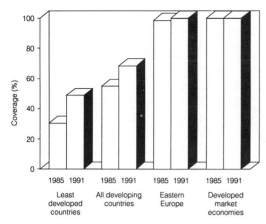

Figure 15.4. Global safe water indicator: population coverage, 1985–1991. Growing numbers of people still remain without access to basic services: 1.5 billion lack access to clean water and 2 billion lack adequate sanitation. Source: WHO (1992).

that mismanagement was a major obstacle to the efficient functioning of government-supplied drugstores. Although the annual stock of drugs supplied by the ministry was too small, the main reason for shortages was the high frequency of private use by health workers and other personnel. This is often the most difficult problem to eliminate, especially in countries where all health personnel are on government salaries. Their salaries are not affected by the quality of their services, and their private use of public resources is a means of supplementing their low income. Traditions of strong family obligations and gift-giving customs, along with poverty and poor health, augment the tendency toward mismanagement (Van de Geest 1983). In several studies and experimental drug distribution programs, it was shown that commercial incentives guarantee better service. Of note is the fact that private hospitals, pharmacies, and even illegal drug vendors seldom run out of drugs (Cassels 1983; Van de Geest 1983).

The problem of drug deterioration and wastage will gradually be solved as more stable products and better monitoring techniques are developed. An indicator to monitor measles vaccine has been developed by the Program for Appropriate Technology for Health (PATH). A red paper disk on the measles vial changes to black following accumulated exposures to high temperatures, warning the health worker that the vaccine has dropped below its minimum required potency (Fig. 15.5) (PAHO 1983).

Table 15.2. Pointers for Recognizing Spoiled Drugs and Supplies

Smell	When some items such as aspirin have been attacked by too much heat and damp, they smell. If a tin smells when you first open it, the aspirins are useless. One needs, of course, to know the normal faint odor of an aspirin container.
Color	Some drugs lose their color when they are spoiled. Make sure you know what color a tablet should be. If it is a different color or colors, do not use it.
Breaking up	When tablets are damp, they break up. You must not use them.
Drying out	Condoms are normally lubricated. If they have dried out, you should not use them.
Melting	Oral rehydration salts (ORS) may melt above 30°C. If you find ORS packets that are dark brown and sticky and will not dissolve, do not use them. Capsules may also melt with heat and as moisture attacks the gelatin. This also signals likelihood of moisture getting to the contents. If you find capsules are stuck together, do not use them; if suppositories, pessaries, creams, and ointments have melted and become runny, do not use them.

Source: Christian Med. Comm. (1983).

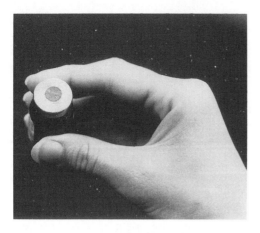

Figure 15.5. Protecting supplies. The red paper disk on the vial of measles vaccine contains a chemical that causes it to turn black following accumulated exposure to high temperatures. Source: PAHO (1983).

With logistical support and supervision organized by an MCH planning unit, many problems can be avoided. Various measures can be taken to improve quantity and quality of supplies:

Control inventory: Establish and monitor detailed accounting system at all levels (date received, condition, quantity, and ongoing record of quantities dispensed) to pinpoint wastage, spoilage, and pilferage.

Improve reliability of transport: Allot enough fuel, make driver accountable, use transport appropriate for weather and geographic conditions; when cold chain is necessary, plan every step in minute detail.

Plan shipments carefully: Include all necessary supplies and parts (avoid sending syringes without needles) and ensure that shipments are equitably distributed and reach peripheral posts.

Establish a reorder system: Base orders on projected need—for example, plan for three months at a time, based on the past six months' usage, and build in an additional three months'

supply. Remember to plan for additional needs for special campaigns.

Establish prescription guidelines and protocol: Avoid overprescribing and waste, and ensure correct use of products. The first step toward this is to establish a national or regional essential drug list.

Monitor storage facilities: Train supervisor to visit facilities regularly to check cold chain equipment, humidity, cleanliness, safety, labeling, and security.

Train staff: Train pharmacists and health workers to be familiar with storage requirements of essential drugs and to recognize common signs of spoilage.

Use appropriate technology: Use protective packaging, room thermometers, PATH measles vaccine indicators, nondisposable blades, and bulk nylon sutures.

Establish an incentive system: Discourage inefficiency and pilferage through community participation in financing and monitoring, rewards for better service, legal profit opportunities, and free or subsidized drugs for staff families.

Cost of Health Care

The degree to which the health of an individual is a collective responsibility and to which services should be financed socially is largely determined by a country's political and social philosophy (Sidel and Sidel 1977; Susser and Cherry 1982). However, human nature being what it is, some payment for medical care or medication undoubtedly may improve compliance and so have a good therapeutic effect. That is, medicine that has to be paid for, even by token payment, is treated with more respect or interest than that which is not.

Medical costs have increased markedly (Benyoussef and Christian 1977; Brice and White 1969; Ginzberg 1969; Hu 1975; Lee and Mills 1983; Newell 1975). If some fees can be paid by the relatively affluent, then there is more hope of improvement and expansion of services for those most in need. Even the most convinced socialists do not all believe in free medication; many countries demand some sort of payment, through insurance or other means. Some countries provide free medical care for children and the aged; others provide free care for those suffering from tuberculosis and venereal disease (Cassels 1983).

Medical care should not be allowed to become farcical. In a certain area, for example, syphilis was diagnosed with unmerited insouciance and became the self-diagnosis of the majority of the population. Many attended dispensaries, and invariably if they had a shilling, they received an injection, and if they had sixpence they were given potassium iodide mixture. If they were ill, they went to the local herbalist. For this, payment was also expected and took the form of cash, a cow, chicken, or a bag of maize. This invisible payment is often forgotten when calculating the cost of health care.

Health care costs are influenced by the greed of the health insurance companies, the elaborateness of the facilities, specialization of services, sophistication of the technology, and the armamentarium of drugs and tests used. The tremendous costs of the supplies, medicine, and medical equipment are borne by consumers, while companies realize high profits. For some children, there are liver transplants, while for others there are only prayers. For some mothers in labor, there is intensive fetal monitoring and for many none at all. The great disparity of services exists where disproportionate resources serve mainly the urban elite at the expense of the rural poor. In some cases, this inequity has been decreased by local contributions of financial and human resources (Jancloes et al. 1982).

Although the concept of health for all is noble and deserving, the danger is that inadequate and inferior services will be provided for the poor, creating the illusion that something is being done when in fact nothing substantive is provided (Mosley 1983). In most developing countries the budget for comprehensive rural health services needs to be increased to prevent "Health for All" from becoming a mere slogan. The budget must reflect commitment rather than promises. Second-class services will not improve the health of the poor. Available services may be basic and low cost but must be effective.

A major obstacle to providing primary health care is obtaining sustainable financing. The Bamako Initiative, which involves thirty-three African countries, including Benin, Barundi, Cameroon, Equatorial Guinea, Guinea, Kenya, Mali, Mauritania, Nigeria, Rwanda, Sierra Leone, and Togo, aims at strengthening or expanding local primary health care services through community involvement. Financing has increased considerably through community management of services, which is mainly achieved through the sale of drugs.

While changes have occurred at the local level through this initiative and more clinics and health posts have been able to be reestablished, there is concern that the financing is achieved through a 200 percent or more mark-up of essential drugs. To saddle the sick not only with the actual cost of their medicines but also with a 200 percent or more additional charge to pay for community health services could be a major step backward (Babb et al. 1993). On the positive side, the Bamako Initiative is confronting the serious problem of the pharmaceutical industry's flooding of poor countries with unnecessary medicines. Initiating a program to supply health posts only with essential low-cost screened drugs is a step in the right direction. Drugs constitute a major cost of most of these programs.

Still, with the worldwide trend to privatization of health care, services for the poor are diminishing. According to the *Lancet*, a World Bank study in Kenya showed that imposing any fee for health services would exclude 40 percent of the population, and these would be the people most in need of services (Lancet 1988; UNICEF 1991).

Some health centers charge minimal token fees for services, drugs, or food rations and use the proceeds for improving local services. Some charge a flat fee that covers anything from a Band-aid to a surgical operation. However, for those who cannot pay, another mechanism must be available so that they are not stigmatized or denied access to care. Although the means test is regarded with disfavor, it exists in some form in every organized society, and without it cases of hardship go unrecognized.

Calculation based on cost accounting must be carefully examined. Often when people want to promote a program, they provide cost-effective data based on the total population rather than on persons served. Through increasing the denominator, the costs per person are minimized and grossly underestimated, resulting in insufficient funding to do the job properly. Costs cannot be an overriding consideration at all times. The eradication of smallpox was cheap at any price. The cost of immunizations such as measles, when calculated in dollars, may seem high, but when calculated in terms of prevention of death and disability is a bargain (Table 15.3). For the most cost-effective programs, measles immunization coverage must be 80% or more. Estimates show that in urban areas when coverage is 80% the number of cases prevented (in thousands) is 14.2, compared to 10.7 when coverage is only 60%. In rural areas when coverage is increased from 60 to 80% the number of cases prevented is even more marked: with 80% coverage 22.6 cases (in thousands) are prevented, whereas when 60% are vaccinated only

16.2 cases (in thousands) are prevented (World Development Report 1993).

Recognizing the shortfall in funding, developing countries are attempting to make the most of natural and/or national resources such as breast milk for infant feeding and are taking steps to maximize their resources. They are containing costs of drugs and supplies that can take up to 40 percent of the national health budget (as against 6 percent of the health budget in developed countries) (WHO 1980). Practices contributing to the high costs are the purchase of unnecessary drugs, overprescribing, and the purchase of expensively packaged brand name drugs.

An essential drug list has been formulated, and local production of essential drugs has begun to decrease dependency on foreign imports. Countries are compiling lists of essential drugs according to their own needs and priorities, based on the WHO list of 220 essential drugs (WHO 1977). Bangladesh now produces about thirty basic preparations, including aspirin, vitamin C, oral rehydration salts, and several antibiotics. Lesotho produces one hundred essential drugs, some of which are exported to neighboring countries. Zimbabwe was forced into developing local drug supplies because of economic sanctions during political change, and as a result chloroquine is now one of the many drugs produced locally (Baumslag 1980).

Other steps that have been taken include better management, supervision, and simple appropriate technology with attention to detail (McMahon et al. 1980; O'Connor 1980; WHO 1980). For example if the dropper for polio vaccine used is not the one supplied, vaccine wastage occurs, and only ten doses may be obtained instead of the usual fifteen. In the surgical field, simple and appropriate technology has been imaginatively suggested. If suture material is needed, unsterile monofilament nylon purchased in bulk is as effective as prepackaged, pre-

Table 15.3. Summary Statement of Savings due to Immunization against Measles

Type of savings	1963–1965	1966–1968	Total
Health and resource			
Cases averted	1,140,000	8,590,000	9,730,000
Lives saved	114	859	973
Cases of retardation averted	380	2,864	3,244
Hospital days saved	65,000	490,000	555,000
Workdays saved	189,000	1,435,000	1,624,000
Schooldays saved	3,775,000	28,450,000	32,225,000
Economic (in dollars)			
Economic benefits	63,192,000	468,351,000	531,543,000
Cost of immunizing persons	43,500,000	64,800,000	108,300,000
Net economic savings	19,692,000	403,551,000	423,243,000

Source: Nat. Commun. Dis. Cntr. (1969).

cut, suture material, and the savings are considerable.

The high cost of medical technology and training of health professionals makes it necessary to use physician extenders and primary care workers. Through self-help and use of community participation (Kroeger 1982; MacCormack 1983), financial and human resources can be mobilized. However, community participation, although generally desirable and effective, can be repressive and opposed by the community (Chowdhury 1981; Werner 1981). Where possible, village-level workers have increased the coverage of the community and reduced preventable conditions. But as village health workers become more experienced, they want more training and may lose their bonds and ties to the community (Rifkin 1980). After training, they may raise their fees and become too high priced for the very poor they were intended to serve (Vaughan and Walt 1983). There are only a few isolated examples of successfully locally financed schemes. The innovative self-financing health and rural development program in Savar, Bangladesh, is one such example (Vaughan and Walt 1983). In Senegal, where coverage has been poor, one community has provided financial and human resources and is in control of the utilization and management, while the government provides the basic health services, technical support, and training. The program has been so successful that it has been extended (Jancloes et al. 1982).

In relatively rich countries where there is segregation by race and economic status, as in South Africa, the unfairness of the resource distribution is reflected in the sixfold higher infant mortality among black people, and the fourteen-fold difference in child mortality as compared with white people. The second-class services and poor standards of living will not be appreciably altered by village-level workers without a change in the social order (Susser and Cherry 1982). While money used sparingly and allocated to priorities can go a long way to reaching those most in need, the basic services of sufficient quality have to be provided whatever the costs.

CONCLUSION

There is no blueprint for the organization of MCH services; each area and each country must develop its own methods. These need to be dovetailed with the existing health services (Roemer 1991). More observation, experimentation, and discussion are needed. Recent worldwide developments in primary health care indicate that MCH activities are among its major elements, bringing together the often separated programs concerned with oral rehydration, immunization, and breast-feeding, with elements concerned with education, community sanitation, food availability, and income generation.

Experiments have been carried out all over the world in methods of organizing MCH services, and there are increasing opportunities for observation and comparison. Nevertheless, it remains true that a disproportionately small amount of money and attention is given to health care compared with the enormous sums contributed to viral, genetic, and surgical research. Delivering a baby in an African hut where there is no light or water helps one to establish priorities and perspective on what is critical. There is more need for concise and practical descriptions of the way ideas involved in the organization and administration of MCH services have been and are being implemented, what are the main difficulties, why they are difficulties, and how they are being met and overcome (WHO 1969, 1980).

A great deal of money, attention, and concentration has been spent on the pathology and biochemistry of nutritional deficiencies. If just one-tenth of this was devoted to exploring the causes of malnutrition and organizing its treatment and prevention, perhaps the world would be in a less sorry state.

REFERENCES

Abel-Smith, B. (1968). What priority health? Tasks and priorities in the organization of medical services. *Israel J. Med. Sci.* **4**, 350.

Arnold, M. F. (1969). Basic concepts and crucial issues in health planning. *Am. J. Publ. Hlth.* **59**, 1686.

Babb S.; Sanders D.; and Werner D. (1993). *Questioning the Solution.* Hesperian Foundation, Palo Alto (in press).

Baumslag, N. (1980). *MCH and Nutrition: A Report on Selected Programs in Zimbabwe, Mozambique, Kenya and Botswana.* Ford Foundation, New York.

Bennett, F. J. (1970). *Community Diagnosis and Health Action.* Macmillan, London.

Benyoussef, A., and Christian, B. (1977). Health in developing countries. *Soc. Sci. Med.* **11**, 399.

Bewes, P. C. (1982). Surgery with limited resources. *Wld. Hlth. Forum* **3**, 58.

Bomgaars, M. R. (1978). Practical evaluation for primary health care programs. In *Manpower and Primary Health Care.* Ed. R. A. Smith. University Press of Hawaii, Honolulu.

Breslow, L. (1969). Some essentials in a national program for child health. *Pediatrics* **44**, 327.

Brice, T. W., and White, K. L. (1969). Factors related to the use of health services an international comparative study. *Med. Care* **vll**, 124.

Brolly, E. H. (1982). Health care data recording system for developing countries. *Trop. Doctor* **12**, 105.

Bryant, J. H. (1969). *Health and the Developing World.* Cornell University Press, Ithaca, N.Y.

Cashman, J. W. (1969). Medical care in the United States *Roy. Soc. Hlth. J.* **3**, 122.

Cassels, A. (1983). Drug supply in rural Nepal. *Trop. Doctor* **13**, 14.

Chowdhury, Z. (1981). The good health worker will inevitably become a political figure. *Wld. Hlth. Forum* **2**, 55.

Christian Med. Comm. (1983). Strengthening and regulating the supply, distribution and production of basic pharmaceutical products. *Contact*, **73**, 1–20.

Churchman, C. W. (1968). *The Systems Approach.* Basic Books, New York.

Cibotti, R. (1969). The integration of the health sector in development planning. *Bol. Ofic. Sanit. Panamer.*, p. 730.

Clavano, N. R. (1982). Mode of feeding and its effects on infant morbidity. *J. Trop. Pediat.* **28**, 287–93.

Djunkanovic, V., and Mach, E. P. eds. (1975). *Alternative Approaches to Meeting Basic Health Needs in Developing Countries.* World Health Organization, Geneva.

Dunlop, D. W., and Caldwell, H. R. (1977). Priority determination for the provision of health services: An economic and social analysis. *Soc. Sci. Med.* **11**, 471.

Feachem, R., et al. (1978). *Water, Health and Development.* Tri-med Books Ltd., London.

Fendall, N. R. E. (1964). Organization of health services in emerging countries. *Lancet* **ii**, 53.

Finau, S. A. (1983). Marketing and primary

health care: Approach to planning in a Tongan village. *Soc. Sci. Med.* **17**, 511.

Ginzberg, E. (1969). Facts and fancies about medical care. *Am. J. Publ. Hlth.* **49**, 785.

Gish, O. (1975). *Planning the Health Sector: The Tanzanian Experience.* Croom Helm, London.

Hart, R. H.; Belsey, M. A.; and Tarimo, E. (1990). *Injecting Maternal and Child Health into Primary Health Care.* World Health Organization, Geneva.

Horn, J. S. (1969). *Away with All Pests.* Middlesex, England.

Hu, T., ed. (1975). *International Health Costs and Expenditures, U.S. Department of Health, Education, and Welfare.* Publication no. (WIH) 76-1067. Washington, D.C.

Huntington, C; Sweeney, R.; and Graham, R. (1992). The shortage of generalist physicians. *Am. Family Physician* **45** (4), 1573–76.

Jancloes, M.; Seck, B.; Vandevelden, L.; and Ndiaye, B. (1982). Priority health care at Pikine (Senegal): Financial contribution and control by the community with governmental support. *Med. Trop.* **42**, 659.

Jelliffe, D. B., and Jelliffe, E. F. P. (1985). *Child Nutrition in Developing Countries: A Handbook for Fieldworkers.* Office of Nutrition, U.S. Agency for International Development, Washington, D.C.

Jelliffe, D. B., and Jelliffe, E. F. P. (1989). *Community Nutritional Assessment in Developing Countries: A Handbook for Field-Workers.* Office of Nutrition, U.S. Agency for International Development, Washington, D.C.

Klarman, H. E. (1967). Present status of cost-benefit analysis in the health field. *Am. J. Publ. Hlth.* **57**, 1948.

Kroeger, A. (1982). Participatory evaluation of primary health care programmes: An experience with four Indian populations in Ecuador. *Trop. Doctor* **12**, 38.

Lancet (1988). Bamako initiative. *Lancet* **2** (8621), 1177–78.

Lee, K., and Mills, A. (1983). *The Economics of Health in Developing Countries.* Oxford University Press, Oxford.

MacCormack, C. P. (1983). Community participation in primary health care. *Trop. Doctor* **13**, 51.

McMahon, R.; Barton, E.; and Piot, M. (1980). *On Being in Charge: A Guide for Middle-level Management in Primary Care.* World Health Organization, Geneva.

Mills, A. (1983). Planning for primary care. *Trop. Doctor* **13**, 18.

Morley, D.; Rohde, J. E.; and Williams, G. (1983). *Practising Health for All.* Oxford University Press, Oxford.

Mosley, W. (1983). *Will Health Care Reduce Infant and Child Mortality? A Critique of Some Current Strategies with Special Reference to Africa and Asia.* Ford Foundation, Jakarta.

Nat. Commun. Dis. Cntr. (1969). *Measles Surveillance Report 7.* National Communicable Disease Center, U.S. Department of Health, Education and Welfare, Washington, D.C.

Navarro, V. (1969). Planning for the distribution of personal health services. *Publ. Hlth. Rep.* **84**, 573.

Newell, K., ed. (1975). *Health by the People.* World Health Organization, Geneva.

O'Connor, R., ed. (1980). *Managing Health Systems in Developing Areas: Experiences from Afghanistan.* Lexington Books, Lexington, Mass.

PAHO (1965). *Health Planning: Problems of Concept and Method.* Scientific Publication no. 111. Pan American Health Organization, Washington, D.C.

PAHO (1982). *Health Conditions in the Americas—1977–1980.* Scientific Publication no. 427. Pan American Health Organization, Washington, D.C.

PAHO (1983). Measles vaccine indicator trial in Peru. *EPI Newsletter* **5**, 2.

Pop. Ref. Bur. (1983). *World Population Data Sheet.* Population Reference Bureau, Washington, D.C.

Reinke, W. A., ed. (1972). *Health Planning.* Department of International Health, Johns Hopkins University School of Hygiene and Public Health, Baltimore.

Rifkin, S. B. (1980). Health care in China: The experts take command. *Trop. Doctor* **10**, 86.

Robinson, P. (1957). Maternal and child health services in South-East Asia, VI. Critical discussion. *J. Trop. Pediat.* **3**, 110.

Roemer, M. (1991). *National Health Services: Comparative Review.* Oxford University Press, Oxford.

Sackett, D. L. (1980). Evaluation of Health Services. In *Maxcy-Rosenau Public Health and Preventive Medicine.* 11th ed. Ed. J. M. Last. Appleton-Century Crofts, New York.

Schofield, F. D.; Tucker, V. M.; and Westbrook, G. R. (1961). Neonatal tetanus in New

Guinea. Effect of active immunization in pregnancy. *Brit. Med. J.* **2**, 785.

Sidel, V. W., and Sidel, R. (1977). Primary health care in relation to socio-political structure. *Soc. Sci. Med.* **11**, 415.

Smith, R. A. (1978). *Manpower and Primary Health Care.* University Press of Hawaii, Honolulu.

Stewart, G. (1959). The importance of programme planning. *Int. J. Hlth. Educ.* **2**, 94.

Susser, M., and Cherry, V. P. (1982). Health and health care under apartheid. *J. Publ. Hlth.* **3**, 455.

USAID (1992). *Child Survival.* Report to Congress. Washington, D.C.

UNICEF (1963). *Children of the Developing Countries.* United Nations International Children's Education Fund, Cleveland.

UNICEF (1967). *The Needs of the Young Child in the Caribbean.* United Nations International Children's Education Fund, New York.

UN (1970). *Trends in the Social Situation of Children.* ECOSCO Document E/CN.5/488. New York.

UNICEF (1991). *1991 Annual Report, United Nations Children's Fund.* UNICEF House, New York.

Van de Geest, S. (1983). Propharmacies: A problematic means of drug distribution in rural Cameroon. *Trop. Doctor* **13**, 9.

Vaughan, J. P., and Walt, G. (1983). Village health workers and primary health care. *Trop. Doctor* **13**, 105.

Werner, D. (1981). The village health worker: Lackey or liberator? *Wld. Hlth. Forum* **2**, 46.

Williams, C. D. (1955). The organization of child health services in developing countries. *J. Trop. Pediat.* **1**, 3.

WHO (1969). Basic Health Services. Mimeographed document. Wld. Hlth. Org. (PHA) **69**, 39.

WHO (1969). *The Organization and Administration of Maternal and Child Health Services.* Wld. Hlth. Org. Techn. Rep. Ser., no. 428.

WHO (1976). *The Primary Health Worker, Working Guide: Guidelines for Training, Guidelines for Adaptation.* Document HMD/74.5. World Health Organization, Geneva.

WHO (1977). *The Selection of Essential Drugs.* Wld. Hlth. Org. Tech. Rep. Ser., no. 615.

WHO (1980). *Guiding Principles for the Managerial Process for Health for All by the Year 2000.* PDWG/REP/3 Annex 3. World Health Organization, Geneva. WHO (1992). *Implementation of the Global Strategy for Health for All by the Year 2000.* 2d ed. World Health Organization, Geneva.

World Development Report (1993). *Investing in Health.* Oxford University Press, New York.

16

Personnel and Training

Hippocratic Oath—To observe the sacred obligation to share in
teaching and training of others.

Health services are labor intensive. Better staff planning and training is a crucial concern in the search for more cost-effective delivery systems. Attempts to redefine personnel roles will be of little use unless preceded by a clear picture of health needs and which service activities are most effectively provided by which type of personnel. Other issues include the best kind of training for health auxiliaries and the way primary care systems should be organized (Baumslag et al. 1978).

Orthodox primary health care systems are typically pyramid-shaped structures administered by physicians or other health professionals (Fig. 16.1). Mid-level workers and village-level health workers are trained to extend scarce professional services by treating simple illnesses and referring more serious cases to central health posts or hospitals.

The traditional priorities of medicine are (or should be) service, teaching, and research, invariably in that order. All over the world, however, the cry goes up that progress in health is limited by a shortage of doctors and nurses (Baumslag and Boston 1982; Bryant 1969; Evans 1981). The most wealthy technologically ad-

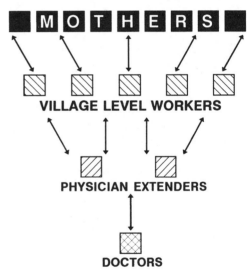

Figure 16.1. The primary health care network. Alone, village-level workers and mothers cannot make a huge impact on mortality and morbitity rates. Adequate support and supervision and a sufficient supply of all types of health workers must be available at the community level for quality family health care, if more than the bureaucracy's image is to be improved.

vanced countries have failed to produce enough health professionals for their own requirements, and they entice trained staff away from countries in much greater need.

Yet at the same time, they offer advice to such poor countries on training programs. The situation has become absurd because of a failure to appreciate the importance of training. Meanwhile, pure research occupies such an exalted status that it commands the largest funds and likelihood of promotion. Even those appointed to teaching posts complain that teaching interferes with their research (Evans 1981; Fendall 1966; Jelliffe and Stanfield 1968; Keynes 1968; King 1966).

Many doctors' and nurses' organizations have so overelaborated their own training programs that only the healthiest and wealthiest can afford their services, except where social justice and so-called socialized medicine invade their preserves. Many of the organizations even resent the idea that there should be different patterns of training, with shorter and more practical programs that could help to relieve the critical inadequacies of medical care. The time has come for drastic reforms in staffing and in the training of health personnel to reach those most in need of health care.

The most famous of all the Hippocratic aphorisms states,

Life is short, art is long, opportunity fleeting, experience treacherous, judgment difficult. The physician must be ready not only to do his duty himself, but also to encourage the cooperation of his patients, of those who are with him, and of his environment.

The first sentence is famous; the second is less famous and less trenchant, but it neatly summarizes the scope of medical care: that it exists not merely to treat disease but to look after people in their environment. If this thought is kept in mind, curricula for training may be made more realistic.

Patterns of medical education are constantly changing. Up to the time of the Listerian revolution, hospitals were primarily places of refuge for the homeless, the destitute, and the dying, not for treatment of the sick. Religious orders provided the majority of such places of refuge. But those who had homes were born, suffered good or ill health, and died in their homes. They were cared for in their homes by their relatives, their retainers, or their patrons; they were visited in their homes by their doctors. The study of medicine was carried out largely through apprenticeship. To observe and to modify home conditions and the practice of home care were integral aspects of the training and duties of the physician.

With the introduction, only a little over a hundred years ago, of antiseptic surgery, anesthetics, bacteriology, biochemistry, and radiology—in fact of all the mechanized adjuncts to medical care— vast changes took place. Medical studies were forced to incorporate more and more of the physical sciences. Specialists and subspecialists burgeoned. Medical training became not only fragmented but confined to institutions, wards, and laboratories, while outpatients were regarded as somewhat of an intrusion and were generally left to junior members of the staff. A hangover from the old monastic tradition that a hospital is an enclosed building has possibly helped to emphasize this tendency.

In about 1900, the development of MCH services in Europe and North America began to reveal anew the need for supervision, advice, and home care. These services were promptly made the responsibility of departments of public health and played no further part in the training of doctors and nurses until comparatively recently. It is gratifying to observe how the isolation of health workers from their patients and families can be modified when they work in the community and deliver care in the homes. In developing countries, by working in the community and in homes, modern practitioners can begin to work with and learn from the traditional healer, the ayurveda, the balmist, the herbalist, and the obeah man. A Sri Lankan study found that a mother's response to treatment for

Table 16.1. Relative Costs of Personnel Development

	Physician	Nurse	Auxiliary	Village-level worker
Thailand	1	5	19	250
Colombia	1	8	25	
Ghana	1			250 (TBAs)
East Africa	1	3	15 (sanitarians) 20 (medical assistants) 20 (nurse assistants)	

Source: Modified from Taylor (1980).

Note: Based on the assumption that medical training costs $30,000.

certain illnesses was better with ayurvedic medicine than with allopathic or modern medicine even though the latter was cheaper (Fernando 1964). This may be because ayurvedic medicine has a more holistic approach.

Although the situation is changing, it is not changing quickly enough for health workers. Many medical students would like to rebel but instead remain silent in view of the relentless pressure and competition. Ornithologists have long recognized that one cannot study birds by examining them in cages, and students, too, wish to move outside their institutions and learn why, where, how, and when problems arise. Nor has change come quickly enough for the numerous disadvantaged families, especially those in the midst of wealthy communities, who are not receiving the health care or education that they need, especially in times of recession, unemployment, and homelessness. Among them are children.

Authorities are slowly beginning to appreciate that it is urgently necessary to deliver the services and to train more people more realistically; to spend less public funds on and devote less attention and personnel to status symbols and more to discovering and helping those in real need (World Bank 1975). Otherwise, there will continue to be understandably widespread dissatisfaction with health services. Every nation that admits responsibility for health care must acknowledge that handing out financial assistance and

free food can be useful but is not enough alone. Where this has been realized, indigenous health workers are being trained as primary care health workers because hospital-oriented medicine has not improved the health of the world's poor.

It is clear that a hospital-oriented, doctor-dependent health care system, as in the Cuban model, is not transferable to other developing countries. It was a luxury showpiece (primary health care allergists etc.) with excellent results, but as the massive assistance from the former Soviet Union has stopped, the system is unable to sustain itself.

It costs fifteen to twenty-five times as much to train a doctor as an auxiliary (Table 16.1) (Taylor 1980). In most developing countries, personnel distribution is skewed; at one end are doctors who are highly specialized and seeing very few patients; at the other end are indigenous practitioners who are not trained but provide most of the care. In between are a few mid-level auxiliary personnel—like a wine glass with an extended base (Fig. 16.2). Most countries have moved to increase the number of community health workers through retraining of indigenous and Westernized health workers and developing mid-level auxiliaries as supervisors and managers, since 80 to 90 percent of illness in the villages can be handled as well or better by auxiliaries (Ronaghy et al. 1983; Smith 1978). Those who cannot be handled by auxiliaries can be referred to appropriate

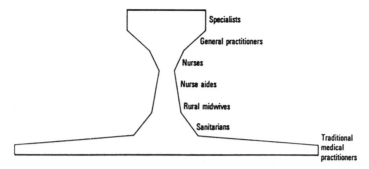

Specialists

General practitioners

Nurses

Nurse aides

Rural midwives

Sanitarians

Traditional medical practitioners

Figure 16.2. Distribution of health care personnel. The lack of mid-level personnel and general practitioners means that many people, especially in rural areas, do not get adequate health care. Source: Modified from Taylor et al. (1968).

specialists through effective regionalization. Emphasis is being placed on relocation, cost-effective interventions, and appropriate technology at the village level. Still, there are many problems to be solved, including adequate supervision and motivation of mid-level workers, transportation for supervision and referral, availability of specialized centers, and turning pilot projects into national programs with some measure of success.

One of the most important, but little heralded, recent developments in medical training has been the organization of the Network of Community-Oriented Educational Institutions for Health Sciences (initiated by the University of Linburg Maastricht, the Netherlands), which involves medical students in the community from the beginning of their studies (Schmidt 1988). Johns Hopkins Medical School has a program for first-year medical students that exposes them to the practical aspects of family medicine. There is a growing recognition of the need for general practice doctors (Huntington et al. 1992; Rosenblatt 1992).

STAFFING

One apparent benefit that has emerged from the socialist countries is the major reorganization that has occurred in health care. Elsewhere in the world, medical services are understaffed. There are complaints that patients have to wait for extremely long periods and doctors have no time to talk to patients and no time to follow up those who fail to keep their appointments. Social workers, dietitians, home economists, health educators, community developers, and volunteers are valuable in reinforcing and supporting roles and in improving the level of living and health. A poor country, however, cannot create all possible types of staff at once; it must determine its priorities. None of these subsidiary workers can replace essential health workers such as physicians, nurses, and medical assistants, but they can increase access to health care and facilitate more equitable distribution of health care resources. Pharmacists in some developing countries are also considered part of the primary health care network, as they often are required to suggest medicines for sick patients and check urine or measure blood pressure.

Nonmedical workers are needed for youth work, delinquency, and adoption, and it is wasteful to remove them from such work. Certainly in the normal pursuit of their duties and in their personal lives, they should try to further individual, domestic, and community hygiene, and they may be helpful in health emergencies. There should be collaboration and understanding between all groups engaged in village improvements, extension work, and community education. But overlapping leads to confusion and waste, so coordination is essential. If health services are paralyzed by a lack of medical personnel, then the most economical solution is to train more doctors, nurses, midwives, but even larger numbers of health workers, to educate the community and constantly review training, functions, and conditions of employment of all types of staff.

Frequently the following complaints are heard: "We cannot get recruits"; "The training is too long and much of it is irrelevant"; "The work is too hard and too dirty"; "They won't take the night work"; "As soon as they are trained they emigrate"; "We are so short of staff and everyone has too much to do, so more of them are leaving"; "They won't stay in government work when they can get five times as much in private practice"; "They are dissatisfied with their pay, housing, transport, promotion, opportunities for educating their children, opportunities for their own further education"; "They have got fellowships to go and work for a Ph.D. in biochemistry so they are giving up this work." These complaints are most pronounced in rural, unserved areas.

There is a serious need for providing incentives and recognizing the special needs of different health workers and their patients (Esman et al. 1980).

Training of Doctors and Nurses

Developing countries, dissatisfied with their lack of qualified personnel and their health care systems inherited from their colonial past, are seeking alternative methods for training and utilizing health care workers at all levels so that they can provide continuity of care and expand and improve primary health care services.

New degree programs for health workers are being developed, and some,

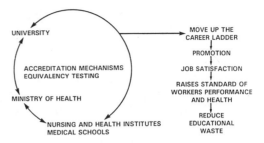

Figure 16.3. Career ladder for upward mobility. Source: Sebina et al. (1985).

paradoxically, are creating problems at the service delivery area. For example, young, inexperienced nurses with a bachelor's degree in nursing are being made supervisors, while enrolled or registered nurses with years of practical experience have no path to promotion. There are a myriad of public health courses offered in the developing countries; they may offer new skills and knowledge, but do not allow for upward mobility in the public health care system. Unless mechanisms are created for providing experienced workers with a good career ladder, good people will leave the system (Fig 16.3). For promotion in the public health care system, health workers are required to have a master's degree or a diploma in public health. In the United States there is one school of public health per 10 million population. Ten percent of trainees in U.S. schools of public health come from developing countries. The training is costly—about $20,000 per year—and if hidden costs such as replacement are taken into account may be as much as $40,000. It has been estimated that one-third of the training is irrelevant. Graduates may not return to their country of origin; they become part of the brain drain. Research may not be relevant for their country, and material learned may not be applicable to their home situation, which can lead to frustration. Most important, only small numbers of individuals may be sent for overseas training; no critical mass of public health experts can be developed to make effective changes in the public health training and services.

The high cost of training public health workers and the loss of experienced staff have led to the creation of more innovative and relevant programs with on-the-job training. The Michigan and Seattle programs in the United States are experimenting with alternatives. The absolute shortage of trained staff will not be solved by using volunteers (often women) and low-paid, low-level health care workers. More resources are needed to develop sufficient numbers of essential health care personnel.

In various parts of the world, experiments in training and organization have been conducted. These include content, site, length, educational techniques, and methods. Some of the beneficial trends in evidence that should be included in the curricula are summarized below:

1. Train for family care, and not leave this mainly to those who have not achieved technical, specialist, or research status.
2. Cut down on the more academic disciplines and basic sciences and provide experience from the earliest years in home and community health (physical, mental, and social).
3. Use hospitals as centers for health care education of the community rather than as isolated institutions.
4. Apply the principles of epidemiology to major local problems—not only communicable diseases—and use a problem-solving approach.
5. Emphasize follow-up to ascertain causes of ill health and to prevent or modify it.
6. Identify all those at risk, and ensure adequate management and support.
7. Teach doctors and nurses how to select, train, cooperate with, and supervise all types of auxiliaries and voluntary helpers and to obtain experience in this area.
8. Conduct part of the training in small community hospitals, health centers, and day care centers where the atmosphere is informal, the equipment is simple, and there is rooming in.
9. Focus on major practical issues such as nutrition, especially maternal and child nutrition.
10. Emphasize the importance of signs and symptoms and of mental and social problems associated with patient care.
11. Train by gaining experience on a community health team, observing the limits and limitations of the various health workers and their roles in education, supervision, and referral (Kasongo Project Team 1983; Werner and Bower 1982; WHO 1981).
12. Raise the status of noninstitutional medicine by involving senior clinicians and by conducting scientific research into community problems.
13. Gain experience with other groups working toward community betterment, such as agricultural extension workers, teachers, police, and religious groups.
14. Use appropriate technology.
15. Cooperate with local herbalists and healers.

A home care service should be an extension of all teaching hospitals, and students should be involved in it during their training. Moreover, experience in pediatric and adolescent services must be available. Medical students should undertake some periods of nursing care in pediatric wards to have a better working knowledge of the service needs.

In the early stages of their training, students must learn to examine and treat patients with meticulous attention to details. In the later stages, they should learn the truly important medico-diplomatic art of dealing with a large pressure of work efficiently, expeditiously, courteously, and cooperatively with other health professionals. Good medicine is obviously not practiced by refusing to see more than three patients per hour and closing the clinic with sixty people waiting who have not been seen at all, but by making the best use of the facilities according to the needs. It is important to organize services so the sickest are seen quickly and by the most trained personnel.

The content of training courses in the medical field needs revision (BMJ 1968). Some still narrowly concentrate on disease patterns found in Western countries. It is possible to meet a consultant in ophthalmology who knows nothing about xerophthalmia and a dermatologist who knows little of the signs and symptoms of protein deficiency. The tendency has been to make medical care more complex and fragmented. The urgent need, however, is to simplify, to coordinate, and to extend.

Nurses

Training of nurses today often concentrates excessively on academic and administrative matters rather than on patient care. Health visitors (concerned with nursing, midwifery, and public health) and public health nurses (concerned with nursing and public health) are so long in training that few can afford to qualify. They can become so scarce that medical services are severely hampered (Dean 1958).

A small core of nurses with post-basic and management training is needed, but modifications in types and grades and of time spent in training are overdue. Practical nurses and nurse aides now assist and even replace registered nurses in hospital care. Visiting nurse associations provide a variety of services for home visiting. But the fact that so many experiments are now being made indicates that the situation is chaotic and the need is desperate. Problems, however, arise with the vast proliferation of new, ill-defined cadres of associates, assistants, and aides

in pediatrics, obstetrics, and in general medicine (Josiah Macy Jr. Fdtn. 1970).

Perhaps the most neglected field in nursing training is that of the educational function of the nurse, especially in hospitals. Wards, particularly children's wards in developing countries, continually admit cases of preventable diseases such as nutritional disorders. Every pediatrician now recognizes the advantages of admitting the mother with the child, but sometimes the nursing staff and the administrators are opposed to the idea. If the mother can be admitted with a child with, say, severe dehydration, a great deal of the parenteral fluids may be replaced orally. The child in a cot will vomit a feed or a fluid poked at him or her by a busy nurse, but a child on his or her mother's lap (with the mother sitting on a low bench or chair) being fed fluids slowly by spoon will become restful and retain the food. A good nurse can calm the mother and the child and can show the mother how to hold, talk to, rest, and feed the child. In the process of the child's treatment, she can give an immense amount of health and nutrition teaching simply, with practical demonstration and encouragement.

In hospitals where the authorities refuse to admit the mother, unrestricted visiting by the parents can be valuable and provide opportunities for parent education. Nevertheless, effort must be made to provide at some accommodation for mothers and always for those who are breastfeeding their babies. Where there is restricted visiting, the task is much more difficult. The nurse can take the opportunity, when the parents come to take their child home or on any other occasion, to give simple information on child care and nutrition and to encourage the parents to bring the child to follow-up clinics or to attend a health center. Efforts must be made to ensure that the primary health care worker is kept informed.

In the same way, outpatient departments provide many occasions for nurses to give useful advice. It is often possible for auxiliaries and volunteers (for example, from women's societies) or lay workers to help with the routine sorting of cards, weighing, and temperature taking, to give the nurses more time for holding short, practical lessons in health education.

Experience in home visiting during the early months of nursing training and in the company of a good health care provider (especially if it concerns a child she has nursed in the hospital) will help familiarize a nurse with what she can do and, above all, how it should be done. The dramatic impact of home visiting cannot be overemphasized. This is now a regular feature of nursing training at the University of Riberao Preto, Brazil, and some other schools.

The more peripheral the worker is, the more comprehensive the approach must be. It is essential to train comprehensive multipurpose auxiliaries, as well as nurses and supervisory personnel. At the same time, problems have to be faced with regard to overloading health workers. Attention to selection of health workers, particularly of community or village health workers, is critical.

Nurses should be trained in the techniques of health education (Williams 1966). Group teaching is often advocated for hospitals, outpatient clinics, and health centers, but unless the teaching is neither mechanical nor impractical, it can be a waste of time. A nurse who is a trained teacher can give classes in schools and to trade unions, agricultural societies, mother's unions, scouts, and guides. Because of practical knowledge of the subject, the nurse will be more successful than lectures or classes given by a teacher who is more experienced in method than in content (Fig. 16.4).

Infant welfare centers were first started in the 1900s in the United Kingdom, France, and the United States. They were directed to give only preventive care, while patients were sent to doctors or hospitals for treatment. Those who worked in areas where they provided the only available medical care soon realized that treatment must come first and should be as efficient as possible. They also saw that preventive work was more effective when combined with curative. An increasing number of MCH enterprises in developing countries have adopted a policy of giving curative as well as preventive treatment. Weighing clinics, under-5 years of age clinics, and mothercraft centers are examples of clinics used as primary centers where all who come are seen and examined. For vulnerable groups, regular attendance must be encouraged. The well are commended, advised, and immunized. Minor disorders are treated at once and advice given. Some cases may be referred to the doctor's clinics, and some children are scheduled for home visits. The seriously ill are sent or taken to hospitals as soon as possible. Nurses with good training and experience have proved admirable at this type of work. They may, in fact, be better than doctors, for they are often more patient and sympathetic. The more sophisticated countries, such as the United States, are beginning to realize the value, the economic advantage, and the absolute need for this type of health worker— for example, for pediatric nurse practitioners (Silver et al. 1968). In the Caribbean, a similar group has developed recently, family nurse-practitioners.

The importance of nursing care cannot be overstressed (Ennever et al. 1969). In areas where malnutrition is rife, the attention to choice, preparation, and presentation of food is far more important than the mere distribution through supplementary feeding programs, as is attention to all the important details of a baby's life that protect him or her from infections. In areas where there is a high death rate from measles and whooping cough, attention to nursing details, as well as to immunization, can reduce mortality.

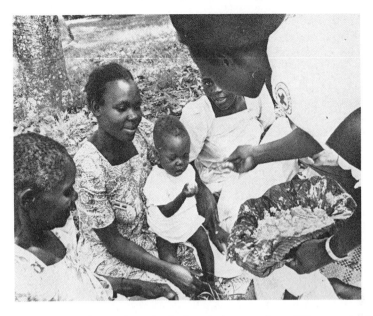

Figure 16.4. Practical experience in the hospital can make a difference. An MCH demonstrator in Uganda gives a weaning food demonstration using locally available, economical, and cultural acceptable mixtures cooked in the traditional way (steamed in banana leaf packets, *ettu*). UNICEF photograph by Peter Larsen.

Occupational therapy on an informal level deserves more attention from doctors, nurses, and other health workers. The subject is too often looked upon as a service provided only if and when a professional occupational therapist visits a ward. However, occupational therapy has a therapeutic value, as well as providing the patient with another interest. Patients do not benefit simply from making baskets or teddy bears. They should be encouraged to improve their independence and self-esteem. Occupation is therapeutic on an informal as well as on a formal level and may lead to better opportunities for income generation on return home if useful skills are learned. Play opportunities for children must be studied also, as these can have an important bearing on recovery.

Midwives

The practice of midwifery is as old as humanity. The mother of the pregnant woman is sometimes the attendant on whom these duties fall, but in every society there are people, usually women, who acquire special skills and reputations for midwifery work.

In the European tradition, the qualified physician of the past generally left obstetric duties to a "wise women," "midwife," or possibly a "male midwife," until the Chamberlaynes introduced obstetric forceps in seventeenth-century England.

It was Florence Nightingale who organized the regular training and registration of midwives in England in about 1870. Their function was to conduct deliveries and recognize abnormalities, and at this they proved themselves excellent and continue to be so. The United States has not encouraged the use and training of midwives. The result has been that in many rural and underprivileged areas, as many as 70 percent of mothers may be delivered without any form of qualified assistance.

Training of midwives must be related to the conditions within which they must practice (Appendixes 5 and 7). A relatively advanced country such as the United Kingdom provides a training of two years, which concentrates on care before, during, and after delivery. But in a developing area where there are few or no other health workers, midwives must be trained more broadly. The training and employment of midwives should be expanded in hospitals, clinics, and homes. Midwives can develop great skills for use in ante- and postnatal clinics, the management of normal cases, the recognition of abnormalities, postpartum home care, and infant and young child care (including nutrition). In Haiti, the training of TBAs reduced neonatal mortality through the provision of antenatal tetanus immunization (Berggren et al. 1983).

In less developed areas babies are often small. Obstetric difficulties are due not so much to disproportion as to anemic, malnourished, and overworked mothers or to untreated diseases, such as worms, pelvic infections, and malaria. Merely admitting the mother to the hospital for a few days at delivery may be expensive and can do little good compared with competent antenatal and postnatal care.

A midwife can be anyone from a completely illiterate TBA to a highly trained obstetric nurse-midwife. All of the various grades in between are valuable, however, and all can be improved by training, supervision, and cooperation. The training of TBA's needs to be individualized to local needs. In less developed areas, some knowledge of midwifery is essential for all health workers, including public health nurses and medical assistants.

Training in the past has concentrated on navigation of the birth canal (Jelliffe 1962). It should instead include nutrition, infant and young child care, related home economics, preparation for and management of breastfeeding (especially before delivery), the organization of ante- and postnatal clinics, home deliveries, and

home visiting and must include some knowledge and understanding of fertility control (Appendix 6).

One outstanding example of the use of rural midwives is the training that originated with the Wolff sisters in the Sudan in the first half of this century. Another example is the instruction of *bidans* (traditional birth attendants) from Trenggannu in Malaysia (Appendix 2) (Williams 1942). Within six months of starting the project, over fifty *bidans* were enrolled; about twenty came to the meeting each week and submitted their baskets, their books, their clothes, their hands, and their patients for inspection, discussion, and instruction. Some of the *bidans* were invited to spend a week or two at the hospital to help with patient care— principally to familiarize them with what the hospital was trying to do, and how it was being done. These *bidans* became a focus of contact with the scattered villages. They welcomed the doctor, nurse, and medical assistants; reported happenings; and encouraged registration. They soon learned not to restrict themselves solely to maternity care but to advise on breastfeeding, weaning diet, and nutrition in general; to look out for cases of fever, diarrhea, worms, skin diseases, and malnutrition; and to encourage care of houses, gardens, water supply, and refuse disposal. Their activities encouraged mothers and children to seek hospital treatment and showed great promise. This experiment, however, was interrupted by the Japanese occupation. It nevertheless represented a good start in a practical program with minimal financial outlay (Williams 1942).

Similar training programs for village birth attendants have been undertaken in many developing countries with the help of WHO advisers and UNICEF equipment (Manguay-Maglacas and Pizurki 1981; Parlato and Favin 1982). The provision of a sturdy bag with equipment and supplies may act both as an initial incentive and as a means of maintaining

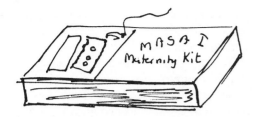

Figure 16.5. Masai maternity matchbox kit: Easy to carry, cheap, and effective. The kit contains soap, blade, and sterile cord tie.

contact and continuing incentive when supplies are renewed. In Guerjerat, India, and Kenya, maternity kits are in use (Fig. 16.5). They cost much less ($.05–$.10) than the UNICEF kit ($46.00) and reach more people. This type of program has also been used for indigenous midwives in the almost inaccessible out islands of the Bahamas.

Where TBAs are trained and their practice encouraged, supervision and evaluation are vital to ensure that good-quality health care is being provided. In Brazil, evaluation of the *parteiras* associated with a hospital at the Federal University of Ceara showed that mothers were delivered in a squatting position, and the cord was tied only after the placenta was delivered. Puerperal infection was absent, fetal distress from prolonged labor was not found, and the frequency of normal deliveries was very high. Much of their success has been attributed to watchful waiting, their knowledge of abdominal massage to speed labor, their ability to recognize a breech or transverse lie, their cleanliness and frequency of hand washing, and the fact that they never do a gynecological examination. Although one of the birth attendants interviewed had over 1,000 deliveries to her credit, she had never seen the genitals of her patients (Araujo 1980).

A study of community-based midwives in rural Greece found their role at the village level to be significant in protecting the health of poor and less-educated mothers. The perception that pregnancy and delivery are natural conditions has changed, and people now tend to seek delivery from specialists. Those who can afford hospital care do so; this has resulted in a decrease in postnatal care and a pronounced negative impact on breast-feeding (11 percent of mothers who delivered at home did not breastfeed compared with 38 percent of those who had hospital deliveries) (Bakoula 1983).

In the Philippines, the TBA *(hilot)* is being used as a stopgap measure until more midwives are trained. In Sudan, untrained midwives had to go underground, as they were considered to be practicing illegally (Mangay-Maglacas and Pizurki 1981). A 1990 survey showed that 60 percent of births in Sudan were assisted by trained health workers, 9 percent by doctors, and 26 percent by TBAs (mainly in rural areas). TBAs used to be the main providers of female circumcision, but they are increasingly being replaced by nurse midwives who have learned to do this as an extracurricular activity (Mahmoud 1992).

The wide variation in type, experience, and practices makes it essential not to accept TBAs as a homogeneous group and to monitor their activities carefully. Even a trained TBA or midwife, however, cannot provide emergency midwifery services. Where there are no doctors, there is now an attempt to train nurse midwives and medical assistants to be able to deal with emergencies.

Auxiliaries

A great range of auxiliary workers is needed, and experiments are being made all over the world in this belated, though highly necessary, aspect of extension programs (Parlato and Favin 1982; WHO 1968, 1970). The delay in developing realistic programs for training personnel has been due to a number of factors.

Before World War II, it was extremely useful to train and use feldschers in Eastern Europe, subassistant surgeons in India, illiterate midwives in the Sudan, and various grades of dressers, dispensers, and hospital nurses all over the world. After the war, many of the newly independent countries seemed to think that these people were "half-doctors" and "half-nurses" and thus incompatible with national dignity because they implied makeshift or "mud-hut" medicine. Many of these extremely practical and useful workers were upgraded or abolished—to the detriment of health services.

The international bodies that were established after 1945 were mainly interested in disease control programs, supplementary feeding, and providing supplies and equipment. Constructive programs such as the establishment of MCH and training services initially received minimal attention. Apparently few people appreciated how much the war had interfered with the normal progress of education and training. For instance, during the three and a half years of the Japanese occupation of Malaya, all education for girls was stopped.

Another factor is that doctors' and nurses' professional societies have been, on the whole, suspicious, disapproving, and economically jealous of any categories of personnel, or their functions, that do not fit in with conventional patterns. This outlook has resulted in a shortage of health staff that interferes with expansion and is damaging to the reputation of the medical and nursing professions. Recently, the tide has begun to turn. In many areas of the world, from New Guinea to New Mexico, experiments are being conducted in the selection, training, and employment of paraprofessional or allied health workers who can perform many of the primary care functions of both physicians and nurses and do so with enthusiasm and skill (Lancet 1970; Greenfield 1969; Parlato and Favin 1982). We are witnessing new human potential and a new mobility in this primary health care revolution. More of these experiments are necessary, with greater expansion of the ideas involved and greater opportunities for comparing their rationale and results.

An advantage of auxiliary programs is that they employ people who are unlikely to join an immediate brain drain, particularly if they are trained locally rather than in a city. Nevertheless, some mobility should be anticipated.

Often auxiliaries are best recruited locally and trained in the region. Slightly older persons are often the best; the main qualifications, however, are enthusiasm and compassion. The types of health workers differ, as well as their educational level, the duration and cost of their training, and their salary (Table 16.2) (Baumslag et al. 1978). Auxiliary training varies from two weeks in the Dominican Republic to three months in Pakistan.

The range of duties of village health workers in primary care projects is broad, and the task and work load may be overwhelming (Table 16.3). Where one worker provides education, another type of village worker provides immunizations. In Tunisia, the front line worker was expected to distribute pills and condoms and also carry out immunizations. In Senegal, the village first aid man performed tasks equivalent to those of a physician assistant in the United States. In Mali the village health worker was assigned an enormous number of tasks that are difficult to provide, let alone supervise.

Multipurpose workers appear to be the trend. The Sine Saloum project in Senegal originally trained three types of health workers: a first aid worker to treat common illness, a hygienist to promote environmental sanitation, and a TBA to provide antenatal and postnatal care and assist at deliveries. But after a few months it become clear that the community could not support three categories of worker, and the project was redesigned. Interestingly, hygienists were excluded because the community considered them the most expendable (or least understandable) group (Parlato and Favin 1982).

Table 16.2. Estimated Costs of Training and Support for Volunteer and Auxiliary Health Workers in Selected Primary Care Health Projects (U.S. $)

Country	Title of worker	Training	Salary
Philippines	Barangay health assistant	$400	$320/year
Pakistan	Village health worker	$200 (3 months) includes $15/month allowance	volunteer
Pakistan	Mid-level worker	$940 (18 months)	
Niger	Village health worker	$150 (15 days), US$50/yr (5 days)	volunteer
	Environmental health worker	$2,000 (1 year) afterward	$1,200/year
	Practical nurse	$2,000 (1 year)	$1,200/year
Jamaica	Community health aid		$1,600/year
	Midwives		$3,500/year
Brazil	Health promoter		$450/year
	Multipurpose auxiliary	6 months	$1,000/year
	Maternal-child health Auxiliary	6 months	$1,000/year
Dominican Republic	Promoter	$56 (2 weeks)	$360/year
	Nurse auxiliary	$56 (2 weeks)	$1,400/year
Cameroon	Mid-level worker	$3,000 (1 year)	
	Village health worker	$500 (2 months)	

Source: Baumslag et al. (1978).

Selection of health workers generally tends to be by the community councils, but often the choice turns out to be a relative of a high official. Nepotism and politics may influence the selection of health workers, and while these people may be able to mobilize sections of the community, they may not inspire confidence. When literacy is a requirement, this often precludes women, and where men are not allowed to examine women, this adds to the problems of access, as is the case in Muslim countries. Furthermore, males do not have as ready access to children. Generally female community workers in their early forties or older are preferred. The Thailand Lampang project has male health workers and is one of the exceptions. Most of the workers are volunteers. In some cases, the government pays them a meager salary. When payment is through the community council, workers retain some allegiance to the community. If paid directly by the government, then they serve the government. Others receive remuneration through the sale of drugs, which may have a detri-mental effect on health promotion be-cause curative medicine becomes the sole focus.

Where untrained traditional healers exist, they may not only compete with the public health care system but they may also do harm, as was noted in a report from Zambia describing a syndrome of cerebral irritability and renal failure following herbal treatment for diarrhea (Maguire and Chawla 1983). Trainers of health care workers may not be adequately trained as educators and may not have assessed community needs or job requirements. They impart a few skills and much information in a hospital setting where they may teach bottle feeding and such nonprimary health care practices.

Without an adequate, well-defined referral system, students are left with an impossible job and, in some cases, an incredible load. Often the countries with the most limited health resources and the weakest infrastructure are those that demand the most of their village health workers (Joseph 1977). Often the least

Table 16.3. Duties of Volunteer and Auxiliary Health Workers in Selected Low-Cost Health Delivery Projects

Afghanistan: Village health worker	Tunisia: Front line worker	Senegal: Village first aid man	Mali: Village health worker
Detect and prevent malnutrition in children	Instruction in use of weaning food	Manage village health unit	Record births, deaths, migration, and marriages
Advise on weaning practices and good storage	Distribute pills and condoms	Diagnose and treat (with drugs) malaria,	Record weights of neonates, infants, and children
Advise on hygiene and sanitation	Immunization shots	conjunctivitis, headaches, cough,	Promote breastfeeding and weaning foods
Provide family planning service	Prenatal screening of mothers	anemia, worms, scabies	Provide iron supplements to pregnant women
Provide first aid	Treat simple wounds	Refer more serious cases	Diagnose and treat early malnutrition
Diagnose, treat and refer:	Screen and treat children at risk of malnutrition	Keep records and manage payments	Refer abnormal pregnancies, serious malnutrition, and severe illnesses to health center
Children's diarrhea Conjunctivitis and trachoma Skin infections Worms Bronchitis and pneumonia	Diagnose and treat, common skin disorders, conjunctivitis, fever, anemia, burns, and wounds	Treat simple wounds	Provide family planning advice
		Assist village chief in birth and death registration	Monitor vaccination status in village
		Assist in vaccination campaigns	Promote hygiene in the home and clean water and sanitation in village
			Vaccinate pregnant women in third month for tetanus
			Provide first aid and oral treatment for malaria
			Distribute appropriate medicines

Source: Baumslag et al. (1978).

educated and least rewarded are expected to have the greatest and widest knowledge and practical burden of work.

Several principles related to the utilization and training of auxiliary health workers should be considered (Mercer 1982; Storms 1979; Werner and Bower 1982):

1. Workers who are selected by and from the communities in which they live are more likely to remain there and also to have a better understanding of the problems of that community.

2. Ongoing training, supervision, and support is essential if the worker is to function effectively.

3. However simple the training, its importance should be acknowledged.

4. A well-defined set of tasks that the worker should be able to perform should be carefully chosen, based on the most common problems. In smaller communities, there will be a narrower range of problems that occur frequently enough so that skills in the identification and management of the problems can be maintained.

5. The auxiliary health worker is often the essential link between the health care system and the community. It is important to strengthen this relationship by treating these workers as important members of the health care

team and to encourage responsiveness and loyalty to the community in which they live and work.

6. The primary goal of all health workers should be to increase the capacity of the community to solve its own problems. The health worker should be dissuaded from adopting the traditional attitudes of medical elitism and demanding unquestioning obedience of a doctor's or other health professional's orders.

7. Training should be related to needs and resources and based on a job description of the health worker, so educational objectives can be defined.

8. Some of the training activities for health professionals and auxiliaries should be carried out simultaneously wherever possible to foster a team spirit.

If the role of auxiliary workers is not carefully defined to complement existing health services, workers may be faced with unfair expectations and an impossible task (Table 16.4). Most of all, resources need to be available. As Mampela Ramphele said, no one can pull themselves up by their bootstraps if they have no boots.

Voluntary Work

Many areas of the world have community development groups, women's clubs, and religious groups whose members can be encouraged to give practical voluntary help in clinics or in home visiting. Some of the members are suitable for recruitment and training as aides or auxiliaries, for they live in and know the community and often show natural leadership and some practical expertise.

Maternal and child health services are particularly suitable for the education and experience they can give, while at the same time receiving help from these women. Most sophisticated countries similarly have women's societies of the same type as the Women's Institute in the United Kingdom. Activities include home visiting (reporting progress, advising attendance at clinics, giving domestic support), working in clinics (keeping cards, helping mothers, taking temperatures, weighing babies, giving out food), and working in hospitals (running a hospital bookstore, writing letters for patients or reading to them, organizing entertainment or occupational therapy). These are often the people who are most useful on health or hospital committees, and their inside knowledge of the needs and resources of the health services makes them invaluable.

There is a tendency for many modern states to take on more of the work of social and welfare services as health and education are too important to be left entirely in the uncertain hands of voluntary effort. The totalitarian societies find that a great deal of their conditioning can be accomplished through these services. But for a more liberal society, the use of volunteers has a number of advantages, and it is these voluntary societies that have often initiated advances in education and in medical care. They have an essential part to play in exploring the needs of communities and experimenting in methods of meeting them. Moreover, by using and guiding voluntary effort, the services may be expanded to reach a greater number of people at minimum cost. The voluntary worker gives priceless assistance and at the same time receives in-service training and education, and so can raise standards of living and of responsibility.

The use of well-prepared national and international volunteers is to be recommended for many types of work, provided there is sufficient supervision and provided activities are part of present and future health service plans (Delano 1970; Keynes 1968). Volunteers may come from the Voluntary Service Overseas and the Peace Corps, as well as nongovernmental organizations (grass-roots or nonprofit groups) such as Wellstart, World Vision,

Table 16.4. Supporting Community Health Workers (CHWs)

	Problems	Solutions
Isolated	Difficult terrain and long distances interfere with communications, support, supplies referral, and retraining. Areas most dependent on CHWs are the most difficult to reach.	Use radio, carrier pigeon, and personal notes if literate or use pictograms if illiterate. Plan for supplies, transport (gasoline), regular supervision, and retraining. Use itinerant trainers.
Overloaded	Too few workers for terrain, too many duties. CHWs are used as a catch-all for everything.	Prioritize tasks. Train more CHWs. Establish referral system.
Disenchanted	Left with curative jobs but no medicines or food supplements, community bypasses them. CHWs stigmatized as "sterilization agent."	Motivate (provide incentives, public recognition). Supervise, provide regular supplies (medicines, food supplements, growth charts). Make sure practice is culturally acceptable.
Unsuitable	Not chosen by or representative of community (political appointees can mobilize, not motivate). Too young (not respected). Wrong sex (males—no access to women and children). Training inflexible (retrained smallpox worker retains disease mentality). Drug profit remuneration encourages only curative practice and even quackery. No allegiance to community if paid by central government.	Community should choose the worker. Analyze possible harmful effects of selection or payment system. Monitor to prevent quackery or to find out if a poor choice has been made.
Great expectations	Government does not follow up (holes dug by community for latrines but no slabs delivered). People expect more than CHW can deliver. CHW expects to gain financially or socially.	Plan with realistic goals and objectives. Before creating enthusiasm, make sure there are means to follow through. Make clear to the community what the CHW can do.
Exploited	Not paid. Payment is only token (inadequate or demeaning).	Agree on regular remuneration in kind or cash, depending on local circumstances. (Mozambique pays in commodities, or people worked land for CHW. Zimbabwe pays minimum domestic wage.)

and the Save the Children's Fund. In every enterprise in the health field, one should consider how to make best use of volunteers.

METHODS OF EDUCATION FOR PROFESSIONAL WORKERS

The methods of education depend on the type of available personnel, facilities for teaching, and requirements of the work. Haphazard training can be avoided through the use of a training plan that follows eight steps:

1. Identify needs and problems to be met by the community health worker.
2. Define major tasks that the trainee will be required to meet.
3. Divide major tasks into specific minor tasks.
4. Indicate knowledge and skills needed.
5. Formulate learning objectives.
6. Formulate evaluation and testing procedure.

7. Plan the logistics of support and supervision procedures.
8. Plan for in-service training based on task analysis and competency.

Lecture-Demonstration Group Discussions

Systematic lectures should be kept to a minimum. Textbooks are expensive, they are soon out-of-date, and they are mainly written for countries with high technology. Journals also are often in short supply and dated. Lectures can, however, point out the relevance of a subject to local conditions, can update facts, figures, and skills, and can add personal experiences within the local context (Rosa 1964). Ideally, they should be intimate and friendly. They are most effective if presented in a participatory form using demonstrations and group discussions that are problem oriented. Students should be given the opportunity to be involved in the teaching.

In some medical schools where systematic lectures have been reduced or discarded, too much lecturing may take place at the bedside, which is difficult for students who want to take notes and can be unpleasant for the patients.

Books, Pamphlets, and Audiovisuals

Where students are literate, it is useful to reproduce and circulate pamphlets or notes adapted to local conditions and problems. It is important to produce teaching materials in the official language of the country. Expatriate staff should be expected to learn the local language.

When dealing with illiterate midwives or auxiliaries, specific instructions should be read to them and referred to in their own language (Appendix 2). Simplified color-coded measures and records can also be adapted for their use (Mangay-Maglacas and Pizurki 1981; Philpott 1980; Shah 1980).

Reading Material

The more advanced categories of students must be encouraged to refer to source material and current periodicals. It is useful to choose a few outstanding articles and to give each student a selected set of photocopied articles to study before each seminar. This material provides a good basis for discussion. Students must also be taught to review the literature critically and efficiently (Riegelman 1981).

Bedside Teaching

Harsh criticisms have been made about the old-fashioned ward round. In fact, a good physician ensures that the patient experiences little discomfort or embarrassment. For pediatric patients, discomfort is to be avoided by every possible means. Grand rounds, when one or two patients are used in demonstrations in a theater before a large audience, must be organized with the greatest consideration to avoid embarrassment. Without objectives, a ward round can become more of a foot-of-the-bed scene than a bedside demonstration.

Physical signs in a child must be studied in small groups with an instructor, possibly in a side room with the mother present. This should not take place without consultation with the nursing staff, so as to make certain of current clinical position and signs.

Regular Observation

A patient admitted to a ward should be seen and observed regularly. The most senior staff member should regularly review patients' care, treatment, and progress. Some students get only a static, textbook picture of disease, because a once-only type of demonstration is given. The way to appreciate the natural history of disease—its onset, progress, complications, and recovery (or termination at autopsy)—is to follow through all these processes and reactions to treatment. Continuing observation in the hospital, outpatient departments, and home care and supervision centers is the only way of developing family- rather than disease-oriented medical care.

The Guessing Game

Another recommended procedure of training is to examine a patient thoroughly on admission before he or she has been worked up with laboratory and other tests. Something can be learned from the physical state of the child as well as the attitude of the mother. It is good practice to guess the age, the weight, the pulse and respiration rate, the hemoglobin, and the temperature before any of these are ascertained mechanically or otherwise. The habit of "guesstimating" will save a number of tragedies that may occur because a low-registering thermometer has been used, or the scales are out of order, or a report has been misplaced—and it will prove extremely useful in emergencies. Such a technique is indispensable for home care, home visiting, and community-side teaching. Throughout training, it is essential to stress the need for extreme gentleness in examination and treatment and for courtesy at all times.

It may seem superfluous to stress these qualities, but too often even experienced pediatricians, obstetricians, and nurses are abrupt in their approach, rough in their handling, and dictatorial and tragically unrealistic in their advice. Working under conditions of great pressure and hardships, sometimes with uneducated, unreasonable, or even callous parents, is infuriating and intolerable. Yet however great the provocation, impatience on the part of the health staff never does any good.

Hospital-bound, laboratory-centered training that characterizes graduate programs in Western countries can be harmful for health professionals in technologically underdeveloped countries who often cannot apply what they have learned to their own countries. The practice of sending health professionals for postgraduate training in pediatrics, obstetrics, public health, or other specialties to Europe and North America needs careful thought because readjustment on return can be traumatic. The traditional status pertaining to (often inappropriate) foreign diplomas and degrees may act as a hindrance to progress in implementing cheaper and more relevant health programs.

In many places, particularly in parts of Africa and in some of the socialist countries, the trend is to make local postgraduate degrees available in the region. Not only is the relevance increased, but the cost is considerably less.

TRAINING OF AUXILIARY HEALTH WORKERS

Although systematic evaluation of the best methods for training primary health care workers is still needed, there is some information as to the best methods and principles of short-term training (Ronaghy et al. 1983; WHO 1977). Because these workers are often semiliterate or even illiterate, they must be taught skills and ideas in ways different from the usual classroom education (Mercer 1982; Storms 1979).

Trainers

Although physicians and nurses most often train auxiliary health workers, they are not always the best choice. For an educational program to be effective, both teacher and student must learn. Trainers must be competent to train, in addition to knowing the subject matter, at both the theoretical and practical levels. Health professionals are not necessarily knowledgeable in training methods and may have only a minimal understanding of the actual field problems of the village-level worker. The best trainers are experienced, competent workers of the type being trained, who can relate well to the needs and problems of the workers. It is particularly helpful if that trainer is the field supervisor after work begins. In any case, it should be remembered that special training for the trainers of auxiliary health workers is usually necessary (WHO 1982).

Training Site

Training should be carried out as close to the actual work setting as possible. It is difficult for individuals who are unfamiliar with a new subject matter to adapt the knowledge and skills they acquire in one setting, such as in an urban hospital (often the most convenient training site), to another work setting, such as their own village. The need for adaptation should be kept at a minimum; thus, the training conditions should be as much like the actual work conditions as is feasible.

Cost of Training

Training is not cheap. In the SINAPS program in Guatemala, training and supervision of voluntary personnel was the most expensive component of the program because of the cost per diem for attendance of personnel at training sessions and additional gasoline required during supervision (Lechtig et al. 1982). This explains why supervision and on-site competency-based evaluation is often difficult although desirable.

Methods

The most important rule to follow in training auxiliaries is to let the trainees do their identified tasks, not just see and hear descriptions (Werner 1982). Learning by experience is how many people, particularly those not highly literate, are accustomed to learning, and frequent repetition helps to consolidate new skills. Some useful methods are case presentations; using actual patients whenever possible (for example, babies, not dolls); small discussion groups; role playing, a valuable technique that allows the trainees to act out what they learn; and the demonstration and practice of the most important skills, including teaching of patients. Probably the worst method for training auxiliary health workers is that most commonly used for the education of professionals: classroom lectures.

Training Content

Health workers working without constant supervision should be trained to take care of the most common problems. General knowledge, while important, cannot replace specific skills such as hygienic practices during delivery; use of at-risk measures for referral (arm circumference and weight); recognition and treatment of common conditions, including malaria, pneumonia, and diarrhea; and teaching mothers to prepare weaning foods. A training curriculum should center around skills most needed in practice. The temptation to provide a wide array of interesting background information, such as the exact anatomy of the intestinal tract, should be scrupulously avoided in most situations. Teaching skills that cannot be utilized should also be avoided; for example, there is no point in teaching people how to prepare and diagnose malaria smears if microscope and laboratory services are unavailable.

THE CURRICULUM IN MCH SERVICES

It may be necessary to examine the training in pediatrics at medical, nursing, and midwifery schools and to improve this considerably (Basalamah et al. 1979; Miller 1973; Walldren 1974; Zais 1976).

The Royal College of Physicians in London lays down rules for the preparation of specialist pediatricians. These do not require any time to be spent outside the walls of institutions. In the United Kingdom alone, there is a great variation in the duration of and attention to pediatric training for doctors; the mean total spent has been estimated to range between 110 and 314 hours. Furthermore, Veeneklaas concluded that "at least half of the pediatric teaching in centers in Europe are not up to standard" (Stapleton 1969); this still holds true today. Great care should be taken before accepting the present position of any university in Europe as one to be copied. The great differences in age structure and in mortality rates makes pediatrics an even more important subject for developing countries (Jelliffe 1962; Jelliffe and Stanfield 1966; Stapleton 1969; Williams 1967; Wise et al. 1968).

Training of doctors for MCH work necessarily entails postgraduate courses. American schools of public health have departments of MCH, but their courses usually include little or nothing in the way of community pediatrics or obstetrics. The schools of public health in the United Kingdom have no departments of MCH. Anyone interested in this area therefore has to learn from various other departments, which include training in communicable disease control, statistics, health education, and hospital administration. The student may have to go outside the school to find training in clinical pediatrics and obstetrics, clinical nutrition, and family planning.

When the American University of Beirut instituted a Diploma in Public Health, all the student physicians followed a course in maternal and child health (Appendix 1). This included three "contact" hours per week for the academic year in MCH and three "contact" hours per week for half the year in nutrition.

Refresher courses can last from one day up to several years. They can be social as well as educational and use many forms of communication. Even at a simple level, they can prove encouraging and exciting and are worth a good deal of effort in time and from personnel, especially when organized in regions other than the capital city and with the cooperation of local people. An example is the course in child health for Grade Two Midwives in Nigeria (Appendix 3). In some programs, peripatetic teams of teachers provide training in the village setting (Vaughan 1983).

CAREER PATHS

To upgrade a medical assistant to the status of medical officer may be to overcome major psychological and educational barriers to progress and promotion. In theory, it seems admirable that this great leap forward should be feasible; in practice, it is fraught with controversy. Nevertheless, it should be considered. The problem is not limited to medical assistants but includes enrolled nurses (students who have undergone 3 years of training in the British system in Africa, many of whom are being discontinued and replaced by nurses with bachelor degrees with little or no experience). Myriads of certificates and diplomas are awarded with no possibility of career advancement, allowing only lateral mobility. Unless there is an infrastructure for health personnel training and development that forges a link between university, ministry of health, and other institutions, especially nursing institutions, for equivalency and accreditation, unnecessary educational waste occurs. Nurses often have to take three similar biochemistry courses to attain higher educational levels. There must be a career ladder to allow upward mobility.

With higher levels of education, all developing countries are experiencing a movement from certificates to degrees. Even "barefoot" doctors want to be trained as "real" doctors (Rifkin 1980). They receive preference for entrance to medical school if they meet the academic requirements. Nurses, medical assistants, and other health professionals with considerable field experience and demonstrated clinical abilities should be given the same opportunities. They should be given medical school admission priority and credit for work done. Judging by the certificates that abound, the situation requires serious attention.

MCH SERVICES

Conditions of Employment

Housing, transport, hours of work, pay and pay increases, promotion, and facilities for education of children must all be considered in detail to avoid hardship and encourage good work. Terms of employment for women, married or unmarried, are of importance; too many well-trained women doctors and nurses are now wasted because of the rigid discriminatory practices that exist. Staff should have breastfeeding breaks and child care facilities. Unnecessarily low standards of service exacerbate the brain drain seen in an extreme form in the Caribbean. In this area, the total number of trained nurses decreased by 543 between 1967 and 1969, and of 100 doctors qualifying at the University of the West Indies Medical School in 1969, 40 emigrated within a year. At that time each doctor cost about $28,000 to train. This "reverse aid" represented a considerable financial loss of over $1 million (Standard 1969). Nurses from developing countries are emigrating to the United States where they are in short supply and get offers of good salaries.

Transport

Satisfied patients and contented staff depend to a considerable extent on transport facilities. Successful integration of hospital, health center, and home care services will necessitate more attention to transport than the usual type of institutional hospital. In 1940, in a remote part of Malaysia, the training of village midwives included learning to ride a bicycle. Whether the health staff should rely on walking, bicycles, cars, motorcycles, elephants, or public transport must be decided according to needs and resources. Whatever decisions are taken, it will be found that efficient work depends largely on adequate transport. To persuade the health staff at all levels, including the physicians, to use transport with skill, economy, and a sense of responsibility is an essential part of training.

Large, elaborate "traveling dispensaries" should be avoided. A car with a couple of boxes of supplies and equipment and a small mobile staff will do more and better work and at much less cost.

A room or two in a house in the village or at the school can be used to examine and treat patients. This can be a better locale for health teaching, record keeping, and maintaining contacts than any mobile clinic. Finally, for hospital and clinic staff who have to travel any distance or who have small children and no child care, a creche, day nursery, or school for their babies and children is invaluable. The creches can also be used to observe children with behavioral and other problems.

CONCLUSION

In spite of the great need for better medical care and more health professionals, today's medical organization is often wasteful, especially in more technically developed countries. There may be several open heart surgery or cobalt units within the same area or staff nurses used to prepare infant formula. At the same time, there is inadequate home care and follow-up; insufficient attention is given to the training and supervision of personnel, and there is insufficient mobility of staff and too few channels of promotion. More attention should be devoted to experiments in the training and employment of auxiliary personnel and their upward mobility. The selection, training, supervision, and evaluation of personnel should be emphasized in graduate courses. Some educators have little training or interest in education. Health workers should understand and practice the principles that they teach. Medical care inevitably makes great demands on personal services, but more informed attention to personnel and training will do much to improve the quality of health services. Two factors must be kept in mind. First, the worker who is responsible for organizing MCH services in a relatively unsophisticated area must have training and experience on a far wider basis than that recommended for the usual pediatric specialist in a sophisticated country. Second, when the time comes that basic education gives less attention to traditional academic subjects and more to human behavior and relationships, economics, and politics, then better students will be available as trainees in health work.

REFERENCES

Araujo, G. (1980). The traditional birth attendant in Brazil. In *Maternity Services in the Developing World—What the Community Needs.* Ed. R. H. Philpott. Proceedings of the Seventh Study Group of the Royal College of Obstetricians and Gynaecologists, London.

Bakoula (1983). The role of the community based midwife in the Greek village. *J. Trop. Pediat.* **29,** 215.

Basalamah, A.; Rosinski, E.; and Schumacher, H. (1979). Developing the medical curriculum at King Abdulaziz University. *J. Med. Educ.* **54,** 96.

Baumslag, N., and Boston, E. (1982). Public Health Training from Concept to Feasibility: Review and Guidelines. Mimeographed report. Tulane School of Public Health, New Orleans.

Baumslag, N.; Rosel, C.; and Sabin, E. (1978). *AID Integrated Low Cost Health Projects.* Vol. 11: *Analysis.* Department of Health, Education and Welfare, Washington, D.C.

Berggren, G. G.; Berggren, W.; Verly, A.; Garnier, N.; Peterson, W.; Ewbank, D.; and Dieudonne, W. (1983). Traditional midwives, tetanus immunizations, and infant mortality in rural Haiti. *Trop. Doctor* **13,** 79.

BMJ (1968). Paediatric teaching for overseas. *Brit. Med. J.* **1,** 465; **2,** 693.

Bryant, J. H. (1969). *Health and the Developing World.* Cornell University Press, Ithaca, N.Y.

Dean, N. M. B. (1958). Health problems of the preschool child in Africa and the role of the public health nurse in their solution. *J. Trop. Pediat.* **4,** 12.

Delano, W. A. (1970). The importance and role of volunteers for development. In *Malnutrition Is a Problem of Ecology.* Ed. P. Giorsky, and O. L. Kline. International Union of Nutritional Sciences, Basel.

de la Pax, T. (1983). The Katiwala approach to training community health workers. *Wld. Hlth. Forum* **4,** 34.

Dixit, H. (1982). Training to meet the health needs in Nepal. *Indian J. Pediat.* **49,** 481.

Ennever, O., Marsh, M., and Standard, K. L. (1969). A community health aide training program. *W. Indian Med. J.* **18,** 193.

Esman, M. J.; Colle, R.; Uphoff, N.; and Taylor, E. (1980). Local Organizations: Intermediaries in Rural Development (mimeographed report). Centre for International Studies, Cornell University, Ithaca, N.Y.

Evans, J. R. (1981). *Measurement and Management in Medicine and Health Service.* Rockefeller Foundation, New York.

Fendall, N. R. E. (1966). Education or research? *Lancet* **i,** 257.

Fernando, M. (1964). Morbidity and medical care in Ceylon. *Ceylon Med. J.* **9,** 26.

Foley, R. P., and Smilansky, J. (1980). *Teaching Techniques: A Handbook for Health Professionals.* McGraw-Hill, New York.

Greenfield, H. L. (1969). *Allied Health Manpower; Trends and Prospects.* Columbia University Press, New York.

Guilbert, J. J. (1982). *Educational Handbook*

for Health Personnel. Offset Publication, no. 35. World Health Organization, Geneva.

Huntington, C; Sweeney, R.; and Graham, R. (1992). The shortage of generalist physicians. *Am. Family Physician* **45** (4), 1573–76.

Jackson, A. D. M. (1966). A survey of paediatric teaching in the undergraduate medical schools of the United Kingdom. *Brit. J. Med. Educ.* **1**, 25.

Jelliffe, D. B. (1955). Pediatric education in relation to child health in subtropical and tropical regions. *Pediatrics* **8**, 398.

Jelliffe, D. B. (1962). Education for child health workers in developing countries. *Postgrad. Med. J.* **38**, 105.

Jelliffe, D. B. (1966). Teaching nutrition pediatrics developing countries. Part 1: Undergraduate training. *Pediatrics.* **38**, 671.

Jelliffe, D. B., and Bennett, F. J. (1963). Different problems in different parts of the world. *Acta Paediat.* (Uppsala), **151** (Suppl.), 13.

Jelliffe, D. B., and Stanfield, J. P. (1968). Para-auxiliaries and medical manpower in tropical pediatrics. *J. Trop. Pediat.* **14**, 199.

Joseph, S. (1977). The Community Health Worker in Developing Countries: Issues in Administrative Structure, Support and Supervision. Paper presented at a symposium on the community health worker, Airlie House, Arlington, Va.

Josiah Macy Jr. Fdtn. (1970). *Annual Report.* Josiah Macy Junior Fundation, New York.

Kasongo Project Team (1983). The Kasongo project. *Wld. Hlth. Forum* **4**, 41.

Katz, F. M., and Fulop, T. (1980). *Personnel in Health Care Studies of Educational Programmes.* Vol. 2. WHO Publ. Hlth Paper, no. 71. Geneva.

Katz, F. M., and Snow, R. (1980). *Assessing Healthworkers' Performance: A Manual for Training and Supervision.* WHO Publ. Hlth Paper, no. 72. Geneva.

Keynes, M. (1968). Personal view. *Brit. Med. J.* **2**, 693.

King, M. H., ed. (1966). *Medical Care in Developing Countries.* Oxford University Press, Nairobi.

Lancet (1970). The future of primary care. *Lancet* **i**, 1325.

Lechtig, A.; Townsend, J. W.; Pineda, F.; Arroyo, J. J.; Klein, R. E.; and de Leon, R. (1982). Nutrition, family planning and health promotion; The Guatemalan program of primary health care. *Birth* **9**, 97.

Maguire, M. J., and Chawla, V. (1983). An association between herbal medicine ingestion and renal failure in Zambian infants. *J. Trop. Pediat.* **29**, 213.

Mahmoud, E. (1992). Statistics and facts need to be checked. *WIPHN News* **11**, 10.

Mangay-Maglacas, A., and Pizurki, H. (1981). The *Traditional Birth Attendant in Seven Countries: Case Studies in Utilization and Training.* WHO Publ. Hlth. Paper, no. 75. Geneva.

Mercer, M. A. (1982). The training of primary health workers. In *New Developments in Tropical Medicine.* National Council for International Health, Washington, D.C.

Miller, G. E. (1973). *Educational Objectives.* WHO Publ. Hlth Paper, no. 52. Geneva.

Parlato, M. B., and Favin, N. (1982). *Primary Health Care: Progress and problems: An Analysis of 52 AID-Assisted Projects.* American Public Health Association, Washington, D.C.

Philpott, R. H. (1980). *Maternity Services in the Developing World—What the Community needs.* Proceedings of the Seventh Study Group of the Royal College of Obstetricians and Gynaecologists, London.

Riegelman, R. K. (1981). *Studying a Study and Testing a Test: How to Read the Medical Literature.* Little, Brown, Boston.

Rifkin, S. B. (1980). Health care in China: The experts take command. *Trop. Doctor* **10**, 86.

Ronaghy, H.; Mehrabanpour, J.; Zeighami, B.; Zeighami, E.; Mansouri, S.; Ayatolahi, M.; and Rasulnia, N. (1983). The middle level auxiliary health worker school: The Behdar Project. *J. Trop. Pediat.* **29**, 260.

Rosa, F. W. (1964). A doctor for newly developing countries: Principles for adapting medical education and services to meet problems. *J. Med. Educ.* **39**, 918.

Rosenblatt, R. A. (1992). Specialists or generalists: On whom should we base the American health care system? *JAMA* **267** (12), 1665–66.

Royal Society of Medicine (1970). Teaching of social and preventive medicine. *Proc. Roy. Soc. Med.* **63**, 387.

Schmidt, H. G. (1988). *Annals of Community-Oriented Education.* University of Linburg, Maastricht, Netherlands.

Sebina, D. B.; Carter, J. P.; and Baumslag, N. (1985). *Towards a Mobile Public Health*

Training Program in Southern Africa. Rodale Press, Gaberone, Botswana.

Shah, K. P. (1980). Appropriate technology in primary health care for better midwifery services. *J. Obstet. Gynaecol. Ind.* **30,** 109.

Silver, H. K.; Ford, L. C.; and Day, L. R. (1968). The pediatric nurse-practitioner program. Expanding role of the nurse to provide increased health care for children. *J. Am. Med. Asso.* **204,** 298.

Smith, R. A. (1978). *Manpower and Primary Health Care.* University Press of Hawaii, Honolulu.

Standard, K., et al. (1969). *Community Health Aide Programme.* University of the West Indies, Mona, Jamaica.

Stapleton, T. (1969). Paediatric education for the 1970s. In *Proceedings of the Sixth Middle East Paediatric Congress,* Athens.

Storms, D. (1979). *Training and Use of Auxiliary Health Workers: Lessons from Developing Countries.* American Public Health Association Monograph Series, no. 3. Washington, D.C.

Taylor, C. E. (1980). Health services in developing countries. In *Maxcy-Rosenau Public Health and Preventive Medicine.* 11th ed. Ed. J. M. Last. Appleton-Century-Crofts, New York.

Taylor, C.; Dirican, R.; and Deuschle, K. (1968). *Health Manpower Planning in Turkey: An International Research Case Study.* Johns Hopkins Press, Baltimore.

Vaughan, J. P. (1983). Village health workers and primary health care. *Trop. Doctor* **13,** 105.

Veeneklaas, G. M. H. (1957). Paediatric education in Europe. *Helv. Paediat. Acta.* **12** (Suppl.), 7.

Walldren, A. (1974). *Curriculum Theory and Curriculum Practice.* WHO Pub. Hlth. Paper, no. 61. Geneva.

Werner, D., and Bower, B. (1982). *Helping Health Workers Learn.* Hesperian Foundation, Palo Alto, Calif.

Williams, C. D. (1966). What is health education? *Lancet* **i,** 1205.

Williams, C. D., and Scharf, J. W. (1942). Preventive paediatrics: An account of health work in Trengganu, Malaya. *Indian Med. Gaz.* 77, 552, 689.

Williams, H. E. (1967). Medical student training in child health in Papua New Guinea. *Aust. Paediat. J.* **3,** 128.

Wise, H. B.; Torrey, E. F.; McDade, A.; and Bostad, H. (1968). The family health worker. *Am. J. Publ. Hlth.* **58,** 1828.

World Bank (1975). *Health Sector Policy Paper.* World Bank, Washington, D.C.

WHO (1968). *Training of Medical Assistants and Similar Personnel.* Wld. Hlth. Org. Tech. Rep. Series, no. 385.

WHO (1970). *Post-Graduate Education for Medical Personnel in the USSR.* Wld. Hlth. Org. Pub. Hlth. Paper, no. 39.

WHO (1977). *Criteria for the Evaluation of Learning Objectives in Education of Health Personnel.* Report of a WHO Study Group. Wld. Hlth. Org. Tech. Rep. Series, no. 68.

WHO (1981). *Guidelines for Training Community Health Workers in Nutrition.* WHO offset publication, no. 59. Geneva.

WHO (1982). *WHO Working Group on Training Trainers (Supervisors) of Primary Health Workers in the Collection and Use of Health-related Information.* WHO/HS/NAT. COM./ 82.382. Geneva.

Zais, R. S. (1976). *Curriculum: Principles and Foundations.* Thomas Y. Crowell Co., New York.

17

Delivering the Services

Medicine has imperceptibly led us into a position to deal with the great social problems of our time. Doctors are the natural advocates of the poor, and social problems are very largely within their jurisdiction.
RUDOLF VIRCHOW, 1849

Since Virchow's time, much has changed. With the rapid technological expansion of medicine, hospitals act as centers of specialist care, and doctors are generally removed from the problems and health care needs of communities. Early in their rigorous training, doctors and nurses are rewarded for recognition of procedures, drugs, and syndromes. Preventive medicine, if taught, is not practiced. Community health care at the primary level is increasingly being provided by mid- and village-level health care workers, often with neither the time nor the experience to address social problems. Doctors may be socially motivated yet lack political organizing skills. Medical schools generally prepare students for accepting, diagnosing, and treating conditions instead of teaching them to effect change through preventive and social measures.

For health workers, the glamour of working in the developing countries with exotic diseases, like bilharzia, trachoma, and kwashiorkor, is soon lost. Too little money, too few health personnel, and inadequate facilities nearly everywhere mean that medical care, often inappropriate to need, reaches only a few. Furthermore, the training of doctors and auxiliary staff has been for individual medicine, not for mass medicine. Antiquated medical curricula and government bureaucracies originally perpetuated the divorce between curative medicine; which is "respectable," and public health, which is a "dirty word." Social medicine and community health were relatively ignored. Under these circumstances, recent medical school graduates cannot be blamed for choosing either to join the brain drain or enter private practice in the cities, thus escaping the necessity of dealing with social problems or fulfilling their role as advocate of the poor (Field 1966).

Recognition of the importance of social factors is derived from studies demonstrating that the causes of common health problems originate from society itself at the macro level and from the family in particular at the micro level and that a strict sectoral approach to health is ineffective (Baumslag et al. 1978; Mosley 1983; Newell 1975).

Although much has been written on the importance of social change and political will of the government to provide egalitarian services (Morley 1983), dramatic changes are still a long way off in most countries. Where, then, does this put the health professional, especially when the evidence is that so many health problems are poverty related? Working under conditions that are primitive may be depressing and may affect the attitude of the health professionals—for example, these people are "lazy" or "no good," or the community may perceive that the health worker "doesn't care" or "knows nothing." Discrimination is ultimately most often related to economics. This may be increased on the basis of a caste system or race, or against the rural poor, and invariably it leads to inappropriate and/or apartheid-type health services that are second class with regard to the number and types of services and health workers. High mortality and morbidity rates bear testimony to this (Susser and Cherry 1982). Yet much can be done to move from hopelessness to hope (Newell 1975). Through careful planning and optimal use of resources, positive gains can be made locally, although national health statistics may remain unaltered. This has been done in many places by individuals whose creativity (even charisma) and resourcefulness have sustained the momentum of a project despite social and political obstacles.

It is not only the European and North American medical schools that are interested now in observing the context in which diseases arise and must be treated or modified; other countries are also becoming aware of the need to consider social medicine as an integral part of medicine. Some countries have addressed the problem through an interlocking series of political, economic, and social measures (Morley 1983): land tenure reform, employment assurance, minimum wage, child labor laws, food security throughout the seasons (price fixing and ration stores, use of local staples, and maximizing the yield), universal education, increasing the age of marriage and decreasing the number of married females, and an extensive network of health care services that encourage maximum community participation and respond to the needs of the people. (For detailed case studies see Morley et al. 1983.) All over the world, people are experimenting to improve the delivery of medical care, and through such experiments, they are obtaining a clear vision of the needs and the urgency. What is evident is that regardless of the social situation, possibilities for change are open to all communities, but no standard method is applicable to all (Newell 1975).

Many programs have successfully extended outreach services through the use of community workers, even where adverse political, social, or economic conditions restrict social services to the poor, disadvantaged, or isolated (Parlato and Favin 1982). Extending the services and involving the people is the first step. Results can be reduced perinatal mortality from tetanus or reduced incidence of low-birthweight babies through at-risk screening. Staff, supplies, and transport may still be severely limited, but an exchange of new ideas may alter the social milieu, encourage optimism, and result in new ways to cope with problems. As a community becomes organized, it becomes politically more visible and gains recognition, support, and new funding priorities. Unfortunately, however, community organization and demands for change can also cause political enmity from autocratic rulers.

The body of knowledge about the components, utilization, organization, costs, and delivery of health care is rapidly expanding although still inadequate; (Yankauer 1969; WHO 1992). Many new approaches are evolving, such as training village-level workers. Other approaches have integrated services, such as water and sanitation, aimed at improving nutrition and health. The combination has a cumulative effect (Gwatkin et al. 1980); improving one factor alone may not have the desired results. Early experimental projects (Danfa, Lampang, and Narangwal) were set up to look at the integration of activities such as family planning, nutrition, and health care within the health services (Baumslag et al. 1978; Parlato and Favin 1982; Taylor et al. 1980). Others have been able to coordinate an intersectoral approach. The Jamkhed project in India is an example.

Regardless of which approach is taken, it is clear that circumstances differ so much among societies that generalizations are never quite applicable to the local environment in which people may find themselves. Food, roads, water, laws, erosion, cultural preferences, practices, and education all have to be considered, and, where there is a village, a consensus obtained. Where homesteads are isolated, it is difficult to feel a sense of community or to organize community participation; working with individual homesteads may be the only way to proceed.

In developing countries health workers, including physicians, must be generalists. They have a unique opportunity to deal with the individual patient from birth to old age, as well as the family and the immediate environment. Neonatal care begins with conception, includes the management of pregnancy and delivery, and continues without interruption to the management of infancy. The artificial barriers between specialties do not apply. The unity of care is beneficial to patient and doctor alike (Barker 1983). Fragmentation of services in the West is an increasing phenomenon. A woman who has a breast abscess is referred to a surgeon, but during pregnancy, to the obstetrician, and at delivery her breasts become the domain of the pediatrician (Baumslag 1973).

Services furthermore may be governed not by the practical considerations or convenience but, in free enterprise societies, by the patterns of practice and by the ability to pay as a primary, commercial profit-making venture (Baumslag 1976). A family practitioner in the United States may see only adults and not children or pregnant women if there are large numbers of pediatricians or obstetricians in the area. The family practitioner may thus not be able to use certain skills, even though trained to do so.

There has been a proliferation of medical specialists and with it, increased health care costs. General physicians (family practitioners) are in short supply. They are specifically trained to prevent costly illnesses and manage health problems inexpensively, whereas a large supply of specialists may result in more frequent and less appropriate use of relatively high cost services (Am. Fam. Phys. 1992).

Much still has to be learned about how to select, train, and teach health workers. The more peripheral the worker is, the greater is the need to be a generalist and the greater is the need to recognize the importance of those "trivia" in behavior that educated or advanced people take for granted. Specialists must be highly trained in a narrow field. At the periphery, on the other hand, we need auxiliary workers who are familiar with local beliefs, practices, and resources and have a number of basic skills and appropriate technology (Shah and Shah 1978).

Whatever we call the peripheral services—family health, maternal and child health, comprehensive or community health, or mothercraft centers—they must include the care and supervision of families, especially of mothers and children, and must aim at including and linking service, teaching, research, and facilities for care in hospitals, health centers, and homes (Am. J. Pub. Hlth. 1970).

In the United States, experimental programs have been initiated to address the health care needs of the underprivileged and the medically indigent, the training of health auxiliaries, and the use of public health nurses at home and clinics. There is a recognition of the need for staff trained for home visiting and follow-up, midwifery services, health education, continuing supervision, and support.

Physicians and nurses are scarce and expensive. Many rural and low-income groups live in deplorable conditions and suffer a lamentable absence of medical services. In spite of some provisions for the medically indigent, it has been calculated that in the United States only 36 percent of families with less than $2,000 per annum received adequate antenatal care in 1983. The situation has worsened with recession, unemployment, and homelessness. Disadvantaged women in rural areas have health care needs that are compounded by poverty, poor sanitation, inadequate water supplies, and malnutrition (U.S. Comm. Civil Rights 1983). There are rural areas in the United States where many women receive no skilled care during childbirth and where the urban poor increasingly are prevented from access to services by lack of insurance, money, or transportation. The training of midwives has been neglected. There is an obvious need to make use of auxiliaries because they can reduce the need for hospitalization and the duration of any hospital stay. Children's hospitals and departments should act as centers of regional child health services (Forfar 1968). Tripartite control (general practitioner, hospital, local authority) should be revised in favor of unification and cooperation (Field 1966) and, wherever possible, through a team approach (Hasler et al. 1968).

Through well-organized services medical care can be improved. Dr. Andreja Stampar in Yugoslavia as early as 1920 pioneered rural medical care. He organized rural health centers, training of village nurses and medical auxiliaries, the follow-up of patients, and the integration of work between hospitals, and he suc-

cessfully coordinated and expanded radiating health centers (Stampar 1966). Another example of well-organized maternal health services was in democratic Costa Rica, where limited resources were used effectively (Field 1966; WHO 1960).

In communist countries such as Cuba, the former Soviet Union, and Mozambique, emphasis has been on child care. However, medical services were not as good as they were believed to be. How much is owed to realistic planning and how much to totalitarian power structure is difficult to determine. Their use of semi-trained staff such as the feldschers has certainly increased the distribution of services to unserved areas (Field 1966), and variations on this theme have been tried in many areas. Good results have also been obtained where child care is a priority, in Sweden, South Korea, Costa Rica, and New Zealand.

Programs that provide services solely for children are very limited because "children are members of families, and family and child health are inseparable" (Susser et al. 1955). Furthermore, "health begins at home; it is there that health is made or broken" (Mahler 1982). Hence with a family-centered service and home visiting, much can be achieved and insights gained.

A number of programs have had excellent results through home visiting, providing home care for newly delivered mothers (Lechtig et al. 1982), ill children recently hospitalized, and the chronically ill. In many developing countries, services at home have included home deliveries. The Domiciliary After Care Program in Singapore was excellent, especially for new mothers (Mahler 1982).

Family health should be integrated into the training and thinking of health workers. The malnourished child should be followed to the home setting, where the health of other siblings and the mother can be determined. Resources should be established and solutions found at the home level. The mother may need rest from continuous pregnancy and lactation, or the siblings may need treatment of infections and malnourishment. The grandmother may have tuberculosis. In many cases, involving the father may be critical, especially if he controls the purse strings and purchases the food. Looking in at home can offer far-reaching preventive measures (Manciaux 1975).

HOME CARE PROGRAMS CENTERED ON HOSPITALS

Home care units have many advantages. They are comparatively cheap to organize. They require only a small staff, usually the main expenditure in hospitals. Patients can be kept under observation in their own homes without the major physical and emotional disruption of a transferral to hospital—of special advantage to children. Contact between the parents and the health staff may be of great benefit to both parties in learning how to improve the environment, nutrition, and child care. A home care service provides opportunities for medical and nursing students to observe and to manage environmental conditions and to observe the correlation between the disease and the environment—human and material.

The disadvantages of home care include the amount of time spent in travel, the difficulty of night work and attendant risks, and the possibility that emergencies may arise for which the provision of services and equipment are not immediately available. All of these factors have to be assessed. On the other hand, the saving of hospital beds, the saving in cost, and the saving in possible emotional disturbance for the child or mother are worth considering. It is remarkable that there are not more experiments along these lines. Systems of district nursing or care of patients in homes are commonly found but rarely in association with teaching hospitals. The Montefiore Hospital in New York City is one of the few hospitals that provides home care for largely chronic cases.

One of the most famous examples of comprehensive rural care is the Kentucky Frontier Nursing Service, started some sixty years ago by the late Mary Breckenridge. Some excellent booklets of standing orders were composed for midwives and nurses working in isolated areas. Other examples of effective comprehensive services have been described in South Africa (Kark and Steuart 1962; Susser et al. 1955). These programs were organized under difficult conditions but were acceptable and effective, and were used for the training of students. Home visiting was an important part of the services (Fig. 17.1).

A home care unit based on the pediatric department of St. Mary's Hospital in London has been in operation for many years and has proved to be most successful. Another example is the Montreal Children's Home Care Program, established in 1964 and organized from and in complete cooperation with the Children's Hospital. A month's rotation through this service is required training for first-year pediatric residents. Only through constant teaching and proving the advantages of home care treatment can the attitudes of the medical profession be changed in regard to this type of treatment.

The cost of a child in a hospital bed is more than sixteen times as much as the cost for home care (Williams 1973*a*). Home care requires no monumental buildings, equipment, or expensive scientific apparatus. It may present difficulties between curative and preventive services because it inevitably undertakes both, but it presents infinite possibilities and should be more widely appreciated. There is no risk of cross-infection as in crowded hospitals; health professionals learn to observe, teach, treat, and adapt; and the home environment often improves as a result of the service (Williams 1973*b*).

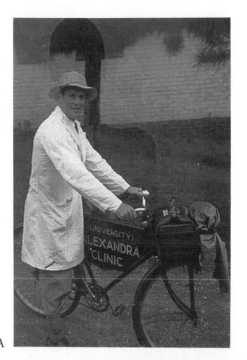

A

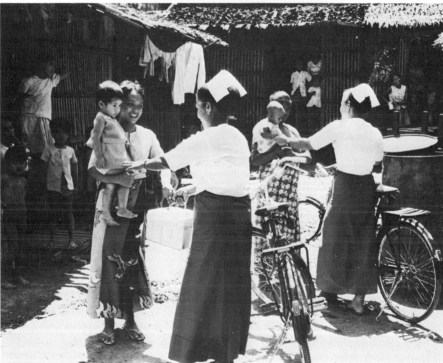

B

Figure 17.1. Home visiting, an important aspect of comprehensive services. (A) A medical student from Alexandria Clinic in Johannesburg, on a bicycle with his medical bag, home visiting the chronically ill. Photograph by N. Baumslag. (B) As part of Myanmar's overall health plan, trained midwives visit mothers and babies in their homes. Bicycles have become a valued part of their equipment. UNICEF photograph by S. N. Pombejr, Burma.

THE FAMILY CLINIC

There is no ideal pattern for MCH services. The best organization is the one that best meets local needs and resources. A good example of well-adapted family care was at a health center in a semirural area near Colombo, Sri Lanka, where a health nurse and two midwives lived (Fernando 1964). The doctor came twice a week to see sick patients and twice a week for family supervision. The population was scattered. It was impossible for a mother to come one day for antenatal care, another day for care of the toddler, and yet another for injections or immunizations. Therefore, each family was encouraged to come once a month at least. The clinic made use of family folders, and when the family presented itself at the clinic, often the whole family situation would be apparent at one glance and could be dealt with at this one visit. This type of organization is suitable to rural conditions. It worked well and appeared to be popular.

An outstanding example of adaptive maternity services originated in the Sudan area seventy years ago. Two midwives from Britain, the Wolff sisters, found a high maternal mortality, largely due to obstructed labor. At that time, most girls were subjected to pharaonic circumcision, which entailed amputation of the clitoris, as well as the labia minora and majora. Many died from hemorrhage or sepsis. Those who recovered often had extensive scarring of the perineum. There was also a high infant mortality from birth trauma, tetanus neonatorum, and sepsis.

Because there were few educated women or girls to be trained as nurses or midwives, the midwives visited around the towns and villages and interviewed the *mukhtars,* or village leaders (Wolff 1926). They found out which women performed deliveries and persuaded some of them to come to Omdurman for a few months' training. They would not take young girls but accepted older women, who often brought their young children with them. All were illiterate. The Wolff sisters taught them to wash their hands, cut their nails, use the simplest equipment, cut the cord with scissors flamed in the fire, and observe strict cleanliness. They also taught them how to perform an episiotomy. They learned how to cut and stitch on old inner tubes before working on actual cases. They were provided with a bottle of antiseptic, eye lotion, and ergot. They learned to distinguish them by taste and smell, as well as by the shape of the bottle, because they could not read labels. They learned to work in the maternity hospital, at antenatal clinics, and at domiciliary deliveries and visiting. After training, they returned home to their own villages. The supervising midwives spent part of the year holding the courses and part in visiting the villages and their former students. The incidence of tetanus neonatorum, sepsis, obstructed labor, and serious perineal damage fell, and in the Sudan now there are many educated women being trained as doctors, nurses, and midwives. But the work of these illiterate midwives was so valuable that this form of training has not yet been discontinued.

PUBLISHED ACCOUNTS OF HEALTH PROGRAMS

There are a number of useful texts available on medical care in developing countries that deal specifically with maternal and infant health (Fernando 1964; King et al. 1978; King 1966; Morley 1973). No one who goes to work in primitive conditions of whatever latitude should be without them. People who have not been forced to adapt can appreciate the pride and satisfaction of adaptation or practical pediatrics. Showing a distracted mother how to hold and feed a sick child not only saves lives but will help to deliver the services so that they may become more acceptable and more widely available.

A classic paper, "Maternal and Child Health in Kumasi in 1937," presents a different method of organization (Williams 1956). Here the hospital admitted maternity as well as pediatric cases, and the antenatal clinics were crowded. In the children's wards, the mothers were always admitted with the children. The daily outpatient clinic was intended mainly for sick children, who numbered up to 250 per day. Of these, 75 percent came from outside the town. But the supervision (and minor treatment) clinics were organized on a neighborhood basis—about eight in a town of 35,000. These were conducted weekly by nurses from the hospital, who also visited in the homes in their own district. It was felt that the advantages of this decentralization were that the nurses enjoyed a variety of tasks: working in hospitals, wards, and outpatient departments; visiting homes; and conducting neighborhood supervision centers. They also had responsibility for minor treatments, for referring patients to the doctor, and for frequent supervision of those at risk. The fact that maternity work (ante- and postnatal care, deliveries in the ward, supervision of TBAs) was included helped to establish continuity of care, as well as the comprehensive approach. These neighborhood clinics were held on a school veranda, in a garage, or in any other sort of shelter.

"A Medical Service for Children under Five Years of Age in West Africa" (1963) and subsequent papers by David Morley have described many innovations adapted by developing countries that could also be adapted by developed countries. "Health Centers in Kenya" (Fendall 1960) gives an excellent account of the organization of a practical network of health services in East Africa. In South Africa, despite the political situation, some in-novative programs have also been developed (Kahn 1958; Kahn et al. 1954). "Recent Experience in Maternal and Child Health in East Africa" (Cook 1966), the report of a seminar held in Uganda, is a mine of information with respect to the health of mothers and children in East Africa and the various types of health work being attempted; it contains reports on "The Ngora Maternity Annex," "A Pediatrics Admission Center," and successful health education in hospitals and health centers).

Uganda

The Ankole Pre-School Protection Program (Cook 1968) in Uganda, established under the direction of the Department of Pediatrics, Makerere, and financed at first largely by Save the Children Fund, is an example of a pilot MCH program that gradually evolved into a permanent and integrated part of the health service. Its objective was not only to give excellent care to a small community but, in a district of over three-quarters of a million widely scattered population, to provide some significant services for all young children and to add to these step by step until a comprehensive service was attained—an example of what WHO has termed a "sequential" program. The program set up mobile teams to back up and greatly increase the range of the established health centers, first with a comprehensive immunization campaign (triple polio, BCG, smallpox, measles) that lasted from 1965 to 1967, covered the entire province, and attained coverage and reattendance rates greater than those of the United States and most European countries. To this were added an intensification of health education, with auxiliary staff trained for the purpose; the commencement of a family planning service; and, once the whole province had been covered by the immunization campaign, the evolution of the mobile teams into a young child clinic service, much among Morley's lines, working both in the existing health centers and at many new sites in community clubrooms. Then an antenatal service staffed by the midwives from the nearest health center was added, with the specific task of detecting and referring at-risk cases to institutional delivery.

Evaluation was by biannual, cross-sectional surveys and by surveillance of hospital records. Only one medical officer was employed in the program; the rest of the staff was made up of paramedical personnel of various levels of training and included experienced medical assistants. The costs of the service, including the research and teaching elements, were consistently low. Communicable diseases that previously took a virtually unchecked toll on child life were enormously reduced. Useful research in methods, for example, jet injection, was carried out. Health workers and medical students observed the program, and some of its features have been adopted in Kenya, Tanzania, Zambia, and Rwanda.

In the Malunda Project developed in Tororo Hospital, Uganda, it was found that treating malnourished children in the hospital and distributing skimmed milk powder did nothing to reduce the number of admissions and readmissions (Harland 1966). Through the combined efforts of the district hospital, district farm institute, and primary school, a program of intensive nutrition education was started. Hospitalized children were accompanied by an attendant (mother, father, or sister), who was carefully taught the beneficial properties of legumes and other protein foods, worked in the hospital garden where these were grown, and went home with seeds. Schools and farm projects were also encouraged to grow, use, and appreciate such "protein gardens." The farm took part in teaching and demonstrating the cultivation and use of rabbits, guinea pigs, pigeons,

chickens, quails, and cattle to farmers and their wives and children. Unfortunately, political unrest has disrupted many of these successful programs.

Other useful project descriptions include the Sukuta Project 39 and the Gbaja Family Health Nurse project in Lagos, Nigeria (Tinubu and Cunningham 1969), which give some practical details about the organization and equipment for initiating a program.

Iran, Turkey, and Malaysia

In Iran an original and imaginative approach was taken in order to provide services to rural poor villages. In 1964 the government of Iran established a system in which newly qualified doctors, assisted by other categories of staff, joined the health corps and took medical care to villages of fewer than 5,000 inhabitants, where 62 percent of the population live. In 1973 the Iranian Plan Organization began training two levels of workers for service in rural areas. Literate village health workers were trained for six months in basic preventive and curative care. Villagers with a minimum of nine years of education were given more extensive training, usually for four years, to become *bedhars*, mid-level workers who act as physician extenders, providing dental care, dispensing antibiotics, and supervising village health workers. Approximately 60 percent of cases were adequately handled by the village worker and 35 percent by the *bedhar*; only 5 percent needed referral to more specialized services (Ronaghy et al. 1983; Ronaghy and Nasr 1970). This service facilitated increased coverage of isolated communities.

In Ankara, Turkey, in order to halt the brain drain and increase the relevance of medical training, community health has been integrated into medical education (Goodman 1964). Under the inspiration of one man, Dr. Ihsan Dogramaci, a 200-bed children's hospital has grown into a general hospital of 1,000 beds, with schools of medicine, dentistry, arts and sciences, physiotherapy and rehabilitation, and nursing (Lancet 1968a). The institution receives three-quarters of its financing from the Turkish government, but it is autonomous in academic and administrative matters. The academic staff is national and all full time, and all senior members have had higher training abroad. In many instances, the brain drain has been reversed. One of the most exciting features of the school is the integrated teaching of basic medical sciences, clinical sciences, and community medicine. During the first year of study, students are introduced to a family care and clinical program. At government health centers, they learn about community medicine in rural areas.

Even relatively inaccessible areas can be reached by extension services. At Gambok, near Kuala Lumpur, a referral hospital was created to serve Malaysian aborigines. Extension services were provided by fifty-nine medical posts and eleven midwife clinics in the deep jungle. A helicopter was used to reach the seventy-five jungle posts, and over a period of three years 250 aborigines, most of them local traditional healers, were trained as health aides (Bolton 1968). Williams and Scharf (1982) as far back as 1942 designed similar experimental programs in a rural area of Malaysia. Similar programs have since been developed in many rural areas.

Singapore

The health history of Singapore is a historical case study of the effectiveness of MCH services. In 1926 the infant mortality rate on the island as a whole was approximately 280. Singapore Municipality started infant welfare centers in 1924. Registration of births and deaths was good and soon became fairly accurate. All newborn babies were home visited, supervision was maintained for up to one year, and sick babies were referred to the government hospitals. In 1938 the infant mortality rate was about 150.

In 1927 maternal and child welfare services had been initiated in the rural areas of Singapore by I. M. M. Simmons, a health visitor. This government service included the supervision and minor treatment of mothers and young children, and good contact and follow-up were maintained with those who had to be referred to dispensaries or hospitals. Within eleven years, the infant mortality rate had been reduced to under 90. Centers with resident midwives and/or nurses had been established in fourteen villages, often at the request of the villagers, who provided accommodation. In 1939 these workers had conducted 3,726 confinements and paid more than 68,000 visits to the homes, and there were nearly 70,000 visits by expectant mothers and children to the centers. The rural population at this time was about 100,000 in an area of 193 square miles. Excellent follow-up was maintained between pediatric wards and the rural health staff.

During World War II, Malaysia was occupied by the Japanese, and all of the services ceased. By 1945 the infant mortality rate had risen again to about 300, but by 1950 these services had been reestablished and the infant mortality rate was again reduced to 90. (In Rangoon and Djakarta, which suffered equally in the Japanese occupation but where the services had not been so successfully restored, the infant mortality rate in 1950 was still about 300.) Since 1945, health care in Singapore Island has shown steady progress. Family planning has been introduced, and more than half the patients at the clinics have come on the advice of the MCH staff. In 1968, the infant mortality rate was 23, and the birthrate had been reduced from 50 in 1950 to 23 in 1968 and to 10.7 in 1981 (Ministry of Health, Singapore 1982). In 1991, the infant mortality in Singapore was 8 per 1,000, one of the lowest in the world (UNICEF 1993). It would be instructive to analyze the expenditures and results of family planning programs in Singapore, where they are combined with MCH, in comparison with other areas where they are not.

Singapore Island has provided extensive MCH services (Table 17.1). Of particular note is the domiciliary after-care Program for mothers who have given birth and have been discharged from government hospitals twenty-four to thirty-six hours after a normal delivery. At each visit, the midwife checks on the general condition of the mother and newborn, looking for symptoms and signs of puerperal sepsis and pyrexia, breast engorgement, neonatal jaundice, gonococcal ophthalmia, and tetanus neonatorum. She teaches the mother, supervises the in-

fant's bath, and advises on personal hygiene, breastfeeding, and other aspects of infant care, including immunization. She encourages the mother to practice family planning. The long-term existence of this service has not only relieved the pressure on hospital beds but also provided important health supervision of women in the immediate postpartum period at much lower cost. More than 72 percent of all women delivered in Singapore utilized these services, giving an average of three visits per woman. Only 6 percent required referral by doctors in the MCH program for further management.

Brazil

Ceara is an impoverished Brazilian state with 6 million people. Almost two thirds of the population live below the poverty line. The leaders are personally and po-

Table 17.1. The Singapore MCH Program

Services for children
    Routine and developmental screening
    Immunization (against diphtheria, pertussis, tetanus, poliomyelitis, tuberculosis)
    Follow-up of children with conditions requiring special care
    Treatment of minor ailments

Services for women
    Family planning (sale of contraceptives at nominal charge, sterilization, abortion, vasectomy clinic for men)
    Domiciliary after-care for newly delivered mother and baby
    Health education

Other services
    Home nursing (for seriously ill, aged, disabled, and nonambulant patients discharged from government
      hospitals)
    Supervision of registered private midwives
    Supervision of central immunization registry
    Assistance to social welfare department (regarding adopted, fostered, and transferred children)
    Registration of births in rural areas

MCH field services
Postpartum nursing	41%
Follow-up on family planning defaulters	15
Home nursing	15
Follow-up on immunization defaulters	14
High-risk premature and other children	7
Follow-up on antenatal defaulters	6
TB, leprosy, and other contacts	2
Other women	0.5

Source: Ministry of Health, Singapore (1982).

Note: Home care services were primarily for first and second deliveries, and tied to family planning incentives. Home care services have recently been dropped from the program and may affect neonatal mortality rates adversely.

litically committed to improving the lives of children. In the three years from 1986 to 1989, infant deaths were reduced by one third, child deaths from diarrheal diseases were cut in half, immunization levels went up to 40 percent, and childhood malnutrition was reduced by one third. A baseline survey (UNICEF 1992) conducted before the program was started revealed that infant mortality was 67 per 1,000 births, that the main causes of death were diarrhea and pneumonia, and that 28 percent of the children were malnourished. Over half the children who died had not seen a health worker.

Providing families with information about basic health information, the importance of breastfeeding, the need for immunization, and how to prevent and treat disease was identified as a priority. But the health services did not have the means to reach the community. The state government appealed to the church, nongovernmental organizations, the mass media, the business community (breastfeeding messages even appeared on bank statements), and the pediatrics society for assistance. The commitment of the Roman Catholic church was decisive, and they provided thousands of volunteers who reached out to the poorest areas of the state.

The 1987 drought was turned to an advantage and 6,000 emergency relief jobs were given to poor women who were trained as community health workers. After the drought, 1,700 of the most promising women were retrained and each was assigned about one hundred families to look after. The Brazilian government now plans to train many more women to increase coverage of nine states based on this effort. Ceara has put into practice the principle of "first call for children" (UNICEF 1992).

India

An innovative approach to enhance child health services is the Integrated Child Development Services (ICDS) program in India, which was started in 1975 to improve the health of children in a more holistic manner than the usual MCH programs. In 1975 there were thirty-three pilot projects, and in 1992 there were more than 250,000 poor villages and urban slums in the project. The government of India provides most of the funds. Food supplements are provided by the states and other special programs are provided by international agencies and NGOs. The program has a village-level focus with courtyard child care centers (anganwadis). These centers offer preschool education for 3- to 6-year-old children and special food supplements for needy pregnant and lactating mothers and young children. They also provide other services such as immunization, growth monitoring, health referrals, women's literacy, and skill training for adolescent girls. Each center serves about 1,000 people in rural and urban areas and 700 in the less populated areas. Each is staffed by the anganwadi worker (AWW), usually a young village woman, and a helper.

Where the ICDS has been in operation for more than 3 years, there are lower infant mortality rates and lower birth rates, the nutritional status is better and mothers receive health care before, during, and after pregnancy. In 1983, it was found that there was tremendous variability in the projects, and better supervision and training was implemented. A special mobile in-service training (MIST) program was developed. Training was village based, hands-on, and skills-oriented, and the different workers in the team (dais, lady health visitors, AWWs, helpers, etc.) learned together. This MIST training was found to be cost-effective, providing more home visits to malnourished children by AWW and better supervision. According to one study, early supplementation of pregnant women with food and iron has lowered the risk of low birth weight to one-third that of infants whose mothers received no supplements. Now in all centers iron, folate, and vitamin A are available. An innovative health and nutrition program was also developed for use in the centers through identifying local feeding and health-related practices that needed changing. Personal communication was found to be the most effective means for changing behavior.

Monitoring of programs was greatly improved with the use of a computerized progress reporting system at the central government and state level. It is standardized and easy to use; it highlights priority activities, checks the accuracy of the field data, and provides readily available and timely feedback. The ICDS program has grown and changed since its inception and has a chance of reaching and serving India's most deprived. By 1997 India plans that ICDS will be present in each of its 5,153 blocks reaching every needy child in the country under 6 years of age (Integrated Child Development Services, 1992, by Pragma Corp., Arlington, Virginia, under USAID/India contract no. PDC5110-I-00-0087-00).

Training Examples

Teaching in the social aspects of medicine is often the most neglected part of the medical and nursing-school undergraduate curriculum. Activities confined to the classroom or visits to sewage farms or slaughterhouses serve only to confirm students in their belief that this is really none of their business. It takes much goodwill and effort to link patient, home, and health services in a teaching situation. This has been achieved in a most impressive way in the medical school of Singapore (Lancet 1968*b*). At least three elements appear to be essential to produce this commendable result: faculty sensitive to the content of social medicine and the best way of getting medical students to respect and learn it, students prepared to expand the parameters of their study, and a health service capable of providing the facts as required. The training in child health in Papua New Guinea is another example of how medical student training can be adapted to different settings and personnel needs (Williams 1967).

In New Orleans, Louisiana, a family planning demonstration program transformed the Department of Maternal and Child Health, School of Public Health of Tulane University, into that of Family Health and Population Dynamics (Beasley et al. 1966; Beasley et al. 1969). The main features of the new approach were cooperation with existing departments of health and hospitals in New Orleans and voluntary societies in other parts of Louisiana. Second, family planning facilities were extended. Records were kept and followed up by reminders and visits so that a very large proportion of postnatal patients were seen and were given information about family planning. At-risk cases were identified and visited. The program was well received. Great emphasis was placed on health education, courtesy, and consideration on the part of all the staff. Third, programs were established for recruitment, training, and supervision of auxiliary health workers, particularly from the more disadvantaged communities. Intensive training sessions for two or three weeks and on-the-job training were provided. These workers were invaluable in providing liaison with nurses and doctors for their own communities.

The training and utilization of auxiliaries has been introduced in many areas. Gradually their work is being extended to apply to antenatal and child care, as well as to postnatal care. These valuable programs show a capacity for rapid extension and effectiveness. Similarly, in New York, the use of the family health worker has been developed as a highly practical approach and form of care (Wise 1968).

In Haiti, community mothercraft centers were organized along the simplest lines to deal with the vast problem of malnutrition, together with the shortage of staff and limited medical services and money. The centers used local equipment and were supervised by local personnel with minimum extra training (King 1969). The mothers looked after the center, provided food and water, cooked the food, and fed the children. They brought their own maize, peas, and beans for grinding at the little hand mill in the center and took the flour for use at home. Each center served a community of 500 to 600 families. Supervision was well maintained in spite of poor roads. These centers serve to illustrate how to simplify health care. Much can be accomplished not in spite of, but because of, simplification.

At the University of the West Indies, Department of Social and Preventive Medicine, Jamaica, a training course for community health workers has been established and a training manual issued. This type of training may provide valuable solutions in a country where conventional medical and nursing training is centered on technology so that many qualified graduates migrate to the United Kingdom and North America (Yankauer 1970).

Established MCH centers can provide a vast field for longitudinal studies. It is gradually being recognized that spot surveys have serious limitations. Only through continued observations can the natural and social history of disease be learned. By following individuals throughout episodes of sickness and health, a better understanding of the cause of diseases and of their interaction emerges. Therefore, it is essential that the scope of MCH includes a system of record keeping that is simple but efficient. Experiments in the organization of services and in methods of training and supervising personnel deserve more attention, more opportunities for observation, and more discussion and assessment.

There are a number of books that de-scribe enterprises to develop health work in various parts of the world (Basch 1990; Wallace and Giri 1990; Werner 1992; Paul 1955; Read 1966). Many of the health programs they discuss are ill-conceived from a medical point of view, as well as from a cultural one, but some have been more successful (Morley et al. 1983; Newell 1975; Werner 1992).

Many of the earlier experiments cited in this book still warrant perusal. There has been an impetus recently to examine health care systems more closely with the view to attaining the goal of health for all by the year 2000. A large number of case studies in primary health care have been reported from many developing countries, and many have innovations that are important to health workers throughout the world (Baumslag et al. 1978; Morley et al. 1983; Newell 1975; Parlato and Favin 1982; UNICEF 1982). In a study conducted by the American Public Health Association on project papers and other documents of Agency for International Development—assisted primary health care projects in fifty-two developing countries, certain trends were found (Parloto and Favin 1982):

1. Coordination is imperative.
2. Community-based facilities are preferable to a fixed base.
3. Change staff from physician dependent to nonphysician dependent.
4. Change medical evaluation education focus from disease oriented to family-based health and environmental protection.
5. Expand the use of traditional healers and midwives.
6. Emphasize the integration of categorical programs.
7. Make use of appropriate technology through a multisectoral approach.
8. Make programs people oriented and effective.
9. Adapt and prioritize health care, but do not compromise it.

10. Provide extensive rather than intensive services.
11. Training must be continuous.
12. Services must be sustainable.

Curative and preventive medicine go hand in hand; they are inseparable. Since many of these programs are rather new, evaluations are few. However, results show that synergistic interventions do make a difference (Baumslag et al. 1978; Gwatkin et al. 1980; Mosley 1983), although the effects may not be immediately evident. Even where there is a social revolution, fundamental changes require conscientious adaptation and cannot be expected overnight.

Newell in 1975 reported on interesting community-based programs including the Jamkhed project in India. Also Morley, Rohde, and Williams (1983) have described and analyzed a number of programs in developing countries that illustrate political commitment, community participation, and program development in a variety of settings, including China, Cuba, Dominican Republic, Nigeria, Philippines, Yemen, and Tanzania.

Ngutu, Zululand

This poverty-stricken population, is beset by many problems in addition to food and water shortages, which include poor roads, difficult communications, and isolated homesteads with no village life (Barker 1983). The hospital was initially not utilized, and the infant mortality was high; one in three infants died. Obstructed labor, fetal death, and vagina-rectal fistulas were reasons for seeking late hospital admission. In attacking the high perinatal mortality, it was established that safe delivery at term, maintenance of infant and maternal nutrition, and prevention of infection were important. Since low birthweight was a major factor, early treatment of maternal malnutrition, anemia, hypertension, and malaria could be preventive. The challenge was also to establish mutual confidence through a system of medicine seen to work, with respect given to traditional methods and thought, and medical care ultimately extended to all. Because trading stores were strategically placed, clinics were held adjacent to them when people came to trade, receive mail, and exchange news. Clinics provided antenatal services to mothers and preventive and curative services to both women and children.

The services were gradually extended, establishing clinics with a resident nurse in some areas and lying-in facilities for low-risk cases. The nurses in the new extended role are given additional training and regular refresher courses in diagnosis, pelvic assessment, decision making, and special care of newborns. A communication network has been set up for advice and referral, and screening criteria for high-risk cases have been developed. Mothers keep their own health cards so they can use the most accessible clinic. For at-risk mothers living far from the hospital, provision is made for their accommodation in small, self-catering facilities, so the mother can stay and await delivery. These women also provide each other with mutual support. Because the hospital serves as a referral center, it is not surprising that 10 to 13 percent of deliveries are by cesarean section, carried out under local analgesia supplemented with narcoleptics. This adaptation was a result of personnel shortages in early days. It is now accepted practice because it is beneficial to both mothers and infants, and mothers can hold their infants even before the stitches are inserted. All newborns and newly discharged infants are expected at a clinic six days later for a check-up.

Although this program operates with very limited resources and in circumstances of severe deprivation, it has lowered the perinatal mortality to 35 per

1,000 infants at the hospital with its network of clinics, as compared with a rate three times higher at hospitals with no peripheral services. However, kwashiorkor and marasmus are still prevalent.

The Jamkhed Project

The Jamkhed Project (Chakravorty 1983; Newell 1975) in Maharashtra State in rural India was developed when it was realized that people kept returning to the hospital with the same complaints and that while medicines could be used for short-term treatment, these services could not be repeatedly extended. There was a need to attend to the social conditions that were inextricably linked to health; addressing the one without the other was next to useless, even if enough drugs and doctors were available.

Discussions with community leaders revealed that food and water, not health, were top priority. In view of this, community kitchens were established, and food was initially begged or borrowed. The digging of wells was started, and farmers who profited donated land for growing food for the nutrition program. Thus, a permanent supplemental food supply was established.

The improvements that this project initiated were many and included the use of tractors instead of animals, small dam and road building, reclamation of land, drain and well digging, hand-pump installation, sapling planting, and house building for the landless. Much of the success was attributed to a team effort, which included 150 illiterate village workers who have been trained and are respected. There has been a marked improvement in the health situation; IMR dropped from 150 per 1,000 to 30 per 1,000 and the percentage of malnourished children from 50 to 30 percent. Significantly, in seven years, not a single diarrheal death occurred.

Mobilizing the community at the grassroots level, the project involved them in a number of important spin-offs, including the organization of farmers' cooperatives for development and leasing of machinery, creating grain and seed banks, and women's clubs. The community kitchen in this program broke down the local caste system. The focus of health services was altered to be viewed as a responsibility of the community. Two-thirds of the costs were obtained from curative services. Drugs, vaccines, and family planning activities were financed by the government. A major constraint was the shortage of staff to provide training for the voluntary health workers. The project served 100,000 persons. Many valuable lessons can be learned from this project.

SINAPS Project

The SINAPS project in Guatemala was developed to test whether certain specific interventions provided to a poor, rural community in an integrated manner would improve the health and nutrition status of mothers and children (Lechtig et al. 1982). The activities selected were so-called cost-effective or "affordable" measures and included immunizations, ORS packages, birth surveillance (weight, growth, development) recorded on birth coupons, nutritional supplementation of malnourished mothers and infants, encouragement of long-term breast-feeding, increased birth intervals through contraception, and improved sanitation through the use of latrines. To deliver these services, rural health promoters and TBAs were trained as primary care workers and were supervised by rural health technicians. Most of the training was in the community and was short term, with frequent refresher courses.

Coverage of the community was achieved through home visits for emergency first aid and for follow-up of malnourished or sick children or children with diarrheal dehydration. Visits were also made at bimonthly intervals for delivery of family planning supplies and collection of data. Community meetings were held every two months for detection of malnutrition and for immunization. With increased coverage there has been an improvement in the health of children in the area. There is evidence that although costs were increased by $1 per person initially, they dropped below the original cost in the second year.

An interesting feature of this program is the birth coupon that the TBAs fill in, which is adapted for use by illiterate workers. Attached to the form is a removable color-coded arm circumference band used for screening of malnourished infants. Training was the most costly item (per diem for trainers), as well as the cost of gasoline for transportation of supervisors. It is hoped that efforts will be increased or at least sustained, but there seems to be no magic quick fix that is affordable even at minimum service levels.

Other Programs

The Russians had their *feldschers*, the Thais their *wechakorns*, the Mexicans their *promotores de salud*, and the Philippines the *katiwalas* (de la Paz 1983). The *katiwala* program grew out of a desperate need in Davao City, Philippines, when a Catholic group decided to start a free clinic in the squatter areas where 75 percent of the children under age 5 were malnourished and tuberculosis was rampant. But the few donated drugs and supplies were insufficient and the services inadequate, and the free clinic was replaced by a cooperative clinic. Through this cooperative, civic-spirited citizens devised a mechanism for payment (1 peso for membership and 0.50 peso for a monthly fee). Drugs were supplied at cost, and a limited amount of financial aid was available for hospitalization. Squatter leaders were elected to advise the clinic. Since services from the public health system were poor (only one public health

nurse for 40,000), traditional healers and *hilots* were the usual health providers. The shortage of trained volunteers in the clinic became a serious constraint, and it became necessary to train primary care workers, the *katiwalas*. The training philosophy adopted was from the doctrine of Paulo Freire: "While no one liberates himself alone, neither is he liberated by others. . . . The best method lies in dialogue." Thus, the *katiwala* learns and teaches in the training programs. The training content is flexible enough to adjust to the needs of participants, and students and teachers learn from each other. Intensive social preparation of the community to receive and support the *katiwala* was found to be essential to the success of the program. Motivation is also critical. Many of the *katiwalas* have become resource mobilizers and linkage builders for their communities, initiating community development projects.

Another interesting experiment in the Philippines is training program developed to meet the needs of unserved areas (Bonifacio 1980; Katz et al. 1980). The program recruits personnel from poorly served areas so they can return for training; for this reason, it emphasizes academic relevance to community problems and circumstances rather than academic excellence. The students are selected by the communities and enter upon a ladder-type program with various points of entry and exit (Fig. 17.2). The first stage of training is the *barangay* community health worker, then on through various health level workers, and eventually, it is envisioned, to an M.D. degree. After each stage of training, students return to the community to carry out the work for which they have been trained. Advancement of students to the next level of training depends on the needs of the community, the health workers' aptitude, and whether they have performed satisfactorily.

This program emphasizes that the clients are the communities, not the stu-

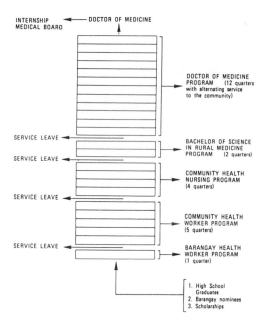

INTERNSHIP
MEDICAL BOARD ← DOCTOR OF MEDICINE

DOCTOR OF MEDICINE
PROGRAM   (12 quarters
with alternating service
to the community)

SERVICE LEAVE ←

BACHELOR OF SCIENCE
IN RURAL MEDICINE
PROGRAM   (2 quarters)

SERVICE LEAVE ←

COMMUNITY HEALTH
NURSING PROGRAM
(4 quarters)

SERVICE LEAVE ←

COMMUNITY HEALTH
WORKER PROGRAM
(5 quarters)

SERVICE LEAVE ←

BARANGAY HEALTH
WORKER PROGRAM
(1 quarter)

1. High School
   Graduates
2. Barangay nominees
3. Scholarships

Figure 17.2. Providing mechanisms for upward mobility of health personnel is essential. A ladder-type curriculum of the Institute of Health Sciences, University of the Philippines, College of Medicine. Source: Bonifacio (1980).

dents, and saturation of the market with particular types of health workers is avoided. Great emphasis has been placed on formative education and remedial learning opportunities. This unique approach to health service development is made possible through agreements between the university and the Department of Health, the sharing of senior staff, and the fact that the director of the training institute is also the director of the regional health services.

CONCLUSION

The scope of MCH services is broad (Fig. 17.3). They must:

- Identify major health problems and priorities.
- Diagnose major causes.
- Target those most at risk: pregnant and lactating women, infants, wean-

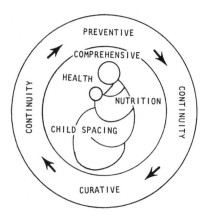

Figure 17.3. Elements for effective MCH services.

lings, single parents low-income groups.

- Assess local resources and local support, government and private.
- Establish measurable goals.
- Extend limited facilities to those most in need
- Provide parallel services for women and infants—services for both on the same day at the same clinic, instead of for infants one day and mothers the next.
- Provide continuity and follow-up. Curative and preventive services go hand in hand.
- Provide comprehensive care. Integrate health, nutrition, and family planning.
- Reach out, make home visits, and provide community instruction and teaching.
- Supervise and support providers of services.
- Evaluate throughout with simple techniques such as mapping, weekly frequency plots, and asking community people.
- Train health professionals.
  Conduct operational research.

If the scope of these services is appreciated in policymaking, they will not only improve the health of mothers and children but will benefit all of family life and improve the effectiveness of all medical services. They will be valuable in solving problems of overpopulation and will raise the standard of living and of responsibility throughout the world. Dr. Andreja Stampar held that *medicine is neither an art nor a science but a social service.* Perhaps it should be all three, as well as a vital component of national development.

REFERENCES

Am. Fam. Phys. (1992). The shortage of generalist physicians. *American Family Physician* 54(4), 1573–1576.

Am. J. Publ. Hlth. (1970). Conference on health services for children and youth. *American Journal of Public Health* 60 (suppl.).

Barker, M. (1983). Reduction in perinatal mortality in developing countries: Experiences from Zululand. *J. Trop. Pediat.* 29, 268.

Basch, P. F. (1990). *Textbook of International Health.* Oxford University Press, New York.

Baumslag, N. (1973). *Family Care, A Guide.* Williams and Wilkins, Baltimore.

Baumslag, N.; Cox, K.; Laskin, M.; and Sabin, E. (1978). *AID Integrated Low Cost Health Delivery Systems.* Vol. 1. Office of International Health, Department of Health, Education and Welfare, Washington, D.C.

Baumslag, N.; Roesel, C.; and Sabin, E. (1978). *AID Integrated Low Cost Health Projects.* Vol. 2. Department of Health, Education and Welfare, Washington, D.C.

Baumslag, N., and Wehrkamp, L. (1976). An analysis of family practice in Georgia and South Dakota. *S. Med. J.* 69, 278.

Beasley, J. D.; Beasley, J. D.; Harter, C. L.; and McCalister, D. V. (1966). Aspects of family planning among low-income, high-risk mothers. In *Advances in Planned Parenthood,* Excerpta Medica International Congress Series, no. 138.

Beasley, J. D.; Frankowski, R. F.; and Hawkins, C. M. (1969). The New Orleans parish family planning demonstration programme. *Milbank Mem. Fd Quart.* 47, 225.

Bolton, J. M. (1968). Medical services to the aborigines in West Malaysia. *Brit. Med. J.* 2, 818.

Bonifacio, A. F. (1980). University of the Philippines College of Medicine, Philippines. The Institute of Health Sciences, Tacloban-Search for a model. In *Personnel for Health Care, Case Studies of Educational Programmes 2.* Ed. F. M. Katz and T. Fulop. World Health Organization, Geneva.

Chakravorty, U. N. (1983). A health project that works—progress in Jamkhed. *Wld. Hlth. Forum* 4, 38.

Cook, R. (1966). Recent experience in maternal and child health in East Africa. *J. Trop. Pediat.*

Cook, R. (1968). The Ankole Pre-School Protection Programme, 1964–7. Mimeographed, Kampala, Uganda.

de la Paz, T. (1983). The Katiwala approach to training community health workers. *Wld. Hlth. Forum* 4, 34.

Ennever, O., Marsh, M., and Standard, K. L. (1969). A community health aide training programme. *W. Indian Med. J.* 18, 193.

Fendall, N. R. E. (1960. Poliomyelitis in Kenya. *E. Afr. Med. J.* 37, 89.

Fernando, M. (1964). Morbidity and medical care in Ceylon. *Ceylon Med. J.* 9, 26.

Field, M. G. (1966) Health personnel in the Soviet Union. *Am. J. Publ. Hlth.* 56, 1904.

Forfar, J. O. (1968). Children's hospitals, children's departments, and hospital child-health community centres. *Lancet* ii, 674.

Goodman, N. (1964). Turkey's experiment in the "socialization" of medicine. *Lancet* i, 36.

Gwatkin, D. R.; Wilcox, J. R.; and Wray, J. D. (1980). *Can Health and Nutrition Interventions Make a Difference?* Monograph no. 13. Overseas Development Council, Washington, D.C.

Harland, P. S. E. G. (1966). The Mulanda Project. *J. Trop. Pediat.* 12, 44.

Hasler, J. C.; Hamphill, P. M.; Stewart, T. L.; Boyle, N.; Harris, A.; and Palmer, E. (1968). Development of the nursing section of the community health team. *Brit. Med. J.* 3, 734.

Kahn, E., and Wayburne, S. (1958). Ten years of Bantu paediatrics. *Proc. S. Afr. Med. Soc.* 4, 253.

Kahn, E.; Wayburne, S.; and Fouche, M. (1954). The Baragwanath Premature Baby Unit—an analysis of the case records of 1000 consecutive admissions. *S. Afr. Med. J.* 28, 453.

Katz, F. M. and Fulop, T., eds. (1980). *Person-*

nel for Health Care, Case Studies of Educational Programmes 2. World Health Organization, Geneva.

Kark, S. L., and Steuart, G. W. (1962). *A Practice of Social Medicine.* Livingstone, Edinburgh.

King, K. W. (1969). *Community Mothercraft Centres in Haiti.* Research Division of Biochemistry and Nutrition, Virginia Polytechnic Institute, Richmond, Va.

King, M.; King, F.; and Martodipoero, S. (1978). *Primary Child Care: A Manual for Health Workers.* Oxford University Press, Oxford.

King, M. H., ed. (1966). *Medical Care in Developing Countries.* Oxford University Press, Nairobi.

Lancet (1968*a*). Round the world. *Lancet* **i**, 137.

Lancet (1968*b*). Round the world. *Lancet* **ii**, 865.

Lechtig, A.; Townsend, J.; Pineda, F.; Arroyo, J.; Klein, R.; and de Leon, R. (1982). Nutrition, family planning and health promotions: The Guatemalan program of primary health care. *Birth* **9**, 97.

McLachlan, G., ed. (1968). Problems and Progress in Medical Care: Essays on Current Research. Mimeographed report, London.

Mahler, H. (1982). Essential drugs for all. Address given by the Director General of the World Health Organization to the 11th Assembly of the International Federation of Pharmaceutical Manufacturers Association, Washington, D.C.

Manciaux, M. (1975). The health of the family. *World Health* (August–September), 4.

Marsden, P. D. (1964). The Sukuta Project: A longitudinal study of health in Gambian children from birth to eighteen months of age. *Trans. Roy. Soc. Trop. Med. Hyg.* **58**, 455.

Ministry of Health, Singapore (1982). *Maternal and Child Health Services, Annual Report 1982,* Primary Health Care and Health Education Division, Ministry of Health, Singapore.

Moffatt, D. (1969). The Ankole Pre-School Protection Programme, 1964–7. Mimeographed. Kampala, Uganda.

Morley, D. (1963). A medical service for children under five years of age in West Africa. *Trans. Roy. Soc. Trop. Med. Hyg.* **57**, 392.

Morley, D. C. (1973). *Pediatric Priorities in Developing Countries.* Butterworths, London.

Morley, D.; Rohde, J.; and Williams, G. (1983).

Practicing Health for All. Oxford University Press, Oxford.

Mosely, W. H. (1983). *Will Primary Health Care Reduce Infant and Child Mortality? A Critique of Some Current Strategies with Special Reference to Africa and Asia.* Ford Foundation, Jakarta, Indonesia.

Newell, K. W. (1975). *Health by the People.* World Health Organization, Geneva.

PAHO (1982). *Health Conditions in the Americas—1977–1980.* Scientific Publication No. 427. Pan American Health Organization, Washington, D.C.

Parlato, M. B., and Favin, M. N. (1982). *Primary Health Care Progress and Problems: An Analysis of 52 AID-Assisted Projects.* American Public Health Association, Washington, D.C.

Paul, B. D., ed. (1955). *Health, Culture and Community.* Russell Sage Foundation, New York.

Read, M. (1966). *Culture, Health and Disease.* Tavistock, London.

Ronaghy, H. A.; Mehrabanpour, J.; Zeighami, N.; Zeighami, E.; Mansouri, S.; Ayatolahi, M.; and Rasulnia, M. (1983). The middle level auxiliary health worker school: The Bedhar project. *J. Trop, Pediat.* **29**, 260.

Ronaghy, H. A., and Nasr, K. (1970). Medical problems of developing nations: An attempt to bring medical care to rural communities in Iran. *Brit. Med. J.* **1**, 295.

Shah, P. M., and Shah, K. P. (1978). Role of the teachers from medical colleges in delivery of health care in rural areas: Development of appropriate technology, training and operational research. In *Delivery of Health Care in Rural Areas.* Ed. Kumer and P. G. I. Chandigarth. India.

Stampar, A. (1966). Serving the cause of public health. In *Selected Papers of Andreja Stampar.* Ed. M. D. Grimek, Monographic series no. 3. University of Zagreb.

Susser, M., et al. (1955). Medical care in a South African township. *Lancet* **i**, 912.

Susser, M., and Cherry, V. P. (1982). Health and health care under apartheid. *J. Publ. Hlth Policy* **3**, 455.

Taylor, C.; Sarma, R.; Parker, R.; Reinke, W.; and Faruqee, R. (1980). *Integration of Family Planning and Health Services: The Narangwal Experience.* World Bank, Washington, D.C.

Tinubu, A., and Cunningham, N. (1969). The

Gbaja Family Health Nurse Project. Mimeographed. Johns Hopkins School of Public Health, Baltimore.

UNICEF (1982). *Assignment Children.* 59/60, UNICEF Supported Programmes in Health Education, Nutrition, Water Supply and Sanitation. Geneva.

UNICEF (1993). *The State of the World's Children.* UNICEF, New York.

U.S. Comm. Civil Rights (1983). *A Growing Crisis: Disadvantaged Women and Their Children.* Clearinghouse Publication 78. U.S. Commission on Civil Rights, Washington, D.C.

Wallace, H. M., and Giri, K. (1990). *Health Care of Women and Children in Developing Countries.* Third Party Publishing Company, Oakland, Calif.

Werner, D. (1992). *Where There Is No Doctor.* Hesperian Foundation, Palo Alto, Calif.

Williams, C. D. (1956). Maternal and child health in Kumasi in 1935. *J. Trop. Pediat.* **2,** 141.

Williams, C. D. (1973a). Health begins at home. *J. Trop Med. Hyg.* **76,** 20.

Williams, C. D. (1973b). Health services in the home. Blackfan Lecture sponsored by Boston Children's Hospital Alumni Association, Boston.

Williams, C. D., and Scharf, J. W. (1982). Preventive pediatrics: An account of health work in Trengganu, Malaya. *Indian Med. Gaz.* 77, 552, 689.

Williams, H. E. (1967). Medical student training in child health in Papua New Guinea. *Aust. Paediat. J.* **3,** 128.

Wise, H. D.; Torrey, E. L.; McDade, A.; and Bostrad, H. (1968). The family worker. *Am. J. Publ. Hlth.* **58,** 1828.

Wolff, M. E. (1926). Report on medical and health work in the Sudan, Ministry of Health, Khartoum.

WHO (1960). *Health Services in the USSR.* Wld. Hlth. Org. Publ. Hlth. Paper, no. 3.

WHO (1992). *Implementation of the Global Strategy for Health for All by the Year 2000.* Second evaluation and eighth report on the world health situation. World Health Organization, Geneva.

Yankauer, A. (1969). Proposals for child health care. *Pediatrics* **44,** 312.

Yankauer, A.; Connelly, J. P.; and Feldman, J. J. (1970). Pediatric practice in the United States. *Pediatrics* **45,** (3), pt. 2.

APPENDIXES

APPENDIX 1. CURRICULA FOR MCH AND FOR NUTRITION TEACHING

The curricula for MCH and for nutrition teaching were as follows:

Curriculum in maternal and child health
Physicians working for DPH

School of Public Health
American University of Beirut,
1960–1964

3 contact hours per week
for 1 academic year

In addition to the course subjects listed below, these students also followed courses in administrative public health, statistics, social science, environmental sanitation, health education, biochemistry, and parasitology. They attended wards and outpatient departments in pediatrics and obstetrics and well-baby clinics. They visited in the area with public health nurses and paid visits in the municipality and in some villages. They also visited in the hospital for contagious diseases.

Course subjects
Reasons for MCH services

History of MCH services
Scope and definitions

Measurements of health
Vital and health statistics
Surveys
Census
Longitudinal studies

Organizations of MCH services—theory and practice, e.g., Europe and the United States

Maternity
Hospitals and health centers
Home deliveries and home visiting
Ante- and postnatal care
Types and sites
Water and other amenities
Building and equipment
Staff quarters
Kitchens and storerooms

Children
Hospitals and health centers
Sick and well children
Home visiting and home care
Mothers and other relatives
Wards and outpatient departments

Laboratories

Transport and follow-up

School health

Sanitation and environment

Routine examinations

Treatment and follow-up

School meals

Health and health education

Vocational training and mental health

Teacher-training colleges

Child development and the factors affecting it

Genetic, hereditary, maternal, drugs, perinatal-environmental, cultural, infective, nutritional, emotional

Common diseases

Patterns of diseases—geographic, environmental, and cultural traditions, customs, work, climate (1) of mothers, and (2) of children:

neonatal
congenital
digestive
nutritional
respiratory
infective,
communicable
parasitic
preventable

Therapeutics

Drugs and equipment

Pharmacopoeia—dietetics

Dental health

Health education (the 5 P's)

Patients and parents

Personnel

Public

Personal (that is, keeping up one's own studies)

Special programs

Orphans, abandoned and neglected children

Day nurseries

Immunizations and disease control (AIDs)

Disabled children

Supplementary feeding

Mental Health

Delinquency, etc. (given by psychiatrist)

Accidents

Training of personnel

Training, supervision, employment, housing, transport, recreation, refresher courses, pay, promotions, and precious mobility between categories

Categories

1. Doctors, nurses, health nurses, midwives
2. Health educators, social workers, nutritionists, community developers, aides and auxiliaries

Patterns of training from various countries

Assistance sociale (France)
Feldscher (Eastern Europe)
Illiterate midwife (Sudan)
Health officer (Ethiopia)

Cooperation with other departments

Administration

Education

Finance

Statistics—Registrar General

Labor

Social assistance

Patterns, availability, uses and abuses

Population

Patterns and problems

Family planning

Legislation

Particularly that affecting women and children

Literature

Textbooks

Journals

Monographs

Pamphlets

Reports

Adaptations (e.g., for village nurses in Tanzania)

Research

Record keeping

Longitudinal Studies

Follow-up—observations and examples

Nutrition

During the second semester a course in nutrition is held, 3 hours weekly

Nutrition for physicians

**School of Public Health
American University of Beirut**

3 hours per week for 1 semester

Introduction and history
Ecology of malnutrition
Food habits, tradition, and culture
Food production, preservation, preparation, composition
Body composition, growth, development and activity
Diet evaluation—given by dietitian

Common types of malnutrition

Their geographical and social distribution

Diagnosis, treatment, follow-up and prevention

Special attention to mild and nonspecific types and their etiology, both from individual and collective aspects.

Infant and child feeding

Milk and milk products

Diets in pregnancy and lactation

Special diets

Special feeding programs

In emergencies

In schools

In orphanages

Supplementary feeding as a continuing policy

Nutrition investigations

Longitudinal studies

Surveys

Food hygiene and food poisoning

Nutrition policies and organization

Legislation

Personnel in nutrition

Doctors, nurses, midwives

Nutritionists, dietitians, etc.

Training—work supervision

Refresher courses

International and voluntary agencies

Literature and periodicals

APPENDIX 2. INSTRUCTIONS TO BIDANS (TRADITIONAL BIRTH ATTENDANTS)

Dr. C. D. Williams, Trengganu, Malaya,* 1940

1. Put your name on the register.
2. When you are in doubt what to do, refer to the Senior Health Nurse. Always follow her advice—and persuade your patients to follow her advice too.
3. Get a basket. Use it for your cases, and see that everything in it is always kept clean and in good order.
4. The basket should be lined with clean cloth. It contains:
   (i) Soap and handbrush made of coconut husk in a tin with lid.

* Now Malaysia.

(ii)   A bottle with ligatures to tie the cord (made from calico) and kept with disinfectant.

(iii) Powder and dressings for the cord.

(iv)   Lotion for the baby's eyes.

(v)   Two bowls, for swabs and for washing hands.

(vi)   A bottle of clean swabs.

(vii) A pair of clean scissors with round ends.

(viii) Two clean towels.

(ix)   A book of forms for notifying the birth.

5. Buy the basket, the towels and the bowls. Nurse will give you the scissors, and will keep you provided with lotion, powder, cord ligatures, and swabs.

6. You must always keep your house and your clothes clean. Keep your hands very clean and nails cut short.

7. Tell the women to come to you for advice as soon as they are pregnant. When a pregnant woman engages you, take her to see the health nurse at an antenatal clinic.

8. See that the patient carries out the health nurse's advice:

(i)   That she eats red rice (i.e., undermilled, not white, rice).

(ii)   That she receives treatment for yaws, worms, or anemia if necessary.

(iii) That she receives treatment for beriberi.

9. Notify the health nurse at once if there is any abnormality *owing to pregnancy,* such as fits, weaknesses, vomiting, swelling of legs, bleeding, fever, depressed nipples, etc.; or *during labor,* such as prolonged labor, hemorrhage, fever, torn perineums, etc.; or *anything the matter with the baby* such as prematurity, discharging eyes, imperforate anus, weakness, inability to suck, etc.

10. When you are called to a delivery, go to the house as soon as you can.

11. Before you deliver the case, see that the woman has a bath, that all the clothes are clean, and that your hands are thoroughly washed with soap and handbrush. Burn the scissors in the fire as you have learned to do. When they are cool use them to cut the cord.

12. Do not place large stones and hot bricks on the abdomen after the baby is born.

13. Do not use a tight cloth or put pressure on the abdomen in the second stage of labor.

14. Do not allow the mother to lie on a couch over a fire for forty days after delivery.

15. When the baby is born, see that the cord is tied and dressed, and that the eyes are washed with lotion in the way that you are taught by the health nurse.

16. Tell the father to register the birth, and you yourself send a notification of birth at once to the health nurse. Anyone in the village who can write may fill up the ticket for you.

17. Visit the house every day until the baby's cord has dropped off and make sure your instructions are followed. If you suspect anything wrong with mother or child, report at once to the health nurse.

18. It is right for the mother to keep quiet and do no work for forty days after the birth. It is wrong for her to stay inside a dark, and often dirty and stuffy house all the time. She should go outside in the sun and fresh air and take the baby with her.

19. Tell the mother to feed the baby herself, not to give *sugi* (rice porridge), *tepong* (flour) or *pisang* (banana) or tinned milk until the baby is 5 months old. The mother is to eat only red rice, not white rice.

20. Tell the mother to attend a welfare center regularly with the baby and have it weighed, and always to follow the advice of the health nurse.

21. If there is any sickness, tell the mother to report at once to the health nurse.

22. Tell the mother to be sure to get the

baby vaccinated before it is 6 months old.

23. The *bidan* must attend the *bidans'* meeting at the clinic at least once a month, and be certain that her basket is always kept in good order.

24. Report at once to the health nurse if you hear of a *bidan* practicing who is not on the register.

25. The Government Health Department does not want to take away your work. The health nurse is there to show you how to improve your methods; as long as you try to carry out her instructions, she will try to help you in your work.

APPENDIX 3. COURSE IN CHILD HEALTH FOR GRADE 2 MIDWIVES, 1969

East Nigeria, Dr. Rainer Arnhold (weekly sessions for 12 weeks)

Objectives of the child welfare project

1. At the end of the course, each participant should be able to recognize the appearance, growth, and development of the normal child, and to recognize the abnormal:
   - (i) Ask the questions giving information about the child's "history."
   - (ii) Examine the child by using eyes and hands and ears.
   - (iii) Inspect the mouth, throat, and teeth.
   - (iv) Know the age at which most children sit, walk, talk.
   - (v) Know the number of teeth in the mouth at a certain age.
   - (vi) Know how much weight a child should gain in a month or a year.
   - (vii) Know how to weigh an infant and a child on scales.
   - (viii) Know the normal bowel habits of the infant.

2. At the end of the course each participant should be able to recognize and treat common childhood diseases:
   - (i) Know the abnormal breathing of pneumonia.
   - (ii) Know the dry skin of dehydration.
   - (iii) Recognize a full or bulging fontanel—or a sunken one.
   - (iv) Recognize a stiff neck, paralysis, or weakness of arm or leg.
   - (v) Recognize a convulsion, or the spasm of tetanus.
   - (vi) Know common skin rashes: scabies, ringworm, chickenpox, smallpox, impetigo, measles.
   - (vii) Recognize whooping cough.
   - (viii) Know the dosage of chloroquine, sulfur, aspirin, piperazine, iron tables, folic acid.
   - (ix) Know the use of soap, benzyl benzoate, and gentian violet in treatment.
   - (x) Know the importance and signs of tuberculosis.
   - (xi) Send the child of a TB adult for examination and treatment.

3. At the end of the course each participant should be able to recognize and send to hospital the seriously ill child:
   - (i) Know the appearance of a child with meningitis, cerebral malaria, strangulated hernia, acute abdominal emergencies, severe dehydration, kwashiorkor.
   - (ii) Give the first dose of medicine for the illness and write a note about it to send with the patient.
   - (iii) Do mouth-to-mouth breathing for the child who has stopped breathing.
   - (iv) Splint for a broken bone.
   - (v) Stop bleeding by pressure.
   - (vi) Give first aid for snake bite.

4. At the end of the course each participant should be able to care for a sick child:
   - (i) Place the unconscious child or the child with convulsions in the right position (on side, head down) to keep him/her breathing and prevent injury.
   - (ii) Give medicine by mouth to a child who refuses it.

(iii) Cool the child with high fever by taking off clothing and "sponging."

(vi) Give enough to drink to the child with diarrhea.

(v) Prepare the diarrhea mixture in the home

(vi) Show the mother how to care for sore skin, sore eyes, draining ears.

5. At the end of the course each participant should be able to start and continue an immunization program, and know how to give immunization injections:

(i) Know the diseases for which vaccines can be used in Nigeria.

(ii) Know the number of injections or doses needed for each disease.

(iii) Know how to store each vaccine properly so that it will remain potent.

(iv) Know how each vaccine has to be given (by injection, mouth, into muscle or skin).

(v) Know which patients must *not* receive a vaccine.

(vi) Know the dangers.

(vii) Tell the mothers about the program and have them come for it.

6. At the end of the course each participant should know the important elements in the local foods, and how to prepare a good diet for a child:

(i) Know the different parts of food: protein (body building), carbohydrates (strength giving), fat (reserve store), vitamins (for growth and health), minerals (for blood).

(ii) Know how to cook a "balanced" meal for a child so that the important parts are included.

(iii) Know what foods are needed by the child.

(iv) Know how to start the first food for the infant at 5 months and food for "weaning" the child.

(v) Know and believe the cause of kwashiorkor and how to prevent it.

(vi) Know how to cook vegetables and other foods so as not to lose important parts of the food.

(vii) Know how to prepare milk feeds and what milk to buy for a good price.

(viii) Know how to feed a motherless infant with cup and spoon.

(ix) Know how to keep milk and cups clean.

7. At the end of the course each participant should be able to organize a children's clinic:

(i) Control patients by using numbered tickets.

(ii) Arrange cards and records so that the needed one can be found without having to look at each card.

(iii) Know the use of an appointment system.

(iv) Space visits to the clinic at proper intervals.

(v) Separate measles, pertussis, and chickenpox patients.

(vi) Separate those coming only for injections from the rest.

(vii) Use ward maid or helper for undressing patients, registration, and other duties which they can perform.

8. At the end of the course each participant should be able to keep records and enter weight on weight curves:

(i) Plot the weights accurately.

(ii) Write in all major illness into the record.

(iii) Write in all immunizations when they are given.

(iv) Identify each card clearly by name, sex, birthday, village, date.

9. At the end of the course each participant should be able to understand and teach basic sanitation for the home:

(i) Know how some diseases are passed from person to person, e.g., typhoid, dysentery, worms, hookworms, scabies, malaria, filariasis.

(ii) Know how to build a proper latrine (depth, cover, place).

(iii) Know the importance of flies and how to keep them away.

(iv) Know how to get drinking water by boiling or fetching it upstream if there is no village above.

(v) Know the good things about wearing shoes.

(vi) Know the need for hand washing.

(vii) Know how to avoid breeding places for mosquitoes around the house.

(viii) Teach these facts to the village mothers alone or in groups.

APPENDIX 4. SAMPLE SCHOOL HEALTH SYLLABUS GIVEN BY HEALTH STAFF, TRENGGANU, MALAYA,* 1940

More usually nurses, auxiliaries, and teachers may give many of these lessons. Guidance and collaboration is needed from other workers (e.g. the agricultural extension service).

Lessons from doctor or hospital assistant (12 lessons)

Anatomy of physiology (2 lessons)
These contain some description of the form and function of the human body. As each structure is described, so its purpose is explained at the same time.

Food (3 lessons)
Provides warmth, energy, and growth. It is the fuel on which the engine runs. What are good foods and why. The importance of growing and preparing food correctly.

Common diseases (4 lessons)
Malnutrition—diseases due to bad food. Beriberi, sore eyes (mainly due to xerophthalmia), and blindness. Diseases due to dirt—yaws and ulcers, worms and diarrhea. Coughs and colds. Explain the work of the hospital, dispensaries, and welfare centers, and the differences between scientific and unscientific medicine.

* Now Malaysia.

First aid (2 lessons)
Cuts, burns, bruises, fractures, bleeding.

Personal hygiene (1 lesson)
Skin, ear, eyes, nose, teeth, clothes, fresh air, spitting, sleep, work, recreation, mental outlook.

Lessons from sanitary inspector (12 lessons)

Hygiene in the home (1 lesson)
What houses are for. How to build them. How to keep them clean and tidy and why. Ventilation. The compound or garden. The water supply and kitchen. The latrine.

Animals that carry disease (2 lessons)
Mosquitoes, flies, cockroaches, rats, bugs, lice, fleas. Dogs (rabies, hydatid). Cows (TB, brucellosis).

Hygiene in the community (3 lessons)
(a) In the town: (b) in the rural area. What the sanitary department does and why. How small or isolated communities can organize their own improvements. What to encourage and why. Education, housing, playing fields, amusements, political, and economic interests. What to avoid and why—violence, gambling, opium smoking, prostitution, extravagance in food and clothing.

Water supply and food inspection (1 lesson)
Water supplies—various sorts. Markets, food, shops, coffee and other drink shops, hawkers. Food storage.

Vegetable and fruit growing (4 lessons)

Animal husbandry (1 lesson)
Care of chickens, ducks and rabbits. Animal proteins. Milking of cows, buffaloes, and goats.

Lessons from health nurse (4 lessons)

Personal hygiene (1 lesson)

How the schoolchild can help in the home (1 lesson)

Teach parents about food and cleanliness. Encourage parents to attend welfare centers or hospital as necessary. Help to keep home, garden, and village clean. Help young children to use latrine properly. Help in garden, in household duties, and in care of animals.

Care of babies and children (2 lessons [for girls])

Source Williams, C. D. (1940). *Experiments in Health Work in Frengganu, Malaya.* Unpublished

APPENDIX 5. SIERRA LEONE: TRADITIONAL BIRTH ATTENDANT TRAINING PROGRAM SYLLABUS

Three-week refresher/training program for village maternity assistants and traditional birth attendants

First week: Maternal care

Monday

Registration

Introduction

The role of the village maternity assistant/ MCH aide/TBA at the village level

Personal hygiene

Reproductive system

Case finding

Inspection of the home regarding its suitability for delivery

Home visiting

Booking patient for antenatal care

Examination of the patient at the first visit

Tuesday

Antenatal clinic; operation of the clinic

Examination during antenatal period

Nutrition during pregnancy

Anemia

Recognition of the danger signs in pregnancy and when to refer to hospital for delivery

Preparation of mother for labor and delivery

Equipment for delivery

Labor—first, second, and third stages; management and danger signs in each stage

Record keeping during labor and delivery

Demonstration of delivery

Wednesday

Care of the newborn

Resuscitation

Care of the umbilical cord—at birth and until the cord drops off (interview participants as to what is used to cut and dress the cord in their districts)

Examination and bathing of the newborn

Care of the eyes

Passage of urine and meconium

Cleaning up after delivery

Thursday

Care in the puerperium

Examination of the mother: breast, abdomen, fundal height, lochia, bladder; urine retention problems

Establishment of breast feeding

Swabbing and vulval toilet

Friday

Care of the premature baby

Feeding of new infants who cannot breast feed

Feeding of the premature infant

The sick baby: diagnosis and management

Saturday

Case demonstration if any

General discussion

Second week: Child care and community health

Monday

The maternal and child health clinic (under-5 clinic)

The need for the infant to be seen regularly, even if well
Immunization: program and needs

The use of antimalarials

The weight chart

Tuesday

Feeding and nutrition

Wednesday

Nutrition (continued)

Breast feeding

Weaning foods

Danger periods in the child's life

The high-risk or at-risk child

Malnutrition: Recognition, prevention, and treatment

Beliefs and customs associated with childbearing and child rearing

Thursday

The common diseases in children: recognition and emergency treatment

Emergency treatment of fever, convulsions, frequent stools, and vomiting

Relationship between some communicable diseases and infections and nutrition

Friday

Community health

Environmental sanitation

Home visiting

Relationship between village maternity assistant, MCH aide, other health and social workers and the TBA in the village (vital registration)

Saturday

Evaluation of the course

Presentation of certificates to TBAs and issuance of UNICEF kits

Closing

Third week: Practicals and family planning

Monday–Friday

Health center practice and observation

Home visiting; family planning

Child spacing and need for this

Continuation of practical experience

Source West, K. M. (1981). Sierra Leone practices of untrained TBAs and support for TBA training and utilization. In *The Traditional Birth Attendant in Seven Countries, Case Studies in Utilization and Training*, Ed A. Mangnay-Maglacas and H. Pizurki. Public Health Paper 75, World Health Organization, Geneva.

APPENDIX 6. SUDAN: TRAINING FOR VILLAGE MIDWIVES

Course content and methods of training

The course as a whole—which is taught in Arabic—is geared to the specific tasks the trained village midwife will be expected to perform upon return to her community. These tasks can be itemized and grouped as follows:

(a) Antenatal care
　(i) diagnose pregnancy by abdominal palpation after the third month, and after taking a careful history;
　(ii) advise pregnant women regarding:
　　—diet and the preparation and preservation of food (with emphasis on local foods)
　　—personal hygiene and the importance of rest and sleep
　　—the antenatal services available and the importance of using them;
　(iii) refer apparently normal pregnant women to the appropriate health facility for routine ante-

natal checks and other available services;

(iv) identity common discomforts of pregnancy and provide treatment for them or refer the patient to the appropriate health facility when discomfort is severe;

(v) identify complications of pregnancy and refer the patient to the appropriate health facility.

(b) Delivery

(i) identify the onset of labor;

(ii) manage apparently normal labor;

(iii) manage normal delivery;

(iv) manage the separation and expulsion of the placenta;

(v) identify deviations from the normal during labor or delivery, provide emergency treatment, and refer the patient to the appropriate health facility.

(c) Care of the newborn

(i) take appropriate care of the newborn, including attention to the cord and breath;

(ii) identify deviations from the normal in the newborn and provide treatment or refer the newborn to the appropriate health facility;

(iii) assist the mother in the initiation of breast feeding.

(d) Postpartum care

(i) advise the mother regarding:
—personal hygiene and simple measures of hygiene in the home
—the importance to herself of an adequate diet and appropriate exercises
—the importance of prolonged breastfeeding
—the resumption of sexual intercourse and of menstruation, and the implications of these with respect to the possibility of future pregnancies;

(ii) observe changes in the uterus, abdomen, and breasts of the mother during the puerperium, identify deviations from the normal, and provide treatment or refer the mother to the appropriate health facility;

(iii) manage breastfeeding.

(e) Infant care

(i) identify conditions that may be detrimental to the welfare of the infant, and advise the parents accordingly;

(ii) identify deviations from the normal in the development of the infant and refer the infant to the appropriate health facility;

(iii) identify infections and disorders common to infancy, and provide treatment or refer the infant to the appropriate health facility;

(iv) advise the mother regarding infant care during the first year of life, including advice on diet and immunization and on the importance of keeping the infant clean and having it examined periodically.

(f) Family planning

While village midwives provide advice to mothers regarding the importance of spacing pregnancies, they are not involved in family planning activities as such. It is envisaged that, as the Ministry of Health/WHO Maternity-Centered Family Planning Project gains momentum, the training program for village midwives will come to include content on family planning.

(g) Other activities

(i) provide health education with respect to home sanitation and the prevention of accidents and communicable diseases;

(ii) participate in public health schemes, including immunization programs;

(iii) report births and infant deaths;

(iv) advise mothers to disallow pharaonic circumcision for their daughters and to seek instead

circumcision proper (circum-
ferential excision of the clitoral
prepuce); perform the circumcision, if requested.

Source El Hakim, S. (1981). Sudan: Replacing TBAs
by village midwives. In *Traditional Birth Attendants
in Seven Countries: Case Studies in Utilization and
Training.* Ed. A. Mangay-Maglacas and H. Pizurki.
Public Health Paper 75. World Health Organization,
Geneva.

APPENDIX 7. OBSTETRIC EMPHASIS IN RURAL AREAS IN THE DEVELOPING WORLD

The following is expected of the midwife working in a rural community:

Antenatal Care

1. Seek out the pregnant women during home visits to other members of the family.
2. Education about the importance of antenatal care is vital. For this to be successful, the midwife should be convinced that it is important and worthwhile.
3. Where ill health is much more prevalent, priority must be given to correction of faulty nutrition and treatment of endemic disease.
4. The midwife assesses the patient's general condition throughout pregnancy and treats medical conditions for which she has been trained or selects high-risk cases for referral.
5. She will anticipate difficulties in labor and select women for hospital confinement.
6. She should be confident in the procedure of external cephalic version.
7. Administration of routine prophylactic therapy and hematinic drugs.

Labor

1. Knowledge of the progress of labor, using the composite partograph, which will help in the early recognition of cephalopelvic disproportion.
2. Competence in breech and multiple deliveries, third-stage management and prevention of postpartum hemorrhage, performing and suturing episiotomies.
3. Perform vacuum extractions, assist with cesarean sections and other operative deliveries, give first aid treatment and resuscitation to cases where there has been unskilled obstetric interference before admission to hospital, perform manual removal of the placenta in emergencies.

The Newborn

1. Competence in endotracheal intubation.
2. Perform male circumcision.
3. Expert knowledge of the care of low-birthweight infants.

Maternal and Child Health

The midwife's role is extended beyond the 28 neonatal days when she is responsible for the infant. When taking care of the under-5s she is expected to know about:

1. Growth and development.
2. Prevention and recognition of communicable diseases.
3. Diagnosis and treatment of minor illnesses.

She also participates in the family planning services.

Source Kwast, B. E. (1979). The role and training of midwives for rural areas. In *Maternity Services in the Developing World—What the Community Needs,* Proceedings of the Seventh Study Group of the Royal College of Obstetricians and Gynaecologists. Ed. R. H. Philpott. London.

APPENDIX 8. INSTITUTE OF HEALTH SCIENCES: INTEGRATED CURRICULUM, UNIVERSITY OF THE PHILIPPINES COLLEGE OF MEDICINE

First Quarter

Courses	Units
Health care A	3
Nutrition A	3

Obstetrics A	3		General chemistry	5
Community hygiene and			Philipino B	3
sanitation	3		Anatomy and physiology B	3
Pediatrics A	3		Total	14
Total	15			

Second Quarter (CCH) *

Courses	Units
English A	3
Fundamentals of anatomy and physiology A	5
Obstetrics	3
Health care B	3
Total	14

Third Quarter (CCH)

Courses	Units
English B	3
Mathematics	3
Sociology	3
Obstetrics C	3
Total	12

Fourth Quarter (CCH)

Courses	Units
Nursing A	3
Biostatistics and community health	5
Logic	3
Psychology	3
Total	14

Fifth Quarter (CCH)

Courses	Units
Ethics A	3
Microbiology	5
Public health A	3
Nursing B	3
Total	14

Sixth Quarter (CCH)

Courses	Units
Ethics B	33
Medical surgical nursing A	3
Public health B	3
Philipino A	3
Total	12

Seventh Quarter (CHN) *

Courses	Units
Nutrition	3

Eighth Quarter (CHN)

Courses	Units
Medical surgical nursing B	3
Mental health and community development	3
National health plan	3
Tropical and communicable disease nursing	5
Total	14

Ninth Quarter (CHN)

Courses	Units
Principles of management in nursing	3
Principles of teaching	1
Nursing perspectives	3
Philippine government	3
Philippine history	3
Total	13

Tenth Quarter (CHN)

Courses	Units
Pharmacology	3
Practicum	12
Total	15

Total units	137

* Integrated curriculum for Barangay Health Worker (BHW); Certificate in Community Health (CCH); Certificate in Community Health Nursing (CHN).

Source Bonifacio, A. F. (1980). University of the Philippines College of Medicine, Philippines: The Institute of Health Sciences, Tacliban—Search for a model. In *Personnel for Health Care: Case Studies of Educational Programmes*, Vol. 2, eds. F. M. Katz and T. Fulop. Public Health Paper 71. World Health Organization, Geneva.

APPENDIX 9. SELECTED REFERENCES, MATERNAL AND CHILD HEALTH

General

Basch, P. F. (1989). *Textbook of International Health*. Oxford University Press, New York.
Berer, M. (1993). *Women and HIV/AIDS: An*

International Resource Book. Pandora (an imprint of HarperCollins Publishers), London.

Cities. Life in the World's 100 Largest Metropolitan Areas. Population Crisis Committee, Washington D.C.

Hetzel, B. S. (1989). *The Story of Iodine Deficiency*. Oxford University Press, New York

International Development Research Centre (1992). *Growth Promotion for Child Development*. Proceedings of a colloquium held in Nyeri, Kenya, May 12–13.

Jamison, D. T., Mosley, H., Measham, A. R., and Bobadilla, J. L., eds. (1994). *Disease Control Priorities in Developing Countries*. New York, Oxford University Press.

King, F. S., and Burgess, A. (1993). *Nutrition for Developing Countries*. Oxford University Press, Oxford, U.K.

Morley, D., and Lovel H. (1986). *My Name Is Today*. Macmillan, London.

Roemer, M. (1991). *National Health Systems of the World*. Oxford University Press, New York.

Sanders, D. (1985). *The Struggle for Health: Medicine and the Politics of Underdevelopment*. Macmillan Education, London.

Seidel, R. (1993). *Notes from the Field. Communications for Child Survival*. USAIS Bureau for Research and Development, Office of Health, Washington, D.C.

Smith, S. E. (1991). *Women and Health: Leadership Training for Health and Development*. McMaster University, Hamilton, Ontario.

Starfield, B. (1992). *Primary Care: Concept, Evaluation, and Policy*. Oxford University Press, New York.

State of the World's Children (1993). UNICEF, New York

UNDP (1992). *Human Development Report 1992*. Oxford University Press, New York

UNICEF (1993). *AIDS: The Second Decade. A Focus on Youth and Women*. UNICEF, New York.

Wallace, H., and Giri, K. (1990) *Health Care of Women and Children in Developing Countries*. Third Party Publishing Company, Oakland, Calif.

World Bank (1990). *Social Indicators of Development 1990*. World Bank, Washington, D.C.

World Bank (1993). *World Development Report on Health*. World Bank, Washington, D.C.

WHO (1992). *Implementation of the Global Strategy for Health for All by the Year 2000*. Second evaluation and eighth report on the world health situation. World Health Organization.

Breastfeeding

International Code of Breast-milk Substitutes (1981). World Health Organization, Geneva.

La Leche League International (1992) *Breastfeeding Answer Book*. Franklin Park, Illinois.

Van Esterik, P. (1992). *Women, Work and Breastfeeding*. Cornell International Nutrition Series no. 23. Cornell University, Ithaca, N.Y.

WHO/UNICEF (1989). *A Joint Statement: Protecting, Promoting and Supporting Breastfeeding. The Special Role of Maternity Services*. World Health Organization, Geneva.

Woman and Child Health

Gordon, G., and Klouda, T. (1988). *Talking AIDS: A Guide for Community Workers*. Macmillan, London.

Institute of Medicine (1991). *Nutrition During Lactation*. National Academy Press, Washington, D.C.

Institute of Medicine (1991). *Nutrition During Pregnancy*. National Academy Press, Washington, D.C.

Jelliffe D. B., and Jelliffe, E. F. P. (1990). *Growth Monitoring and Promotion in Young Children: Guidelines for the Selection of Methods and Training Techniques*. Oxford University Press, New York.

Measham D. (1990). *Toward the Development of Safe Motherhood Program Guidelines*. World Bank, Washington, D.C.

Proceedings of the Sixth International Women and Health Meeting (1990). Philippines Organizing Committee, Quezon City, Philippines.

Tew, M. (1990). *Safer Childbirth? A Critical History of Maternity Care*. (1990). Chapman and Hall, London

UN (1990). *The Situation of Women 1990. Selected Indicators*. United Nations, Vienna.

UN (1991). *The World's Women. Trends and Statistics, 1970–1990*. United Nations, New York.

USAID (1992). *Child Survival*. Seventh Report to Congress on the USAID Program. U.S.

Agency for International Development, Washington, D.C.

Women's Health: Across Age and Frontier (1992). World Health Organization, Geneva.

APPENDIX 10. FREE AND LOW-COST INTERNATIONAL HEALTH NEWSLETTERS

ACTION FOR CHILDREN
UNICEF Publications, 3 UN Plaza, New York, NY 10017
A joint publication of the NGO Committee and UNICEF. Events and new developments in the field of health.
AFRICA RECOVERY
DPI, Room S-1061, United Nations, New York, NY 10017
Discussion of general development topics, aid, and government responses.
AIDS ACTION *
Appropriate Health Resources and Technologies Action Group (AHRTAG), 1 London Bridge St., London SE1 9SG, U.K.
Information exchange on AIDS prevention and control.
APHA INTERNATIONAL HEALTH
SECTION NEWS
American Public Health Association, 1015 Fifteenth St., N.W., Washington, DC 20005
Organizational news.
APPROPRIATE TECHNOLOGY
IT Publications Ltd., 103–105 Southampton Row, London W1B 4HH, England
Agriculture, aquaculture, food processing, small-scale industry, community development, waste utilization, energy, and health.
APPROPRIATE TECHNOLOGY FOR
HEALTH NEWSLETTER
Strengthening of Health Services Division, World Health Organization, CH 1211 Geneva 27, Switzerland
ARI NEWS (Acute Respiratory Infections) *
Appropriate Health Resources and Technologies Action Group (AHRTAG), 1 London Bridge St., London SE 1 9SG, U.K.
ASIAN WOMEN AND CHILDREN
Press Foundation of Asia, Third Floor, S&L Building, 1500 Roxas Blvd. Manila, Philippines
MCH issues in Asia.
BOILING POINT *

Note Asterisk indicates publication is free to developing countries only.

Intermediate Technology Development Group, Fuel and Food Programme, Myson House, Railway Terrace, Rugby CV21 3HT, U.K.
Provides information on the design, construction, and appropriate materials for stove making, materials test reports, cooking practices, the fuel crisis, and conservation programs in various countries.
CAJANUS *
Caribbean Food and Nutrition Institute, University of West Indies, Kingston 7, Jamaica
Nutrition issues pertaining mainly to Caribbean countries.
CBR NEWS
Appropriate Health Resources and Technology Action Group (AHRTAG), 1 London Bridge St., London SE1 9SG, U.K.
Information on equipment and aids relating to disability, emphasizing community-based rehabilitation for the disabled.
CENTER FOCUS
University of Hawaii School of Public Health, International Center for Health Promotion/Disease Prevention Research, 1960 East-West Rd., Honolulu, HI 96822
CHILD LINK
Attn: Child Link editor, Pathfinder, 2324 University Ave. W, Suite 105, St. Paul, MN 55114
On serving children with special health care needs.
CHILDREN IN THE TROPICS
Centre International de l-Enfance, Chateau de Longshamp, Bois de Boulogne, 75016 Paris, France
AIDS, mother-child interaction, respiratory ailments, disability, traditional medicine, sex education, diarrheal disease, immunization, nutrition.
COMMUNITY EYE HEALTH
International Centre for Eye Health, 27–29 Cayton St., London EC1V 9EJ, U.K.
Aspects of blindness and eye care, with up-to-date information on ophthalmic practice and opinion. For specialists and nonspecialists in eye care.
CONTACT *
Christian Medical Commission, 150 Route de Ferney, CH 1211 Geneva 20, Switzerland
Varied aspects of Christian community involvement in health.
COORDINATOR'S NOTEBOOK
Consultative Group, % UNICEF—PDPD/A-6M, 866 UN Plaza, New York, NY 10017

Strengthen and extend existing information networks to improve child care and enhance early childhood development in developing countries.

DECADE WATCH

United Nations Development Program, Division of Information, 1, UN Plaza, New York, NY 10017

Water and sanitation.

DEVELOPMENT EDUCATION EXCHANGE PAPERS

Freedom from Hunger Campaign, Action for Development, Food and Agriculture Organization, Via Terme di Caracalla, 00100 Rome, Italy

DEVELOPMENT FORUM *

United Nations, P.O. Box 5850 GLPO, New York, NY 10163-5850

On development, peace, and ecology.

DHS NEWSLETTER

(Demographic and Health Surveys)

Institute for Resource Development (IRD)/Macro, 8850 Stanford Blvd., Suite 4000, Columbia, MD 21045

DIALOGUE ON DIARRHOEA *

Appropriate Health Resources and Technologies Action Group (AHRTAG), 1 London Bridge St., London SE1 9SG, U.K.

On diarrheal disease.

DISASTER PREPAREDNESS IN THE AMERICAS

PAHO, 525 23d St., N.W., Washington, DC 20037

Latin America. Covers the practical approaches to disaster preparedness and international assistance.

DRUG INFORMATION BULLETIN *

Pharmaceutical Unit, World Health Organization, CH-1211 Geneva 27, Switzerland

International transfer of information on drugs.

ECOFORUM AND NEWS ALERTS * (supplementary bulletin)

Environmental Liaison Centre (ELC), P.O. Box 72461, Nairobi, Kenya

Strategies relating to environment/development interaction and sustainability.

EDUCATION FOR HEALTH: PROMOTING HEALTH AROUND THE WORLD

Division of Health Education and Health Promotion, World Health Organization, Avenue Appia, 1211 Geneva 27, Switzerland

International health education and health promotion.

EPI NEWSLETTER (Expanded Program for Immunizations)

PAHO, 525, 23d St., N.W., Washington, DC 20037

EPIDEMIOLOGICAL BULLETIN

PAHO, 525 23d St., N.W., Washington, DC 20037

Epidemiology and related topics.

ESSENTIAL DRUGS MONITOR

WHO, CH-1211 Geneva 27, Switzerland

Essential drugs, supplies, and policies in developing countries.

FAMILY HEALTH INTERNATIONAL PUBLICATIONS

Attn: Publications Assistant, Family Health International, P.O. Box 13950, Research Triangle Park, NC 27709

FAMILY PLANNING ENTERPRISE

Enterprise Program, John Snow, Inc., 1100 Wilson Blvd., Ninth Floor, Arlington, VA 22209

Profiles of innovative, successful models.

FOOD AND NUTRITION

Food and Agriculture Organization, United Nations, Subscription Department, Food Policy and Nutrition Division, FAO, Via delle Terme di Caracalla, 00100 Rome, Italy

Issues of food and nutrition.

FOOTSTEPS TO HEALTH

TEAR Fund, 100 Church Rd., Teddington, Middlesex TW11 8QE, U.K.

Practical advice on specific diseases, health education, planning priorities, and general development issues.

GATE

German Appropriate Technology Exchange, GTZ/GmbH, P.B. 5180, Dag Hammarskjold-Weg 1, D-6236 Eshborn 1, Federal Republic of Germany

GLIMPSE *

International Center for Diarrhoeal Disease Control, Bangladesh, G.P.O. Box 128, Dhaka, Bangladesh

Latest developments and research in diarrheal diseases.

HAI NEWS

Health Action International Network, International Organization of Consumers Unions, P.O. Box 1045, 10830 Penang, Malaysia

Promotes the safe, rational, and economic use of drugs worldwide.

HEALTH ACTION

Catholic Hospital Association of India, P.O. Box 2126, Gunrock Enclave, Secunderabad, A.P. 500 003, India

Promotes technologies for the prevention of disease and the promotion of health.

HEALTH NEWS AND VIEWS

Family Health Division, Ministry of Health, P.O. Box 992, Gaborone, Botswana

HEALTH AND POPULAR EDUCATION

Diagonal Oriente 1604, Casilla 6257, Santiago 22, Chile

Popular Education and Primary Health Care Network News.

HEALTH TECHNOLOGY DIRECTIONS

Program for Appropriate Technology in Health (PATH), 4 Nickerson St., Seattle, Washington 96109-1699

Focuses on specific topics with detailed practical advice on diagnosis and management.

HEALTH FOR THE MILLIONS

Voluntary Health Association of India, 40 Institutional Area, South of I.I.T., New Delhi 110 016, India

Approaches to comprehensive primary health care in India, emphasizing the integration of health issues with development.

HEALTH POLICY AND PLANNING

Journals Subscription Department, Oxford University Press, Walton Street, Oxford OX2 6DP, England

Journal on health and development.

HEALTHY CITIES

The Editor, "Healthy Cities," Normanton Grante, Laughan Ave., Aigburth, Liverpool 17, U.K.

Supports public policies promoting health in the cities of the world.

HK REPORT

Helen Keller International, Inc., 15 West 16th St., New York, NY 10011

Information on combating blindness worldwide.

IBFAN ACTION NEWS*

International Baby Food Network, 3255 Hennepin Avenue, Suite 230, Minneapolis, MN 55408

Up-to-date news of the international baby foods campaign.

IBFAN AFRICA NEWS

P.O. Box 34308, Nairobi, Kenya

Nutrition, breastfeeding, contaminated milk issues, IBFAN training courses, and country reports.

IDD NEWSLETTER

International Council for the Control of Iodine Deficiency Disorders, % Dr. J. T. Dunn, Box 511, University of Virginia Medical Center, Charlottesville, VA 22908

On iodine deficiency disorders.

IDRC REPORT

International Development Research Center, Box 8500, Ottawa, Ontario K16 3H9, Canada

Agriculture, health, information, and social sciences research.

INSIGHT

Helen Keller International, Inc., 15 W. 16th St., New York, NY 10011

HKI programs.

INTERCOM

UNICEF, 3 United Nations Plaza, New York, NY 10017

Emphasizes communication of ideas between policymakers and implementers internationally.

INTERNATIONAL CHILD HEALTH FOUNDATION NEWSLETTER

International Child Health Foundation, P.O. Box 1205, Columbia, MD 21044

On oral rehydration treatment.

INTERNATIONAL DATELINE

Population Institute Communication Center, 777 United Nations Plaza, New York, NY 10017

Population planning, family planning, contraceptives, women's rights, and mother and child health.

INTERNATIONAL HEALTH NEWS

National Council for International Health, 1701 K Street, N.W., Suite 600, Washington, DC 20006

General analysis of international health issues.

IPPF MEDICAL BULLETIN

International Planned Parenthood Federation, Regent's College, Inner Circle, Regent's Park, London NW1, U.K.

Information on clinical aspects, issues, and developments in family planning.

IRC NEWSLETTER

International Reference Centre for Community Water Supply and Sanitation, P.O. Box 93190, 2509 AD, The Hague, Netherlands

On water and sanitation.

IRCWD NEWS

International Reference Centre for Waste Disposal, Ueberlandstrasse 133, CH-8600 Duebendorf, Switzerland

Waste disposal and low-cost sanitation.

ITIR NEWSLETTER

Intermediate Technology Information Ring, Nudestraat 4, 6701 CE Wageningen, Netherlands

Ophthalmology and related fields.

L.I.F.E. NEWSLETTER*

League for International Food Education, 915 Fifteenth St., N.W., Suite 915, Washington, DC 20005

On the entire food cycle.

MCH NEWS PAC

Pacific Basin Maternal-Child Health Resource Center, University of Guam, P.O. Box 5143, UOG Substation, Mangilao, Guam 96923

MOTHERS AND CHILDREN *

Clearinghouse on Infant Feeding and Maternal Nutrition, American Public Health Association, 1015 Fifteenth St., N.W., Washington, DC 20005

Infant feeding and maternal nutrition.

MUSTAQBIL (FUTURE)

UNICEF, P.O. Box 1063 Islamabad, Pakistan

Development issues affecting children.

NETWORK

Family Health International, Research Triangle Park, NC 27709

Family planning and family health.

NEWSLETTER FROM THE SIERRA MADRE

Hesperian Foundation, P.B. Box 1692, Palo Alto, CA 94302

Promtoes community-based self-care.

NFI BULLETIN

Nutrition Foundation of India, B-37, Gulmohar Park, New Delhi, India

Nutrition research, news, and issues in India.

NIPCCD NEWSLETTER

National Institute of Public Cooperation and Child Development, 5 Siri Institutional Area, Hauz Khas, New Delhi 110 016, India

NIPCCD activities.

NU

International Child Health Unit, Department of Pediatrics, Uppsala University, ICH University Hospital Entrance II, S-751 85 Uppsala, Sweden

News on health care in developing countries. Provides a forum for discussion on current health care issues and information exchange focused on developing countries.

NUTRITION NEWS

National Institute of Nutrition Tarnaka, Hyderabad 500 007, India

Mainly for doctors.

ONCHO UPDATE

Edna McConnell Clark Foundation, 250 Park Avenue, New York, NY 10017

On oncerciasis (river blindness).

ORT TECHNICAL LITERATURE UPDATE

PRITECH Project, (Technologies for Primary Health Care), 1655 N. Fort Meyer Dr., #700, Arlington, VA 22209

On oral rehydration therapy and related health issues.

OUTLOOK

Program for the Introduction and Adaptation of Contraceptive Technology (PIACT), 4 Nickerson St., Seattle, WA 98109-1699

Information on contraceptive and reproductive health issues.

POPULATION HEADLINERS

Economic and Social Commission for Asia and the Pacific (ESCAP) Population Division, UN Building, Bangkok 10200, Thailand

Articles on family planning, breastfeeding, literacy, and population and family health.

POPULATION REPORTS

Population Information Program, Johns Hopkins University, 624 N. Broadway, Baltimore, MD 21205

Reviews important issues in Population and family planning.

PROJECT INFORMATION MEMO

Program for the Introduction and Adaptation of Contraceptive Technology (PIACT), 4 Nickerson St., Seattle, WA 98109-1699

Abstracts on recent developments in reproductive research and contraception.

RDI NEWS

Relief and Development Institute, 1, Ferdinand Place, London NW1 8EE, U.K.

All aspects of disaster relief, particularly famine, sudden impact disasters, and refugees.

REDES

W. K. Kellogg Foundation, Malecon 28 de Julio 489, Of. 801, Miraflores, Lima 18, Peru

W. K. Kellogg Foundation–assisted projects. Covers agriculture, health, and education.

REFUGEE REPORTS

Refugee Reports Subscriptions, Sunbelt Fulfillment Services, P.O. Box 41049, Nashville, TN 37204

News service of the U.S. Committee for Refugees.

SAFE MOTHERHOOD

Division of Family Health, World Health Organization, 1211 Geneva 27, Switzerland

Maternal health issues and activities worldwide.

SCHISTO UPDATE

Edna McConnell Clark Foundation, 250 Park Avenue, New York, NY 10017

Schistosomiasis.

SENTINEL—HEALTH AND ENVIRONMENT INTERNATIONAL

Monitoring and Assessment Research Centre, 459 Fulham Rd., London SW10 0QX, England

On industrial and environmental health and safety.

SYNERGY

Liaison Officer (International Health), Association of Universities and Colleges, 151 Slater St., Ottawa, Ontario, Canada

Canadian international health initiatives.

STUDIES IN FAMILY PLANNING

Population Council, One Dag Hammarskjold Plaza, New York, NY 10017

Family planning and related health and development issues.

TDR NEWSLETTER

Special Programme for Research and Training in Tropical Diseases (TDR), World Health Organization, CH 1211, Geneva 27, Switzerland

Research on TDR.

TIBS NEWS

Informative Breastfeeding Service, 16 Gray St., St. Clair, Port of Spain, Trinidad

Breastfeeding and other child health information for mothers.

TRACHOMA UPDATE

Edna McConnell Clark Foundation, 250 Park Avenue, New York, NY 10017

On trachoma.

UNHCS HABITAT SHELTER BULLETIN

United Nations Centre for Human Settlements, P.O. Box 30030, Nairobi, Kenya

Concerned with human settlements at international and national levels.

URBAN EDGE

World Bank Publications, P.O. Box 37525, Washington, DC 20013

Practical articles on all aspects of urban development.

VITAMIN "A" NEWS NOTES

Helen Keller International, 15 West 16th St., New York, NY 10011

Information on vitamin A activities internationally.

VOICES RISING *

Women's Programme, International Council of Adult Education, 229 College St., Suite 309, Toronto, Canada M5T 1R4

Links women in adult education and those organizing for social change.

WATERLINES

Intermediate Technology Publications Ltd., 103–105 Southampton Row, London WC1B 4HH, England

On appropriate water technology, water supply, and sanitation methods.

WIPHN NEWS

Women's International Public Health Network, 7100 Oak Forest Lane, Bethesda, MD 20817

Publishes a newsletter for women in public health and related fields. Provides information to improve the status, nutrition, and health of women.

WOMEN NEWS

United Nations Secretariat, Branch for the Advancement of Women, Vienna International Centre, P.O. Box 500, 1400 Vienna, Austria

WORLD HEALTH

Magazine of the WHO, World Health, WHO, Avenue Appia, 1211 Geneva 27, Switzerland

General public health.

WORLD HEALTH FORUM

WHO, Distribution and Sales, 1211 Geneva 27, Switzerland

Journal of health development.

WORLD IMMUNIZATION NEWS

Task Force for Child Survival, Suite 1, 1989 North Williamsburg Dr., Decatur, GA 30033

Technology, policies, and general articles on immunization and infant health.

WORLD NEIGHBORS IN ACTION

World Neighbors International Headquarters, 5116 North Portland Avenue, Oklahoma City, OK 73113

A "how-to" publication.

XEROPHTHALMIA CLUB

27–29 Cayton Street, London EC1V 9EJ, U.K.

Source Based on an Appropriate Health Resources and Technologies Action Group (AHRTAG) Resource List.

INDEX